W9-AZV-633

Advancing Nursing Science Through Research

To my family, L. J., R. J., and J. A., for their love
and encouragement.

Advancing Nursing Science Through Research

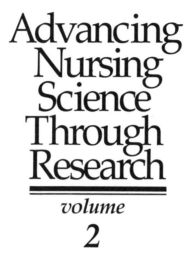

volume
2

edited by

Linda E. Moody

SAGE PUBLICATIONS
The International Professional Publishers
Newbury Park London New Delhi

Copyright © 1990 by Sage Publications, Inc.

All rights reserved. No part of this book may be reproduced or utilized in any form or by any means, electronic or mechanical, including photocopying, recording, or by any information storage and retrieval system, without permission in writing from the publisher.

For information address:

SAGE Publications, Inc.
2111 West Hillcrest Drive
Newbury Park, California 91320

SAGE Publications Ltd.
28 Banner Street
London EC1Y 8QE
England

SAGE Publications India Pvt. Ltd.
M-32 Market
Greater Kailash I
New Delhi 110 048 India

Printed in the United States of America

Library of Congress Cataloging-in-Publication Data

Moody, Linda E.
  Advancing theory for nursing science through research / Linda E.
Moody.
    p. cm.
  Includes bibliographical references.
  ISBN 0-8039-3811-X (v. 1). — ISBN 0-8039-3812-8 (v. 2)
  1. Nursing—Philosophy. 2. Nursing—Research—Methodology.
  [DNLM: 1. Nursing Research—methods. 2. Nursing Theory.   WY 20.5
M817a]
RT84.5.M66 1990
610.73'01—dc20
DNLM/DLC
for library of Congress   90-8259
                                                                  CIP

FIRST PRINTING, 1990

Sage Production Editor: Diane S. Foster

Contents

Acknowledgments

My heartfelt appreciation is expressed to Lois Malasanos, Dean, College of Nursing, and Nita Davidson, Assistant Dean for graduate studies in nursing, at the University of Florida, for the opportunities, challenges, and guidance they have provided me as a faculty member in the graduate program.

A note of deep gratitude is expressed to colleague-friends at the University of Florida and around the country for providing inspiration, wise counsel, and an ever-willingness to exchange and critique ideas: Sally Hutchinson, Gene Anderson, Nancy Diekelmann, Christine Tanner, Kathleen McCormick, William Holzemer, Gloria Clayton, Patricia Moccia, Moira Shannon, Pheobe and Arthur Williams, Janice Thompson, Molly Dougherty, Margaret Wilson, Kathleen Smyth, Hossein Yarandi, Diane LaRochelle, and Patricia Benner.

And a special note of gratitude is expressed to all the contributors and reviewers, especially Sally Hutchinson and Pamela Brink, who were instrumental in helping me bring this project to fruition.

I am deeply indebted to the editors at Sage, especially Christine Smedley, Diane Foster, and Susan McElroy, who generously applied their special skills and talents toward the completion of this work.

—Linda E. Moody

Preface

The eight chapters in Volume 1 of this book were designed to be used as a text for the first graduate-level theory course in nursing while the eight chapters in Volume 2 of the text support a theory-research course at the doctoral level that focuses on research methods for theory building in nursing science. This book is as much about research as it is about theory: The major thesis of the text is that the process of theorizing and the process of research must be linked and explicated in order to advance scientific knowledge.

The underlying philosophy of the book is based on a number of beliefs about nursing, about theory, about the relationship of theory to practice and research, and how research, as one epistemic method of knowing, will assist in addressing significant clinical problems and advancing scientific theories. These beliefs are presented in the Preface to provide an orientation to the philosophy undergirding both volumes.

Societal conditions demand improvement in the delivery and distribution of health care services, and nursing can play a vital force in effecting positive changes in a variety of roles and settings. Research is not only aimed at the discovery of scientific truths—theory building through research is one effective strategy for advancing theory for practice and improving health care to consumers.

Although a statistical approach is used most often to test interventions and develop predictive theories for practice, not all problems, concerns, or issues in nursing can be analyzed in this way. The methods of hermeneutical inquiry, conceptual analysis, sociolinguistic inquiry, case study, and other nonstatistical approaches, which are presented in Volume 2, may also yield theories for understanding or explanation of the events studied.

Because of the nature of the complex human phenomena that nursing must address, the discipline needs to accept and promote the use of multiple theoretical and research paradigms. Further, nursing research needs to proceed in orderly directions, generating knowledge built on previous knowledge in order to provide the scientific basis for nursing practice and nursing education. The process of accumulating knowledge for a discipline is dynamic and as such there are no permanent, immutable truths.

Theorizing is not reserved for academicians—good practitioners are often some of the best theorists in that their hunches provide the basis for developing propositions that can be empirically tested. Theories provide us with a vision: Good theories expand our vision and guide our thinking, our practice, and our research. Theories also serve as heuristic devices by which we can discover new knowledge or revise old ways of thinking. In this way, the theoretical is utilitarian but how useful it is depends on the quality of the theory. In assessing a theory, the issue is not whether a theory can be proven but how useful it is in puzzle-solving or in assisting us in solving important problems that the discipline of nursing must address.

Complex human phenomena require research methods that will provide valid and reliable measures of the concepts being studied. To dismiss human problems that demand our attention because we do not yet have the measurement or analytic tools is to ignore an important challenge. A claim by many in nursing is that researchers have used research methods that have been so narrowly focused ("reductionistic") that the essence of the human problem was overlooked or missed. The real issue in science is not whether the research perspective is reductionistic, because all scientific studies require that the phenomena be conceptually reduced to permit valid and reliable measurement and analysis of their fundamental constituents. The issue at stake, regardless of research approach, is whether the *level of reduction* for the phenomenon under study was appropriate. The nature and scope of the research question should guide the level of reductionism necessary to adequately study the phenomena of interest, and the research design and methods should be selected accordingly.

The process of theory building through research is a dialectic one. That is, it proceeds as a nonlinear series of events that are dependently or causally related, regardless of the level of refinement of the theory or conceptual model. Theory-directed research and research-directed theory proceeds best when the link between the theory and the research is formally defined by the investigator.

The process of scientific discovery requires creativity and caring for and commitment to puzzle-solving; from this it can be inferred that the conventional notion of "detached objectivity" in science is neither possible nor desirable. Scientific research involves an interaction between the scientist and the object of investigation, and what the scientist observes is directly related to the nature of that interaction. Scientists engage a subject of study by interacting with it through means of a particular frame of reference or theoretical perspective: What is observed and discovered in the object (i.e., its objectivity) is a product of this interaction and the study protocol through which it is operationalized. Therefore, because it is possible to engage objects or events of study from various theoretical perspectives or worldviews, it is clear that studies of the same objects or events may yield different research outcomes. In fact, the worldview of the researcher provides the language that permits the research question to be asked in the first place. This viewpoint affirms the importance of explicating the relationship of the theoretical perspective and the research.

Theory, regardless of level of refinement, always serves to guide the researcher in the formation of questions and to influence the research methods, data collection, and interpretation of results. Because scientists tend to see the world in terms that are derived from their own mental sets it is essential to acknowledge how one's worldview or theoretical perspective influences the mode of research inquiry and the outcomes of the research. Progress in nursing science is best advanced when the researcher identifies the theoretical notions underpinning the research and attempts to formalize the link between the theory and all phases of the research.

Finally, in terms of the discipline of nursing, although science and research are key elements in the structure of the discipline of nursing, they do not stand alone. Nursing's mission of addressing health issues of social significance and providing quality health care to all can be achieved only through a synthesis of the sciences and the humanities. We must continue to advance nursing—the art and science of caring—through artful and scientific means.

PART I

Statistical Research Approaches for Theory Building

1

Randomized Clinical Trials

LINDA E. MOODY

The use of clinical trials is one preferred path of inquiry for building predictive-level theories.

Much has been written in the nursing literature during the last decade about the need for research that addresses the effectiveness of various nursing interventions in the treatment of human responses to illness. Also suggested are studies that examine methods that will reduce risks for disease and promote health. Priorities for these research domains were discussed in Chapter 3 (in Volume 1 of *Advancing Theory for Nursing Science Through Research*). The use of randomized clinical trials is a major research strategy that has been recommended to advance clinical knowledge. The focus of this chapter will be on the use of randomized clinical trials as an appropriate path of inquiry to advance knowledge for nursing interventions to hasten development of middle-range, or prescriptive-level, theories.

Key Terms and Concepts

This chapter is based on the premise that the reader has an understanding of major research designs and basic research concepts, such

AUTHOR'S NOTE: The author wishes to acknowledge Dr. Hossein Yarandi for his helpful critique of this chapter.

15

as experimental design, sampling methods (random assignment) and sampling issues, control and experimental groups, causality, multicausality, middle-range or predictive-level theory, probability, bias, placebo, Hawthorne effect, manipulation, double-blind, validity and reliability, instrumentation, selection-maturation interaction, selection-history interaction, selection-instrumentation interaction, statistical inference, effect size, and replication.

Many of these terms and concepts will be reviewed throughout this chapter. However, if you have been away from the subject for a while, you will find it beneficial to review Chapters 3, 5, 7, and 8 in Volume 1.

The Concept of Causality

Experimental studies are conducted in order to determine cause and effect. The assumptions underlying causality derive from the logical positivist philosophy. Positivists, such as David Hume and John Stuart Mill, noted that causality cannot be observed but can be inferred when certain conditions are established. In order to be able to establish cause and effect, the necessary and sufficient conditions for causality must be met (Cook & Campbell, 1979). Criteria for causation are as follows:

(1) There must be a strong correlation between the proposed cause and the effect—that is, when X changes, so does Y. This is known as *covariation*. A number of observations will be needed to establish covariation.

(2) The proposed cause (X) must precede the effect (Y) in time. In other words, there must be *causal direction*.

(3) The proposed cause must be *necessary* for the effect to occur. The effect does not occur unless the proposed cause occurs first. This criterion is referred to as *nonspuriousness*. We need to be sure that other variables that cause changes in Y are not responsible for the effect of X on Y. *Spurious associations* occur when two variables are correlated but are correlated because of the influence of another variable.

(4) The proposed cause must also be *sufficient*—that is, requiring no other factors—for the effect to occur.

Causal relationships are expressed in the form of testable propositions, or hypotheses, and are derived from past research and theory. (For a complete discussion, see Chapter 5 in Volume 1.) Experimental studies attempt to demonstrate causality and increase predictive ability. As you might expect, meeting these necessary and sufficient conditions to demonstrate causality is practically impossible, especially in the real world, where multiple factors are involved in causation. Therefore, it is important to recognize the existence of partial causation and view causality in probabilistic terms.

Multicausality

In scientific circles, the more accepted notion of causality is that multiple factors or variables are involved in the causation of a particular effect or effects. Because of these complex interrelationships, it is virtually impossible that a single theory would be able to explain all the factors involved in causation. Causation may be examined further according to the level of causal factors. Three levels were proposed by Cook and Campbell (1979):

(1) *Molar* causal laws relate to large and complex objects or events.
(2) *Intermediate* mediation considers causal factors operating in between molar and micro levels.
(3) *Micromediation* examines causal relations at the level of small particles such as atoms.

The positivists' notion of necessary and sufficient conditions for causality do not hold for the perspective of multiple causation. Because nursing is concerned with human responses and other complex phenomena or events, most problems must be considered from the perspective of multiple causation and probability.

Probability and Statistical Inference

Research phenomena in nursing require that the notion of causality be viewed in relative terms of probability, specifically, statistical probability. The use of inferential statistics permits us to infer whether relationships observed in a sample are likely to occur in a larger population of concern. When the investigator concludes that the results are statistically significant, it means that the results obtained from the study are unlikely to have been caused by chance, according to some specified level of probability, usually $< .05$ or $< .01$.

Types of Relationships in Hypotheses

Hypotheses specify the relationship between two or more variables. The most common types of relationships expressed in hypothetical statements are depicted in Table 1.1.

TABLE 1.1

Type	Relationship
Null	No relationship is presumed to exist.
Inferential/ Correlative	A relationship is presumed that deals with the degree of influence of one variable on another.
Direct/ Inverse	A specific correlative relationship is presumed where one variable has a predictable association with another: One variable increases as the other increases (direct) or one increases while the other decreases (inverse).
Causal	Changes in one variable are presumed to result from variations in another.

The value of the null hypothesis is that the relationship is not pre-judged or that a commitment to a specific relationship is suspended. Thus the probabilities are left open to emerge from empirical testing. Inferential and correlative relationships can be tested prior to moving toward causal relationships. Causal relationships demand the highest burden of proof. The time-honored method in science is to select two groups and introduce the proposed causal variable to the experimental group and not to the control group. Most scientists view causation as a labored and lengthy process of gaining adequate empirical support for hypotheses.

Predictive-Level Theories

As discussed extensively in Chapter 2 (Volume 1), the building of middle-range, or predictive-level, theories, referred to by Dickoff and James (1968) as situation-relating to situation-producing, will derive from well-designed experimental studies that address "why" or "what will happen if" type questions. It is this kind of explanatory knowledge that is needed to advance the scientific base of nursing practice. And the use of randomized clinical trials is one preferred path of inquiry for building predictive-level theories for practice.

Major Types of Research Designs

The research design provides the structure or map to guide the researcher in a systematic inquiry of the study variables of interest.

Box 1.1. Types of Research Designs

I. OBSERVATIONAL STUDIES. There are various types of observational studies, some may be prospective or retrospective. No deliberate intervention is made by the investigator.

Cross-sectional

　Observation studies at a single point in time

　Cohort (prospective or retrospective)

Longitudinal

　Case control (retrospective)

　Cohort (prospective or retrospective)

　Historical (retrospective)

　Trend (prospective or retrospective)

II. EXPERIMENTAL STUDIES. All experimental studies are *prospective* and at least one intervention (*independent variable*) is manipulated.

True Experimental

　Randomized controlled trials Subjects are randomly assigned to concurrent groups; the study is designed to determine if the intervention has the expected effect on the experimental group.

　Single case study Responses of an individual are compared under different treatment conditions, with the individual acting as his or her own control.

Quasi-experimental　Subjects are not assigned randomly to groups or trials in which comparison groups, if any, are not concurrent.

Time series (prospective)

In research, two broad types of designs or studies are recognized, *observational* and *experimental.* Within these two broad types, designs may be further classified according to time frame, whether retrospective or prospective, and by type of study, as shown in Box 1.1.

Observational Studies

The majority of studies in nursing have been observational. To be more specific, 56% of nursing practice studies during the decade

1977-1986 were cross-sectional, retrospective studies that involved a single data collection point; only 9% were experimental (Moody et al., 1988). These findings highlight the need to go beyond the single, snapshot study in order to build explanatory knowledge for the discipline. Another valuable design is trend analysis, which is longitudinal. It may be prospective or retrospective and data are collected at several points throughout the study. The trend analysis design has many uses in nursing and should be used more often when the experimental approach is not appropriate.

Experimental Studies

The specific purpose of an experimental design is to determine cause and effect. The *independent* variables are expected to be the causal factors, while the *dependent* variables (or *response* variables) are designated as the effects of the independent variables. Experimental designs are usually more scientifically rigorous than other methods of research, and the researcher is actively involved in the control and manipulation of the research environment. The following conditions must be met in the design of the true experimental study:

(1) The investigator has *control* over at least one dependent variable.
(2) There is *manipulation* of a least one independent variable.
(3) There is *random assignment* of subjects or units to the experimental and control groups.

The primary advantage of the true experiment is the control the investigator has over variance, which facilitates empirical testing of the relation between the independent and dependent variables and permits causal inference.

The other major type of experimental design, the quasi-experimental study, differs in only one respect from the true experimental study in that, for ethical or other reasons, there is no random assignment to the control or experimental groups. Because of this, the ability to deduce causal inference from the quasi-experimental study is not as strong as with the true experimental design. In this chapter, we will focus on types of randomized clinical trials. Another experimental design, the time-series design, has a number of uses in nursing research and is discussed fully in Chapter 4 of this volume.

Randomized Clinical Trials

A randomized clinical trial, also known as a clinical trial, is a type of experimental design. A clinical trial is a prospective study comparing the effect and value of one or more interventions against a control in human subjects (Friedman, Furberg, & DeMets, 1985, p. 2). The discussion in this chapter will be limited to human experimentation. Selection of the randomized clinical trial design as a mode of inquiry indicates that the researcher has posed a Level III (predictive) research question (see Chapter 4, Volume 1). Level III research aims address the effects of interventions on the dependent (response) variables, as presented in the example below from a proposed clinical trial (Moody, Martin, & Notelovitz, 1989).

The goal of this three-year randomized clinical trial (RCT) for post-menopausal women, 50-69, is to determine effective preventive treatments to improve the health status of aging women who are at risk for osteoporosis, atraumatic fractures, and cardiopulmonary problems. Because calcium replacement is considered standard preventive treatment for post-menopausal women, the study design is a standard-treatment controlled, repeated measures design with random assignment to one of four treatment groups: Group A-45 minutes of aerobic treadmill training thrice weekly for 18 months (AE) and estrogen, progesterone, and calcium replacement (EPCR); Group B- AE and calcium replacement; Group C- EPCR only; and, Group D- standard treatment (CR-calcium replacement only). The primary study aims are to analyze main and interactive effects of the four treatments on these dependent study variables, which are indicators of health status in post-menopausal women:

1. bone mineral density (BMD) of the femur and spine as measured by dual energy x-ray absorptiometry and bone fragility as measured by patellar bone modulus (PBM) ultrasound;
2. pulmonary fitness as determined by spirometry (FVC, FEV25, MVV) and maximal inspiratory pressure (MIP);
3. cardiovascular fitness as indicated by blood pressure, maximal oxygen uptake (VO2max) and blood lipids (HDL2, HDL/LDL ratio).
4. psychologic response (mastery and quality of life) as measured by the Health Risk Assessment Tool (HRAT) scales.
5. symptom response (depression state and fatigue) as measured by the HRAT scales.

Related to the primary study aims, the multivariate analysis will determine significant covariates, specifically, personality factors and protocol adherence that may affect the dependent variables and will use multiple analysis of covariance in assessing treatment effects on the dependent variables. Studies such as this are needed in nursing to provide health counseling and interventions that are scientifically based.

Historical Perspective

Although use of experimental studies in nursing dates back to the 1950s, randomized clinical trials, in the strict sense of the term, have only been used since the 1980s. The value of randomized clinical trials has been increasingly recognized by nursing, medicine, and grant-funding agencies, such as the National Institutes of Health, National Center for Nursing Research. A randomized clinical trial is a true experiment that compares the effect and value of intervention(s) in an experimental group of human subjects against a control group of human subjects who do not receive the intervention(s). The control group must be sufficiently similar in key aspects to the experimental group so that differences in outcome may be correctly attributed to the intervention(s) (Friedman, Furberg, & DeMets, 1985, p. 2). The clinical trial may employ more than one intervention and the intervention may be a preventive action, diagnostic or therapeutic agent, device, regimen, procedure, instruction, or some other variable.

Clinical trials are appropriate when there is some evidence to indicate that a new or different treatment or intervention would be more beneficial, safer, more cost-effective, or less harmful than the current or standard method. As Friedman, Furberg, and DeMets (1985) point out, the results of some treatments are so dramatic that no clinical trial is needed, as was the case when penicillin was used to treat pneumococcal pneumonia.

The clinical intervention must not have been used to the extent that it is commonly accepted as standard treatment because it would then be considered unethical to conduct a clinical trial. The preferred clinical trial is one that is randomized and double-blind. Randomization reduces the potential for bias in the allocation of subjects to the intervention group or to the control group. Through randomization, all subjects are equally likely to be assigned to either the intervention or the control group so that comparable groups are produced. More will be said about the randomization process in the discussion on sampling.

Although there are a number of clinical trials in nursing of high quality, a large number have deficiencies in design, conduct, analysis, presentation, or interpretation of results (Moody et al., 1988). It is the intent here to provide the fundamentals needed to ensure a successful clinical research trial.

Ethical Issues in Experimentation

The ethics of clinical trials have long been debated with different arguments, ranging from the obligation of the health care provider to the patient to individual welfare versus the public good. Questions of random assignment to intervention groups often plague the investigator, and when to terminate a clinical trial can become an issue of concern. The current consensus is that properly designed and conducted clinical trials are ethical and they can address important health questions without compromising or impairing the welfare of the participants.

Again, to avoid an ethical problem, the clinical intervention must not be the preferred treatment or be accepted as standard treatment because it would then be considered unethical to conduct a clinical trial. Other ethical issues can be prevented through the use of randomized double-blind procedures.

For example, an investigator may be tempted to assign the sicker patients to a particular intervention, in the hope that the patients will benefit. However, this will create a selection bias and make interpretation of the results difficult. Friedman, Furberg, and DeMets (1985) note that objection to random assignment is not appropriate unless the investigator has cause to believe that a preferred therapy exists. And, in that case, a trial should not take place. The use of a placebo is acceptable if there are no reasons to believe that one therapy is better than another.

Randomization reduces the potential of bias in assigning subjects to either the intervention group or the control group. Through randomization, all subjects are equally likely to be assigned to either the intervention or the control group so that comparable groups are produced.

The other major ethical issue of concern in clinical trials is that of informed consent. The U.S. Department of Health and Human Services has established guidelines for informed consent (Code of Federal Regulations, 1983) that are implemented on the local level by an institutional review board (IRB). An example of an IRB-approved informed consent form for subjects is shown in Box 1.2. Subjects must be told that they are free to withdraw at anytime without penalty and must be told of their chances of receiving a placebo or the standard or usual care. Potential side effects of the intervention and potential effects of delayed treatment need to be fully explained in terms the subject can understand. The participant should be told that results of the study will not be released until the study has ended. When there is conflict during a study about what is good for the research versus what is good for the participant, the needs of the participant should always predominate. Use of a study protocol, as depicted in Box 1.3, will assist in the conduct and completion of an ethical clinical trial.

Linking Theory and Research

In order to develop predictive-level theory, the researcher must link the theory with the research design and explicate a theoretical perspective that is derived from past research. In Chapter 7 (Volume 1), we presented a process for developing a conceptual map or theoretical perspective to guide the design, conduct, and analysis of the study. The reader is referred to this chapter for a discussion of how to explicate the theory-research link. The importance of this process for theory building cannot be overstated.

Designs for Randomized Clinical Trials

Six types of research designs for the randomized clinical trial are recognized by Friedman, Furberg, and DeMets (1985). The basic types of designs are parallel, withdrawal, crossover, factorial, group allocation, and equivalent. Each of these designs will be discussed here and illustrated with examples from nursing research. Conventions of notation will be used to illustrate certain designs. For example, "X" is used to denote experimental manipulation (intervention or treatment), "O" denotes observation or measurement, and "R" indicates randomization.

Parallel Design

The parallel randomized clinical trial is the most basic experimental design. It is also the least expensive, most uncomplicated, and

Box 1.2. Example of an IRB Approved Informed Consent Form

SOURCE: Moody, Martin, & Notelovitz, 1989.

INFORMED CONSENT TO PARTICIPATE IN RESEARCH

J. HILLIS MILLER HEALTH CENTER
UNIVERSITY OF FLORIDA
GAINESVILLE, FL 32610

You are being asked to volunteer as a participant in a research study. This form is designed to provide you with information about this study and to answer any of your questions.

1. TITLE OF RESEARCH STUDY
   Clinical Trial to Improve Health in Aging Women

2. PROJECT DIRECTOR
   Name: Linda Moody, Ph.D, R.N.
   Telephone Number: 904/392-3524

3. THE PURPOSE OF THE RESEARCH
   This study will examine which of the four treatments below, has the greatest effects on bone mass density, lung function, blood fats, and, overall fitness of postmenopausal women, aged 50-69. By taking part in this study, you agree to be assigned by chance to one of these four treatment groups:
   Group A: members of this group will do aerobic exercise training on a treadmill for 45 minutes three times a week for 18 months and take estrogen, progesterone, and calcium carbonate therapy;
   Group B: members of this group will take estrogen, progesterone, and calcium carbonate therapy;
   Group C: members of this group will do aerobic exercise training on a treadmill for 45 minutes three times a week for 18 months and take calcium carbonate therapy;
   Group D: members of this group will take calcium carbonate therapy alone.

4. PROCEDURES FOR THIS RESEARCH
   Baseline Tests
   a. When the study begins, you will be asked to complete a questionnaire about your diet, exercise, health problems, medical history, and personality profile. To confirm your eligibility for the study and to obtain information about your health status, these medical tests will be done:
   Chest and spine x-rays, electrocardiogram, physical examination (which includes a Pap smear and an endometrial biopsy), blood pressure, weight, skinfold measurements, a bone density test of your spine and hip, a bone-fragility test of your kneecap, a mammogram, and a lung function test.
   You will also have a treadmill exercise test to measure your maximal oxygen uptake. Your heart rate, heart rhythm, and blood pressure will be monitored during this test. Strenuous exercise, food, and caffeine are prohibited for 8 hours

prior to this test. The exercise testing will be maximal, continuing until you no longer increase your oxygen uptake or until you feel a state of exhaustion.

b. Blood will be drawn from a vein in your forearm (about 2 tablespoons or 10 milliliters) so that a complete blood count, hormones, and cholesterol and other blood fats can be measured. It is important that you not eat or drink anything other than water, 8 hours before the blood sample is drawn.

c. The total time for all the initial tests will take about *3-4 hours*. If the above tests indicate that you are eligible, you will be assigned by chance to one of the four groups by choosing an envelope with a group assignment on it.

If you are not in an exercise training group or the estrogen and progesterone group, we will assist you in obtaining the appropriate treatment from your local physician if the study shows that these treatments are effective and appropriate for you.

d. All women in the four study groups will be provided with calcium supplements to take for the entire time of the study.

Study Procedures

a. If you are assigned to one of the exercise groups, you agree to train on a motorized treadmill *three times per week for 45 minutes per session for 18 months*. The training protocol will be gradual, according to the American College of Sports Medicine guidelines, in order to permit you to reach your maximal exercise potential by the 18th session.

If you are not in one of the exercise groups, you agree to *not enroll* in a formal exercise program and to *not start* an aerobic exercise program until the study ends.

b. Every *year*, you will have these tests done:
   –physical examination, including Pap smear and endometrial biopsy
   –mammogram

c. Every *six months*, you will have these tests done in order that we may determine the effects of the treatments:
   –blood cholesterol
   –lung function tests
   –blood pressure, weight, height, skinfold fatness tests
   –bone mass density and bone fragility tests
   –completion of a questionnaire to assess your symptoms and well-being
   –treadmill exercise testing

d. Every *two months*, we will telephone you to discuss these topics related to the research:
   1. Any side effects from any of the drugs or exercise
   2. Any side effects from exercise training, if you are in the exercise group
   3. Any problems in following the exercise or drug therapy programs based on your group
   4. Any new health problems noted

e. At the *end of the study*, you will have *all* the tests repeated that you had done when you first entered the study so that we will be able to assess the effects of treatment.

5. POTENTIAL RISKS OR DISCOMFORTS

If you wish to discuss any risks or discomforts you may experience, you may call the Project Director listed on page one of this form. You are free to withdraw from the study at anytime.

The measurement of your hip and spine bone density exposes you to minimal ionizing radiation or x-rays. Exposure to x-rays is measured in millirems. The total exposure from the spine and hip measurements is about 75 millirems per year. The x-ray exposure from the mammogram, chest and spine x-rays is about 475 millirems. For comparison, a person's average exposure to the sun and other natural sources of radiation is about 100 millirems per year.

The maximal graded exercise testing on the treadmill is associated with a small risk of heart and circulatory problems. The risk for serious heart beat disturbances is 4.8 per 10,000; heart attacks, 3.6 per 10,0000; and, deaths, .5/10,000. Maximal exercise testing may result in leg muscle soreness, but this usually disappears within 48 hours.

The exercise training on the treadmill is a low risk activity and will be restricted to 70-85% of your maximal heart rate as measured on your most recent exercise test. Exercise training of this type is consistent with guidelines for exercise programs established by the American College of Sports Medicine. The small risk of bone or muscle injuries will be minimized because we will use a graded exercise training program.

There are no known risks or pain associated with the physical examination, skinfold tests, bone fragility tests, and, administration of the health questionnaire. The Pap smear and endometrial biopsy may cause some mild lower abdominal cramping, which usually disappears in 15-30 minutes.

The risks of drawing blood from a vein include discomfort at the site of needle insertion; possible bruising and swelling around the insertion site; rarely an infection; and, rarely, faintness.

Past studies have shown that estrogen, progesterone, and calcium replacement can help increase bone mass density in postmenopausal women. While not all the evidence is in on the benefits and risks of taking estrogen and progesterone together, there are some potential risks and side effects that you should know about.

Side effects from estrogen and progesterone therapy may include: monthly bleeding, tenderness or breast enlargement, irritability, depression, weight gain, slight rise in blood pressure, and fluid retention. There is a rare chance that women at risk for heart disease are more likely to develop a blood clot in the lung or have a stroke. You will be screened at the beginning of the study for these risk factors and excluded from the study if these risk factors are present.

These side effects may occur when taking calcium carbonate: abdominal gas and bloating. When the study begins, the Project Directors will advise you as to how to minimize any side effects you may have from these drugs. Your blood pressure, weight, and blood fats will be measured every six months and you will be asked about drug tolerance every two months to help reduce any side effects or risks from the estrogen, progesterone, or calcium. If health problems are noted, you will be advised to withdraw from the study and seek appropriate treatment from your local physician.

According to the National Institutes of Health Consensus Development Conference on Osteoporosis (1984), the risks to women in this study who receive the standard treatment of calcium supplements alone or exercise and calcium supplements are judged to be minimal during the study period.

6. POTENTIAL BENEFITS TO YOU OR TO OTHERS

The benefits you will derive by taking part in this study over the 30-month period are as follows:

a. Six (6) physician-supervised maximal exercise tests with measurement of maximal oxygen uptake and heart-lung function.
b. Six (6) measurements of spine and hip bone mineral density and bone fragility.
c. Free supervised exercise training if you are assigned to one of the training groups for eighteen (18 months).
d. Free estrogen and progesterone therapy if you are assigned to one of the training groups.
e. Free supply (1500 mg/day) of supplemental calcium during the entire study.
f. Twenty-five dollars ($25) when you finish the initial study tests and $25 for each year of the study that you complete, for a maximum of $100.

When the study ends, we will assess your physical condition and risk factors and make recommendations for your treatment and follow-up that are based on the study findings. We will send these recommendations to your local physician who can provide the appropriate treatment. If you do not have a local physician, we will assist you in locating one. If you wish to join an aerobic walking group after the study ends, we will assist you in locating one that is appropriate for your age and medical condition.

7. ALTERNATIVE TREATMENT OR PROCEDURES, IF APPLICABLE

The procedures used in this study pose minimal risk to the subjects. Estrogen, progesterone, and calcium carbonate have been used in previous studies, in combination and as single drugs, to increase bone mass density but questions remain about dose-response and combination therapy. The dose-response of aerobic training to increase bone mass density has not yet been determined. Based on past research, there are no known, scientifically-based alternative preventive therapies that could be used in this study that would decrease the risks to subjects and at the same time allow the researchers to answer the study questions.

Box 1.3. Example of A Study Protocol

SOURCE: Adapted from Friedman, Furberg, and DeMets (1985).

Background of the Study

Research Objectives
  1. Primary research question and response variable
  2. Secondary research questions and response variables
  3. Subgroup hypotheses

Study Design
  1. Study population
      a. Inclusion criteria
      b. Exclusion criteria
      c. Sample size estimates
  2. Enrollment of subjects
      a. Training of research team
      a. Informed consent
      b. Assessment of eligibility
      c. Baseline examination
      d. Intervention allocation
  3. Intervention
      a. Description and schedule
      b. Measures of adherence
  4. Follow-up visit description and schedule
  5. Ascertainment of response variables
      a. Training
      b. Data collection
      c. Data monitoring and quality control
      d. Data analysis

Study Termination Policy
  1. Criteria for termination

Organizational Considerations
  1. Participating investigators
  2. Study administration
      a. Committees and subcommittees
      b. Policy and data monitoring committee
  3. Budget Process

most frequently used design. Subjects are randomly assigned to the experimental or the control group and "pre" and "post" measurements are taken on both groups. The parallel design can be depicted as follows:

$$R \ O_1 \quad X \quad O_2$$
$$R \ O_1 \qquad O_2$$

When there are only two groups, it is referred to as a two-arm study; a three-arm study would employ three groups. An example of a two-arm, parallel study by Gill et al. (1988) is depicted in Box 1.4 in which the two groups were the infants who received (NNS) and those who did not (ONNS).

The Withdrawal Design

In the withdrawal design, the randomized clinical trial is implemented on subjects who are already on a regimen. This design is considered to be a special case of the parallel design. For example, subjects with chronic lung disease who have been on long-term IPPB therapy are randomly assigned to one of two groups. One-half are gradually withdrawn from the therapy or the therapy is gradually decreased and discontinued. The other half remain on the standard IPPB therapy and the outcomes of both groups are compared.

Crossover (Counterbalanced)

The crossover randomized clinical trial uses each subject to serve as his or her own control in that subjects start on one treatment and then switch (crossover) to another. In using this design, the assumption is made that there are no residual effects from one treatment period to another. Two methods to decrease the residual or carryover effects of treatment include (a) the provision of "washout" time or time between treatments to allow the treatment effects to clear so that the subject will return to baseline or starting condition, or (b) the second treatment is given twice (A/B/B), or the treatments may be given twice and alternated for both groups over four periods (A/B/A/B or B/A/B/A).

An example of the crossover design is the study by Doering and Dracup (1987) in which cardiac output was measured by thermodilution in 51 adult postcardiac surgical patients using three positions:

Box 1.4. Effect of Nonnutritive Sucking on Behavioral State in Preterm
Infants Before Feeding

SOURCE: Gill, N. E., Behnke, M., Conlon, M., McNeeley, J. B., & Anderson,
G. C. (1988). *Nursing Research, 37*: 347-350.

To describe the effect of nonnutritive sucking (NNS) on behavioral state
(BSt) in preterm infants before feedings 24 infants were randomly assigned
and studied before each of their first 16 bottle feedings. Twelve received
NNS by pacifier for 5 minutes; 12 did not receive a pacifier (ONNS). BSt
was measured with a 12-category scale for 30 seconds before the 5-minute
period (BSt1) and for 30 seconds after (BSt2). Sleep states decreased for
both groups. BSts considered more optimal for feeding increased more
during NNS (86 versus 46). Restlessness states were three times less
frequent after NNS (23 versus 68). Differences between groups were
nonsignificant at BSt1, but were significant at BSt2, p < .001. In the absence
of self-regulatory feeding policies based on early hunger cues, NNS for 5
minutes prefeeding is simple, brief, and suitable for implementation in
busy neonatal intensive care units. Nonnutritive sucking was an effective
modulator of behavioral state for this sample.

---

supine, right lateral, and left lateral. To control for sequence (crossover) effects, patients were assigned by coin toss to one of two
position sequences: supine-right-left or supine-left-right. In all, 26
subjects were tested using the former position and 25 were tested
using the latter position. After the first position of the sequence was
tested, a waiting period of at least 15 minutes was observed to allow
for the restabilization of hemodynamic parameters. After returning
to baseline, two cardiac output readings were taken and averaged.
The same procedure was repeated for the second and third positions.

Factorial

The factorial randomized clinical trial can be thought of as a
parallel four-arm study. Two interventions are compared with a
control in a single experiment. The factors are different aspects of the
intervention and all factors are given. An example of a factorial study
is shown in Box 1.5 in which the researchers randomly assigned
infants to a control group or one of three experimental conditions to
test the effects of sensory stimulation on healthy infants.

Box 1.5. Developmental and Temperament Outcomes of Sensory
          Stimulation in Healthy Infants

SOURCE: Koniak-Griffin, D., & Ludington-Hoe, S. M. (1988). *Nursing
    Research, 37*, 70-76.

This experimental study was designed to assess the longitudinal effects of
a home-based program of unimodal and multimodal stimulation provided during the infant's first 3 months on 4- and 8-month developmental
status and temperament of normal, full-term infants. Unimodal stimulation was administered in the form of a stroking procedure. A multisensory
hammock was used to offer multimodal stimulation. Intervening with
rocking hammocks and similar types of devices has previously been found
to produce a soothing influence on premature infants. Stroking may lead
to increased activity and alertness, decreased crying, and enhanced motor
development. Sensory stimulation programs are based on the theory that
there is a sequential development of the senses and the somatosensory
system is the earliest system to mature. Eighty-one healthy, full-term
infants were randomly assigned to a control group of one of three experimental conditions: daily administration of a cephalocaudal stroking procedure; placement on a multisensory hammock that provided auditory,
vestibular, and tactile stimulation during expected sleep cycles; and a
combination of the prior two treatments. All interventions were provided
during the first 3 months of life. Infants in the control group received the
natural stimulation provided in their home environments without additional supplementation. Four- and 8-month assessments were done using
the Bayley Scales of Infant Development and the Revised Infant Temperament Questionnaire. There were no significant treatment effects on
weight or psychomotor development. Although infants receiving unimodal stimulation obtained lower 8-month cognitive development scores
than infants in other experimental and control groups, their scores were
within the normal range. Control group infants achieved the most opti-
mum mood and distractibility scores at both 4 and 8 months. Although
the findings have implications for both nursing practice and research,
nurses who care for child-rearing families must carefully evaluate the
potential effects of sensory stimulation programs on development of
full-term, healthy infants before advocating their widespread application.
Further research should be directed to determine which aspects of unimodal and multimodal stimulation are most salient in facilitating or
inhibiting specific aspects of cognitive development and temperament
among infants of varying ages. Longitudinal studies would assist in
assessing long-term effects of early sensory stimulation.

Box 1.6. Self-Reported Factors Influencing Exercise Adherence in
        Overweight Women

SOURCE: Gillett, P. A. (1988). *Nursing Research, 37,* 25-29.*

The purpose of this study was to determine the effect of intensity-controlled, graded dance exercise and selected components of behavior modification on exercise adherence in overweight middle-aged women. Thirty-eight moderately overweight women, aged 35 to 58, participated in a 16½-week dance exercise program. Using a schedule generated from a table of random numbers, participants were randomly assigned to an experimental group (*n* = 20) that received intensity-controlled, graded exercise and individual and group reinforcement, or to a control group (*n* = 18) that exercised at a moderate intensity typical of commercial fitness classes and received no special reinforcement. Before exercise training began and at the completion of 16½ weeks, a structured, open-ended interview was conducted. Ninety-four percent of the women in both groups adhered to the program, an exceptionally high adherence rate for this population. Eight participant-identified factors seemed to have influenced exercise adherence: group homogeneity, carpooling and social networks, pleasurable feelings associated with increased energy and fitness, leader with a health-related background, time limitation of exercise program, commitment to an established goal, desire to change body image, and desire to change health status and improve physical health.

---

*This study is an example of the use of both quantitative and qualitative data analysis. According to Downs (1988, p. 3), it is also a classic example of an occurrence of the Hawthorne effect in research.

Group Allocation

The group allocation design for a randomized clinical trial is also a special case of the parallel design. In this design, the focus is on the group rather than the individual, and the groups are randomized for treatment. Special methods exist for analyzing individual data, if required. This design is commonly used in educational programs or health-promotion and wellness programs, when groups are assigned various interventions. An example of group allocation is depicted in Box 1.6.

Equivalent

The equivalent design is an extension of the parallel design, except for the difference in expected direction of treatment effects. In the equivalent design, the researcher is not so much interested in comparing the efficacy of the interventions but in assessing the effect that the interventions have on quality of life. This design has been used to assess quality of life for women who have had a radical mastectomy or a lumpectomy with chemotherapy.

Research design summary. The research design provides the researcher with a map for implementing the study, so it is critical to expend adequate time and efforts to plan a sound research design. The researcher needs to have a good understanding of the use of research designs and statistical methods and the ability to communicate with the biostatistician early in the planning phase of the project. The biostatistician will be able to provide better assistance if the clinical researcher explains the significance of the research problems and past research conducted in the field.

It is beyond the scope of this chapter to provide the particulars for each of the major designs discussed above. For those interested in complete details of the design, conduct, and analysis of randomized clinical trials, refer to Fleiss (1986), Friedman, Furberg, and DeMets (1985), or Meinert and Tonascia (1986) as well as the other sources listed at the end of this chapter.

Measurement Considerations

The most elegantly designed clinical trial will not offset the detriment caused by inexact measurement. Before clinical trials are initiated, the researcher must determine whether it will be possible to measure the response variables of interest in the study. Fleiss (1986, p. 1) expands on this point:

> The requirement that one's data be of high quality is at least as important a component of proper study design as the requirement for randomization, double blinding, controlling for prognostic factors, and so on. Larger sample sizes than otherwise necessary, biased estimates, and even biased samples are some of the untoward consequences of unreliable measurement that will be demonstrated.

A number of instruments and instrumentation methods have been developed within nursing and from other disciplines that will assist the researcher in obtaining valid and reliable measurements on the response variables. Refer to Chapter 8 in Volume 1 for more information on measurement, locating instruments, and instrumentation.

In some cases, the researcher may have to develop an instrument or devise instrumentation to measure the response variables. If this is the case, sufficient time and resources must be allocated to develop and test the validity and reliability of the instrument or instrumentation procedures before the clinical trial begins.

Variance in Experimental Design

Theoretically speaking, the true experiment is the ideal study design in that it measures relationships among variables with the most precision, rigor, and control. Kerlinger (1986, p. 284) elaborates on the importance of achieving control over variance in order to gain this precision:

> By constructing an efficient research design the investigator attempts (1) to maximize the variance of the variable or variables of his substantive research hypothesis, (2) to control the variance of extraneous or "unwanted" variables that may have an effect on his experimental outcomes, and (3) to minimize the error or random variance, including so-called errors of measurement.

An easy way to remember this critical point is through what Kerlinger has coined as the MAXMINCON principle: *Maximize experimental variance, minimize error variance, and control extraneous variance.*

Maximizing experimental variance. Experimental variance, also called systematic variance, refers to the variance of the dependent (response) variables that results from the independent (intervention or manipulated) variables of the substantive hypothesis. For example, experimental variance is the variance in the response variable (blood pressure) due to the independent (intervention) variables, A (biofeedback) and B (aerobic exercise), and *attribute* or *prognostic* variables, weight and gender. Although experimental variance in some cases may mean only the variance due to a manipulated variable, Kerlinger (1986, p. 287) includes attributes or risk factors, such as age, sex, and intelligence, in experimental variance. Thus, in order to maximize systematic variance, the researcher must design the study so that the interventions are as different as possible.

Controlling extraneous variance. The researcher must be able to control the influences of independent variables extraneous to the purposes of the study; that is, extraneous variables must be minimized, isolated, or eliminated. There are a number of ways to control extraneous variance.

(1) Eliminate the extraneous variable. If we are concerned about the effect of intelligence and adherence to a dietary regimen, we might decide only to select subjects from one intelligence level, say, standard scores from 90 to 110. Or if we study the effects of interventions on blood pressure and are concerned about the influence of racial membership, we might choose to study only one racial group. The principle here is to eliminate the effect of a possible influential independent variable on a response variable by selecting subjects so they are as homogeneous as possible on that independent variable. A disadvantage of this method is that the researcher loses generalization power. For example, if we only study one gender or one racial group, then our findings are limited.

(2) Randomize to control extraneous variance. Theoretically, this is the only way to control extraneous variance and maximize generalizability of the findings. If randomization has been followed, then the intervention groups can be considered statistically equal in all possible ways. It does not mean that the groups are equal in all the possible variables, but the probability of their being equal is greater. The principle followed here is to, whenever possible, randomly assign subjects to experimental groups and conditions and randomly assign conditions and other factors to experimental groups.

(3) Build the extraneous variable into the design. Building a variable into an experimental design "controls" the variable, because it becomes possible to extract from the total variance the influence of the dependent variable. For example, assume that gender was to be controlled for but it was not expedient to study only one gender. You might want information on the actual differences between genders on the response variable or be interested in the interaction between gender and one or more of the other variables. Thus you would add gender, as another independent variable, to the design. This method permits statistical extraction of the variance contributed by the variable, gender, and extraction of the between-gender variance. The principle of this method is to control the extraneous variable by building it into the research design as an attribute or prognostic variable. This will yield important information about the effect of this variable on the variance of the dependent variable and its potential interaction with other independent variables.

(4) Match subjects. The basic principle underlying this method is to split a variable or factor into two or more parts, such as low risk or high risk, and then randomize within each level. The variable on which subjects are matched must be substantially related to the response variable or the matching of subjects will be a waste of time. It is also difficult to match on more than two variables because it is usually impossible to find an adequate number of subjects. Kerlinger (1986, p. 289) notes that, when there is a substantial correlation between the matching variable(s) and the dependent variable (preferably > .50 or .60), then matching reduces the error term and increases the precision of an experiment. If subjects are used with different treatments, such as in repeated measures or randomized block design, there is substantial control of variance. With matching, random assignment to an intervention group should still be done because matching does not substitute for randomization.

(5) Use of statistical methods. Instead of matching, there are statistical methods, such as analysis of covariance, along with complete randomization, that may be preferable methods of variance control. Statistical methods control variance in that they assist in isolating and quantifying systematic, extraneous, and error variances. One last point is that the statistical methods cannot be isolated from the type of research design—they must be used together appropriately. If matching is used, an appropriate statistical test must be used, otherwise the matching effect, and the control of variance, will be misspent.

(6) Minimizing error variance. Error variance is the variability of measures due to random fluctuations. Theoretically, when measurement conditions are ideal, random fluctuations are self-compensating, that is, up and down, down and up, and so forth, so that, on balance, the mean error variance is zero. Error variance is usually associated with errors of measurement, which may occur in cases of respondent fatigue, guessing, lack of concentration, or transient health states of subjects. Random fluctuations in instrumentation systems may contribute to error variance. Factors related to individual differences among subjects may add to error variance; when individual differences cannot be accounted for as systematic variance, they are lumped under error variance.

There are two approaches to minimizing error variance: reducing errors of measurement through controlled experimental conditions and increasing the reliability of measures. The more uncontrolled the conditions of a clinical trial, the more the determinants of error variance can operate. Reducing error variance can be done by carefully establishing controlled conditions, by giving specific and clear instructions to subjects, and by excluding situational factors that are extraneous to the purpose of the clinical trial. Increasing the reliability of the measures will reduce error variance.

An important reason for reducing error variance is to permit systematic variance a chance to be revealed and quantified. The problem of error variance can be expressed mathematically:

$$V_t = V_b + V_e$$

where V_t is the total variance in a set of measures; V_b is the between-groups variance, which is due to the influence of the experimental variables or the intervention; and V_e is the error variance (in analysis of variance, the within-groups variance and the residual group variance) (Kerlinger, 1986, p. 290). Thus, for a given amount of V_t, the larger V_e is, the smaller V_b must be. This example illustrates the importance of the MAXMINCON principle. Consider further the following equation:

$$F = \frac{V_b}{V_e}$$

For the numerator of the preceding fraction to be evaluated as being a significant departure from chance expectation, the denominator should be an accurate measure of random error. It is clear in this example why the systematic variance is maximized (V_b); random error is minimized (V_e); and extraneous variables are controlled.

Reliability

A discussion of the major concepts of reliability will be reviewed in this section. Also refer to Chapters 5 and 8 in Volume 1 for more detailed information on reliability. After the measurement process, that is, assigning numbers to objects or events, two issues are at stake: reliability and validity. The quality of the data depends in part on the dependability or reliability of our measurement methods. *Reliability* refers to the stability, consistency, predictability, dependability, and precision of the measuring instruments. In other words, if we repeat the measurements using the instruments, how likely are we to obtain similar results? With all measurement, we can calculate a mean, standard deviation and a variance. The variance calculated is the total obtained variance, also known as the sum of squares, and it includes systematic and error variance. *Reliability* is defined through error variance: the more error, the greater the unreliability; the less error, the greater the reliability. Thus, by estimating error variance, we gain an estimate of the reliability. Kerlinger (1986, p. 408) provides two equivalent definitions of reliability:

(1) Reliability is the proportion of the "true" variance to the total obtained variance of the data yielded by a measuring instrument.
(2) Reliability is the proportion of error variance to the total variance yielded by a measuring instrument subtracted from 1.00, the index 1.00 indicating perfect reliability.

A useful formula for determining reliability is as follows:

$$r_{tt} = \frac{V_t - V_e}{V_t}$$

where r_{tt} is the reliability coefficient, V_t is the total obtained variance, and V_e is the error variance.

In some clinical studies, the researcher may have a response variable that is qualitative in nature, such as condition improved, no change, or condition worsened. Cohen's kappa statistic (Cohen, 1977) is the measure of reliability for this type of qualitative data.

Related to reliability are two other terms, *sensitivity* and *specificity*, that the researcher must be concerned about if a diagnostic test is used to measure a dependent (response) variable. *Sensitivity* of a test measures the ability of the test to correctly confirm the presence of a disease or prognostic factor or to avoid a false negative. *Specificity* is the ability of the test to correctly confirm the absence of the disease or prognostic factor or to avoid a false positive.

In summary, the quality of the data depends on the reliability of the measurement instruments as well as their validity. The principle of MAXMINCON also applies in terms of achieving adequate reliability.

Validity

Validity refers to authenticity or truth value and, as related to measurement instruments, we are most concerned about *construct* (theoretical) validity. Construct validity, and other forms of validity, were discussed in Chapters 5 and 8 in Volume 1. However, specific to the design and conduct of randomized clinical trials, two types of validity are of concern: internal validity and external validity.

Internal validity refers to the relationship between the response variables and the independent variables, that is, did the independent variable have a true effect on the response variables or is there some other variable that intervened? Put another way, internal validity addresses how much truth value there is to the hypothesis or seeks to determine whether a more plausible explanation exists to explain the findings. There are several factors that may influence or threaten internal validity.

Threats to internal validity. Threats to internal validity may operate jointly and consequently; if internal validity is not supported, the results cannot be generalized beyond the study. Each of these threats to internal validity, first noted in the original work of Campbell and Stanley (1963), are summarized below.

(1) Maturation. Maturation of subjects occurs with passage of time when events occurring between sets of measurements of a variable distort the influence of the intervention variable on the response variable. Random assignment and completion of the study in as short a time as possible will help minimize effects of maturation.

(2) History. Historical events, all known as secular effects, may occur during the experiment to influence the effects of the intervention on the response variable. Again, random assignment will assist in minimizing the effects because all groups will then be exposed to similar events.

(3) Testing. This is defined as the effect of testing on retesting scores. To avoid subjects becoming test wise, build in a second control group that is tested the same number of times as the experimental group so you can determine the effect of subjects becoming test wise.

(4) Instrumentation error. Instrumentation refers to the lack of reliability in measurement of the response variable. Other than selecting or developing a valid and reliable method for measuring the response variable, minimize error by keeping scorers "blind" as to which subjects belong to the experimental or control group. In addition, adequate training in the use of instruments or instrumentation will help minimize error.

(5) Statistical regression. This means that there is a tendency for subjects who have responses at the extremes of a distribution to have less extreme scores when retested. This occurs when subjects are

chosen for a study because of their extreme scores, and the problem can be minimized by random assignment.

(6) *Differential selection.* This refers to systematic differences in the allocation of subjects to study groups. To avoid major differences in groups, the researcher uses random assignment or matching. When these methods do not work, an uneven distribution may result and affect the response variable. An example would be if a researcher was testing the effect of exercise on pulmonary function and found that 55% of subjects in the treatment group had asthma while only 8% of those in the control group had asthma. In this situation, the researcher will not be able to correctly assess the effect of the intervention because of the high number of subjects in the treatment group with asthma and its potential effect on the response variable, pulmonary function.

(7) *Experimental mortality.* Experimental mortality, also known as differential loss of subjects, causes problems in interpreting the relationship between the independent variable and the response variable. For example, if subjects in the intervention group who are less healthy or are responding less well than those who stay in the study, the researcher may overestimate the effect of the intervention. Other than having an excellent rapport with the subjects, spending time with those who express concern or are disgruntled, keeping appointments within the time frame, helping subjects appreciate their contribution to the study, providing incentives or monetary awards to those who finish (within ethical guidelines), little can be done to prevent experimental mortality.

External validity pertains to the representativeness or generalizability of the study findings. In other words, can the study results be applied to other populations or in other contexts or were the findings simply a function of the specific population studied?

Threats to external validity. A number of factors may affect external validity. They are briefly discussed here.

(1) *Reactivity.* Reactivity refers to the responses of subjects being studied. The classic example of reactivity is the "Hawthorne effect," which was observed in a study of the effects of manipulating working conditions of employees at the Hawthorne plant of Western Electric Corporation. Employees improved their production rates significantly, regardless of the condition manipulated, simply because they were involved in a study. The study involvement led to increased morale of the workers, hence increased production. Another type of reactivity is when subjects try to estimate the preferred response and try to please or outwit the researcher.

(2) Novelty. The novelty of study participation may also contribute to subjects' responding more positively or more negatively than if they were not being studied. Thus some subjects may not present a typical experience. To control for the novelty effect, some investigators use a control procedure rather than no intervention for the control group. The researcher may place subjects in the control group on a waiting list for delayed treatment, so they too are exposed to the novelty of being studied.

(3) Testing. If pretesting is used in a study, the results will be less generalizable to a population that has not been pretested. For example, if subjects are pretested with an attitude inventory, they may have time to reflect on their attitudes and respond differently on retesting than subjects who have never taken the inventory.

(4) Joint effects of reactivity and manipulation. The joint effects of reactivity and being selected for an intervention group may decrease the generalizability of findings. For example, if a researcher is testing the effect of biofeedback on reducing nausea from chemotherapy and the control group has sicker patients or more advanced disease than the treatment group, their response would be expected to be considerably worse than subjects who receive the intervention. Thus it would be difficult to generalize the findings because the groups are not comparable.

(5) Multiple treatments. In clinical trials, subjects may be involved in more than one intervention or several protocols during a relatively short period of time. At the same time, the investigator may be unaware of subjects who are involved in other studies or who engage in self-care or other treatments that might affect the study outcome. Obtaining a complete health history and gaining the subject's cooperation early in the study can help minimize the problem of multiple treatments. Periodic checks to confirm the subject's commitment to the study will also help reduce this problem.

(6) Selection bias. When subjects who want to receive a particular study intervention enroll in the experimental group and are compared with subjects in a control group who do not want the intervention, a selection bias occurs that causes problems in interpretation and generalization of the findings. Those seeking the intervention may be sicker, they may be more motivated, they may be socioeconomically advantaged, or they may differ in some other factor from the control group to make the groups noncomparable. Thus random assignment is the way to avoid selection bias.

Procedures for Randomization

The randomized control trial is the benchmark against which all other designs are compared. Clinical trials have three distinct advantages over other methods (Friedman, Furberg, & DeMets, 1985, pp. 35-36):

(1) Randomization removes the potential of bias in the allocation of subjects to the intervention or control group.
(2) Randomization tends to produce balanced or comparable groups, that is, the measured or unknown prognostic factors and other characteristics of the subjects at the time of randomization will be, on average, balanced between the groups.
(3) Randomization ensures the validity of statistical tests of significance in that it is possible to ascribe a probability distribution to the difference in outcome between treatment groups receiving equally effective treatments and thus to assign significance levels to observed differences.

Ideally, neither the investigator nor the subject knows in advance which group or intervention will be assigned to whom: This is referred to as *double-blind randomization* (also known as masking). If the investigator knows, but the subjects do not, it is a *single-blind randomization*. A number of methods for randomly assigning subjects may be used. The most commonly accepted randomization procedures will be discussed here. Two broad types of categories of randomization are recognized: fixed allocation randomization and adaptive randomization.

Fixed Allocation Randomization Procedures

With fixed allocation randomization procedures, the interventions are assigned to subjects with a prespecified probability, usually equal, and the allocation probability is not altered throughout the study. There are three standard procedures for fixed allocation randomization: simple randomization, blocked randomization, and stratified randomization.

(1) Simple randomization. This is the most basic form of randomization and several procedures can be used. One way is to toss an unbiased coin each time a subject is eligible to be randomized. If the coin turns up heads, the subject is assigned to group A; if it turns up tails, to group B. With this procedure, one-half of subjects should be in group A and one-half in group B.

Another method is the use of a random digit table in which the equally likely digits 0 to 9 are arranged by rows and columns. The researcher randomly selects a certain row or column and observes the sequence of digits in that row or column. For example, group A might be assigned to those subjects for whom the digit was even, and group B to those for whom the next digit was odd. With this method, each subject has an equal chance of being assigned to A or B.

For studies with large sample sizes, a more expedient method is to use a random-number-producing algorithm, which is available on most computer systems. Using a uniform random number generator, a random number, in the interval from 0.0 to 0.999, is produced for each subject. The researcher assigns subjects to group A with probability P and subjects to group B with probability 1-p. If the random number is between 0 and P, the subject is assigned to A; otherwise, to group B. If equal allocation is not desired, that is, P = 1/2, then P can be set to the desired proportion. This method can also be adapted to more than two groups. For equal allocation, the interval is divided into thirds and assignments are made respectively. For example, for equal allocation for three groups A, B, and C, the intervals would be A = 0-0.333, B = .334-666, and C = .667-.999. The drawback to this method is that imbalances may occur with small samples. Therefore, the method is best used with samples greater than 30 (Friedman, Furberg, & DeMets, 1985, p. 53).

(2) Blocked randomization. Blocked or permuted block randomization was proposed by Hill (1971) to prevent imbalance in the number of subjects assigned to each group. For example, if subjects are randomly assigned with equal probability to groups A or B, then for each block of even size, four, six, or eight, one-half of the subjects will be assigned to A and the other half to B. The order in which the interventions are assigned in each block is randomized. The process is repeated for consecutive blocks of subjects until all are randomly assigned. To illustrate, suppose a researcher wants to be sure that, after every fourth randomized subject, the number of subjects in the intervention group is equal. Using a block size of four, there are six possible combinations of group assignments: AABB, ABAB, BAAB, BABA, BBAA, and ABBA. One of these six is selected at random, let us say, AABB. The four subjects are assigned accordingly and the process is repeated until the sample size is fulfilled. The number in each group will not differ by more than b/2 when b is the length of the block. Thus blocking will produce more comparable groups if the type of subject recruited for the study changes during the entry period. For example, Friedman, Furberg, and DeMets (1985) point

TABLE 1.2

Factors in Stratified Randomization

Age	Sex	Cardiovascular Risk
1. <60	1. Male	1. Low risk
2. 60 or >	2. Female	2. Moderate risk
		3. High risk

out that subjects from different sources may vary in severity of illness. One source, with more seriously ill subjects, may be used early in the study and another source, with less ill subjects, later in the study. If the randomization were not blocked, more of the seriously ill subjects might be randomized to one group. A disadvantage of blocked randomization is that the data analysis should reflect the blocked randomization. That is, if blocked randomization is ignored in the analysis, the study will likely have less power then it would have with the correct analysis, and the true significance level is actually less than computed (Friedman, Furberg, & DeMets, 1985, p. 56).

(3) *Stratified randomization*. A goal of allocation is to achieve groups that are comparable in selected characteristics, such as prognostic or risk factors that correlate with subsequent subject response or outcome. For any study, especially small studies, there is no guarantee that all baseline factors will be similar for the groups. Imbalances in prognostic factors can be dealt with prospectively or retrospectively. Stratified randomization is a prospective method to achieve comparability between the study groups for prognostic factors. This process involves measuring potential subjects for the selected factors prior to the study, determining the stratum to which each belongs, and randomizing within that stratum. Within each stratum, the process may be simple randomization, but in most, it is blocked. Blocked randomization is a special stratification that stratifies over time whereas stratified randomization refers to stratifying on factors other than time (Friedman, Furberg, & DeMets, 1985). An example is shown in Box 1.7 for a block size of 4, and the three factors age, sex, and cardiovascular risk. The design has $2 \times 2 \times 3 = 12$ strata (Table 1.2).

Small studies are more likely to require stratified randomization because, in large studies, the magnitude of the numbers increases the

Box 1.7. Stratified Randomization with Block Size of Four				
Strata	Age	Sex	Cardiovascular Risk	Group Assignment
1	<60	M	1	ABBA BABA....
2	<60	M	2	
3	<60	M	3	
4	<60	F	1	
5	<60	F	2	
6	<60	F	3	
7	60>	M	1	
8	60>	M	2	
9	60>	M	3	
10	60>	F	1	
11	60>	F	2	
12	60>	F	3	

SOURCE: Friedman et al. (1985), p. 47.

chance of obtaining comparable groups (Friedman, Furberg, & De-Mets, 1985, p. 58). As the number of factors is increased, the strata increase markedly. For example, increasing the age factor by 1 (< 60, 60 to 70, and 70 or >) increases the strata from 12 to 18. Therefore, only critical variables should be selected for stratifying and they should be kept to a minimum. Increased stratification in small studies may defeat the purpose if the subsamples are small, or even unavailable, within each stratum. Friedman, Furberg, and DeMets (1985) explain that, for studies with 100 or fewer subjects, stratifying the randomization by using two or three prognostic factors may achieve greater power, but, for larger studies, stratification at the time of analysis will achieve an equivalent expected power. Another factor to consider in multicenter trials is that subjects may vary from center to center in terms of prognostic factors and type of care provided. Stratifying by center permits individual center analysis as well as comparison of trends by center with the overall study results.

Adaptive Randomization Procedures

The fixed allocation procedures just described are nonadaptive strategies, as contrasted to adaptive procedures, in which the allocation probabilities change as the study progresses. Two types of adaptive procedures are commonly used: baseline adaptive randomization and response adaptive randomization (Friedman, Furberg, & DeMets, 1985, p. 59).

Baseline adaptive randomization procedure (the biased coin method). This procedure attempts to balance the number of subjects in each group based on the previous assignments without considering subject responses. The purpose of the algorithm is to randomize the allocation of subjects to groups A and B with equal probability as long as the number of subjects in each group is equal. Friedman, Furberg, and DeMets (1985, p. 59) further note:

> If an imbalance occurs and the difference in numbers is greater than some prespecified value, the allocation probability (P) is adjusted so that the probability is higher for the group with fewer subjects. The investigator can determine the value of the allocation probability he wishes to use. The larger the value of P, the faster the imbalance will be corrected, while the nearer P is to 0.5, the slower the correction.

An allocation probability of $P = 2/3$ is suggested when a correction is indicated, because most of the time $P = 1/2$. Hence the name, "biased coin method." A major advantage of this procedure is that it guards against a severe baseline imbalance for important prognostic factors. For example, if age is a prognostic factor and study group A has more older subjects than group B, the allocation plan is such that the next several older subjects would be randomized to group B, which has fewer older subjects.

A disadvantage of this method is the complex statistical analysis, which calls for computer simulation of the assignment of subjects to groups by considering all possible sequences of assignments that could have been made in repeated experiments using the same biased coin allocation rule where no group differences are assumed to exist (Friedman, Furberg, & DeMets, 1985, p. 61). This simulated replication generates the significance level of the statistical test to be used, assuming that no group differences exist.

Response adaptive randomization. With this method, the response of subjects to the intervention is considered in determining future allocation of subjects. Two models are commonly used, Play the Winner and the Two-Armed Bandit, that assume that the researcher is randomizing subjects to one of two interventions and the primary response variable can be assessed relatively quickly. In the first method, Play the Winner, the first subject may be assigned by the toss of the coin, and the second subject to the same group as the first subject, if the response to the intervention was successful; if unsuccessful, the second subject is assigned to the other group. The investigator stays with the winner until a failure occurs and then switches.

The other method, the Two-Armed Bandit, continually updates the probability of success as soon as the response outcome for each subject is determined. This information is used to adjust the probabilities of being assigned to either group such that a higher proportion of future subjects would receive the superior or more successful intervention.

Both of these methods were developed in response to clinical investigators who expressed ethical concerns about the randomization process. Friedman, Furberg, and DeMets (1985) point out that, although these methods maximize the number of subjects on the superior intervention, the potential imbalance will result in loss of power and require more subjects to be enrolled than with the use of a fixed allocation with equal assignment probability. Another limitation is that many clinical trials do not have response variables that occur immediately or they have no single outcome variable that permits rapid assessment of response to the intervention. These methods also assume that the population from which the subjects are recruited is stable over time. If the nature of the study population changes and these changes are not accounted for in the analysis, the reported significance levels could possibly be severely biased. Because of these difficulties, these methods are not often used.

Summary of Randomization

The procedure for randomization depends on a number of factors. Here is a summary of guidelines that will assist in achieving the objectives of randomization for large or small studies.

(1) Blocked randomization should be used in large studies that involve more than several hundred subjects.

(2) In large, multicenter trials, randomization should be stratified by center.

(3) For large studies, randomization stratified on the basis of prognostic factors is usually unnecessary because randomization usually makes the study groups quite comparable for all risk factors. If necessary, stratified analysis can be used once the data have been collected.

(4) For small studies, the randomization should also be blocked. If the study is part of a multicenter trial, it should be stratified by center. Because the sample size is small, a few strata for important

factors may be defined to assure balance for those factors. For many risk factors, adaptive stratification techniques should be used and accounted for in the analyses.

(5) For small studies, stratified analysis can be done post hoc even if stratified randomization was not done; this will suffice in most cases (Friedman, Furberg, & DeMets, 1985, pp. 64-65).

For more detailed information on randomization procedures, consult Friedman, Furberg, and DeMets (1985), Pocock (1979), and Fleiss (1986).

Sampling Considerations

Sample size needs to be determined early in the planning of a clinical trial. Sample size is one of the most important considerations in clinical trials because the number of subjects influences whether the investigator will have the statistical power to discern whether the intervention had the intended effect. This point is emphasized by Friedman, Furberg, and DeMets (1985, p. 83):

> Clinical trials should have sufficient statistical power to detect differences between groups considered to be of clinical interest. Therefore, calculation of sample size with provision for adequate levels of significance and power is an essential part of planning.

Often, studies with low statistical power are abandoned and the interventions are never adequately evaluated, resulting in a loss of potentially beneficial treatments. Because of this, an estimate of the required sample size will assist in achieving sufficient statistical power. Sample size estimates are based on mathematical models that *approximate* the true, but unknown, distribution of the response variables. Before discussing the details of estimating sample size, a brief review of key statistical concepts of hypothesis testing are presented.

Statistical Concepts Related to Sample Size

Understanding the process of estimating sample size requires an appreciation of the essential statistical concepts of hypothesis testing, significance level, and power. For purposes of illustration, the discussion will focus on studies with one intervention group and one control group. To construct hypothesis testing, the researcher must identify the response variables and determine the type of response variable:

(1) *dichotomous response variable*—success or failure, presence or absence of some risk factor, expressed in terms of event rates
(2) *continuous response variable*—blood pressure, weight, height, or the like, or change in blood pressure, weight, height, or the like
(3) *time response variable*—length of time for an event or response to occur, such as failure or occurrence of a clinical event (survival analysis is commonly used as a time response variable).

When the response variable is dichotomous, event rates in the intervention group (P_I) and the control group (P_c) are compared. For a continuous response variable, such as mean weight loss, the true but unknown mean level in the intervention group (U_I) is compared with the mean level in the control group (U_c). For a time response variable, such as survival data, a hazard rate, λ, is usually compared for the two study groups or is used for sample size estimation. Friedman, Furberg, and DeMets (1985, p. 85) note that sample size estimate for response variables that do not exactly fit into any of the three categories can be safely estimated by using the one category into which each response variable fits best.

Hypothesis Testing

First, we will discuss hypothesis testing in a clinical trial with two groups for a dichotomous response variable (event rates). The same principles apply for the other two categories of response variables. The researcher does not actually know the true values of the event rates but the clinical trial will provide estimates of the event rates, for both groups, denoted by P_I and P_c. The researcher will test whether or not a true difference exists between the event rates of subjects in the intervention and control groups. The conventional way to state this is in the form of the null hypothesis, H_0. The null hypothesis states that no difference between the true event rates exist, and it is typically expressed as follows:

$$H_0 : P_I - P_c = 0$$

The objective is to test the null hypothesis and decide whether or not to reject it. The null hypothesis is presumed true until empirical

evidence provides support to reject it. Because we only have estimates of the true event rates, it is possible that, even if the null
hypothesis were true, the observed rates between the two groups
might be different due to chance alone. If the observed differences in
event rates are large enough by chance alone, the null hypothesis
might be rejected incorrectly. Rejecting the null hypothesis when it
is true is called a Type I error. The Type I error, referred to as the
significance level, is denoted by α. The researcher wants to avoid
making a Type I error. The probability of observing differences as
large as, or larger than, the actual differences observed, given that
H_0 is true, is called the "P-value," or P. The decision rule is to reject
H_0 if $P < \alpha$. The level of α chosen is traditionally 0.01 or 0.05,
depending on the power needed and the sample size that will be
available for the study. The smaller the α, the larger the sample size
will have to be, as demonstrated later in our example.

   If the null hypothesis is not true—that is, it is correctly rejected as
false—then there must be an alternative hypothesis, H_A, that must
be true, where

$$P_I - P_c \neq 0.$$

The observed difference can be small just by chance alone even if the
alternative hypothesis is true, so the researcher might, on the basis
of a small observed difference, fail to reject H_0 when it should be
rejected. Failing to reject H_0 when it should be rejected is a Type II
error, or a false negative result. The probability of a Type II error, β,
is dependent on the specific value of the true but unknown difference
in event rates between the two groups as well as the sample size and
α. The probability of correctly rejecting H_0 is denoted by 1-β and is
called the power of the study. The term *power* in this case means the
ability of the study, in quantitative terms, to find true differences of
various values of δ. Because β is a function of α, the sample size, and
1-β, is also a function of these parameters. The plot of 1-β versus δ
for a given sample size is called the "power curve" (Figure 1.1).

   On the horizontal axis, values of δ are plotted from 0 to an upper
value, δ (0.25). On the vertical axis, the probability, or power (1-β),
of detecting a true difference is shown for a given significance level
and sample size. In this example, a sample size of 200 (100 in each
group), a one-sided significance level of 0.05, and a control group
event rate of 0.5 (50%) were assumed. From the example, you can see
that, as δ increases, the power to detect δ also increases: If δ = 0.10,

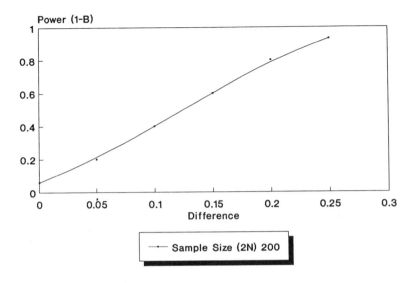

Figure 1.1. A Power Curve

SOURCE: Adapted from Friedman, Furberg, and DeMets (1985).

the power is about 0.40; when $\delta = 0.20$, the power is almost 0.90. For most clinical trials, researchers like to have a power of 0.90 or 0.95, or, put another way, a 90% or 95% chance of finding a statistically significant difference between the event rates, given that a difference, δ, actually exists.

If the significance level is .05 or .01 and the power is 0.90 or 0.95, then the only remaining factors to vary are δ and the total sample size. At this point, the clinical researcher must decide the minimum difference (δ) between groups that can be used to judge the difference as clinically important. Previous research may assist in providing statistics for δ to support this judgment.

Before calculating the sample size, the researcher must decide if there is interest in differences in one direction only (one-sided test), such as improvements in intervention over control, or an interest in differences in either direction (two-sided test), testing whether the intervention is better or worse than the control. In making this decision, Friedman, Furberg, and DeMets (1985, p. 86) note that the researcher must be ever mindful that a new intervention has the potential for harm as well as benefit. If an investigator finds evidence during a study to indicate that an intervention is harmful, the clinical trial should be terminated or, if the design permits, modified.

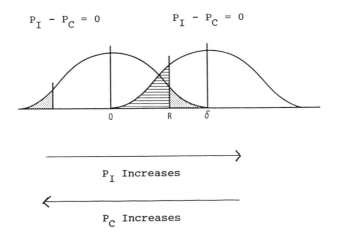

$$P_I - P_C = 0 \qquad P_I - P_C = 0$$

0   R δ

P_I Increases

P_C Increases

Figure 1.2. Frequency Distributions from Clinical Trials: Example 1

For a one-sided hypothesis test, the significance level should be half of what would be used for a two-sided test, so that both tests require the same degree of scientific evidence to judge a treatment effective. For example, if we use the .05 level for the two-sided test, then for an equivalent one-sided test we would use .025.

Figures 1.2 and 1.3 illustrate two frequency distributions when $P_1 - P_c = 0$ and when $P_1 - P_c$ actually equals some difference to be detected, δ. Figure 1.2 (Bulpitt, 1983, p. 101) represents a study in which there were sufficient numbers of subjects in the trial to ensure that a result, R (just compatible with the null hypothesis), has a Type II error of 10%. A Type II error is represented by the lined area and a Type I error is depicted by the dotted area. In this study, the result R lies just within the results expected with the null hypothesis, and the sample for the trial was sufficient so that the distribution for the main objective $P_1 - P_c = \delta$ does not overlap the distribution of results for the null hypothesis to a great extent. The lined area (10%) represents the Type II error, or the probability of concluding that a given difference is not present when in fact it is. The power of the trial is said to be 90%.

Figure 1.3 (Bulpitt, 1983, p. 101) represents a trial in which there were so few subjects that a result R (just compatible with the null hypothesis) has a Type II error of 80% and a power of only 20%. There is a large degree of overlap of the two distributions.

In selecting samples, if a randomization strategy is used, the intervention and control groups will be more likely to have an equal

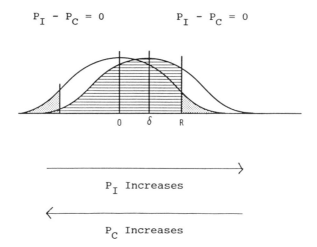

Figure 1.3. Frequency Distributions from Clinical Trials: Example 2

number (N); here, the total sample size will be referred to as 2N. The total sample size, 2N, is a function of the significance level, α, the power, 1 – β, and the size of the difference in response (δ) between the two groups. A change in either α, 1 – β, or δ will cause a change in 2N. If the magnitude of the difference δ decreases, then the sample size will have to be increased to ensure a high probability of detecting that difference. Note too that, if the estimated sample size is larger than can be obtained, then one or more parameters will need to be modified, and the parameter is usually the value selected for δ, because the significance level is typically set at .05 or .01. The other choice is to decrease the power, 1 – β, of the study. Friedman, Furberg, and DeMets (1985, p. 87) recommend that, if any of these alternatives are unsatisfactory, one should consider abandoning the trial.

Estimating Sample Size

Estimating sample size needs to be done early in the planning of the clinical trial. A number of formulas can be used to determine an estimate of the sample needed to achieve the desired statistical power (Bulpitt, 1983; Friedman, Furberg, & DeMets, 1985; Marks, 1982a; O'Brien & Lohr, 1984). Based on the above discussion, the estimate of the sample size will depend on the objective of the clinical trial: whether the effect of a new intervention (I) is better than the control or standard treatment (C); whether the new intervention is comparable with the control or standard treatment; or whether the new intervention is better or worse than the control. This may be thought of in terms of the one-sided or two-sided hypothesis tests that we discussed earlier. The sample size calculation should be based on the specific test statistic that will be used in the study to compare experience outcomes. For example, if the primary response variable is the occurrence of an event during the study period, the null hypothesis is compared with the alternative hypothesis, respectively:

$$H_0 : P_c - P_I = 0$$

$$H_A : P_c - P_I \neq 0$$

The estimates of P_I and P_c are $\hat{P}_I$ and $\hat{P}_c$:

$$\hat{P}_I = \frac{r_I}{N_I} \quad \text{and} \quad \hat{P}_c = \frac{r_c}{N_c}$$

where r_I and r_c are the number of events in the intervention and control groups and N_I and N_c are the number of subjects in each group. The usual statistical test for analyzing a binomial or dichotomous response such as event rates is provided in the formula (Friedman, Furberg, & DeMets, 1985, p. 88):

$$Z = (\hat{P}_c - \hat{P}_I) / \sqrt{\overline{P}(1-P)(1/N_c + 1/N_I)}$$

where $\overline{p} = \dfrac{r_I + r_c}{N_I + N_c}$. The square of the Z statistic is algebraically equal to the chi-square statistic, which is often used. For large values of N_I and N_c, the statistic Z approximates a normal distribution with mean 0 and variance 1. If the test statistic Z is larger in absolute value than the critical Z_a (also called the constant Z_a), the researcher will reject H_0 in the two-sided test. The probability of a standard normal random variable being larger in absolute value than Z_a is α. For a one-sided hypothesis, the constant Z_a is chosen so that the prob-

TABLE 1.3

Z_a for Sample Size Formulas for Various Values of a

	Z_a	
a	One-Sided Test	Two-Sided Test
0.10	1.282	1.645
0.05	1.645	1.960
0.025	1.960	2.326
0.01	2.326	2.576

SOURCE: From Friedman et al. (1985, p. 89)

ability that Z is greater (or less) than Z_a is α. For a given α, Z_a for a two-sided test is larger than for a one-side test (Table 1.3).

Thus the sample size required for the design to have a significance level α and a power of $1 - β$ to detect true differences of at least δ between the event rates P_I and P_c is expressed by this formula (Friedman, Furberg, & DeMets, 1985, p. 89):

$$2N = \frac{2\left\{ Z_\alpha \sqrt{2P(1-P)} + Z_\beta \sqrt{P_c(1-P_c) + P_I(1-p_I}} \right\}^2}{(P_c - P_I)^2}$$

where $2N$ is the total sample size (subjects) with $\overline{P} = \frac{(P_c = P_I)}{2}$; Z_α is the critical value corresponding to the significance level α; and Z_β is the value of the standard normal value not exceeded with probability B. Z_β corresponds to the power $1 - β$. For example, if $1 - β = 0.090$, $Z_\beta = 1.282$. Values of Z_α and Z_β are shown in Tables 1.3 and 1.4.

Using an example to illustrate, a nurse-researcher is testing the effects of a behavioral intervention in a two-year blood pressure reduction program and comparing it with a control group who have expressed a desire to lower their blood pressure but are not enrolled in a special program other than the usual bimonthly doctor visits. The dichotomous response variable, event rate, is determined by the percentage of subjects who have attained their normal blood pressure at the end of the two-year program. The sample will be randomly assigned to equal intervention and control groups. The event

TABLE 1.4

Z_B for Sample Size Formulas for Various Values of Power (1-B)

1 - B	Z_B
0.50	0.00
0.60	0.25
0.70	0.53
0.80	0.84
0.85	1.03
0.90	1.282
0.95	1.645
0.975	1.960
0.99	2.326

SOURCE: From Friedman, Furberg, and DeMets (1985, p. 89).

rate (percentage who attain normal blood pressure) in the control group the first year is expected to be at 15%. The researcher hopes that the intervention will increase the annual rate to 20%. If the assumptions are correct for the annual rates, then at the end of the two-year study, about 30% of the subjects in the control group will have attained normal blood pressure while 40% of the subjects in the intervention group will have succeeded in attaining their normal blood pressure. The study is set at

$$P_c = 0.30, \ P_1 = 0.40, \text{ and, therefore,}$$

$$\overline{P} = \frac{(0.3 + 0.4)}{2} = 35$$

The study is designed as a two-sided test with a 5% significance level and 90% power. From Tables 1.3 and 1.4, the two-sided 0.05 critical value is 1.96 for Z_α and 1.282 for Z_β. Substituting these values into the sample size formula given above yields: $2N = 952.3$. Rounding to the nearest 10, the total sample size would be 960, or 480 for each group. Sample size estimates for a variety of values of P_1 and P_c, using this same formula, are depicted in Table 1.5. Note that, as the difference in rates between groups increases, the sample size decreases. As the power increases, the sample size also increases.

TABLE 1.5

Approximate Total Sample Size for Comparing Proportions in Two Groups

True Proportions		$a = 0.05$ One-Sided		$a = 0.05$ Two-Sided	
			Power		
P_C Control Group	P_I Intervention Group	1-B 0.90	1-B 0.80	1-B 0.90	1-B 0.80
0.60	0.50	850	610	1040	780
	0.40	210	160	260	200
	0.30	90	70	120	90
	0.20	50	40	60	50
0.50	0.40	850	510	1040	780
	0.30	210	150	250	190
	0.25	130	90	160	120
	0.20	90	60	110	80
0.40	0.30	780	560	960	720
	0.25	330	240	410	310
	0.20	180	130	220	170
0.30	0.20	640	470	790	590
	0.15	270	190	330	250
	0.10	140	100	170	130
0.20	0.15	1980	1430	2430	1810
	0.10	440	320	540	400
	0.05	170	120	200	150
0.10	0.05	950	690	1170	870

SOURCE: From Friedman, Furberg, and DeMets (1985, p. 90).

When the investigator selects a more rigorous significance level, the required sample size estimate will increase. Note also that studies that have small event rates, that is, 10% or less (< 0.1), necessitate large sample sizes unless the interventions are so powerful that the response outcomes are markedly changed (Friedman, Furberg, & DeMets, 1985, p. 92).

Sample Size Adjustment for Nonadherence

The clinical researcher will always have to address the problems encountered when subjects in the control and/or intervention groups do not adhere to the study protocol. Subjects' lack of adherence to protocol will affect the power of the study and the sample size needed to demonstrate a significant difference in the response variable. When a subject in the intervention group fails to comply and is no longer subject to the effects of the intervention, the subject is referred to as a "dropout." Similarly, a subject in the control group may initiate use of the intervention at some point in the study and thus may receive any benefit or harm; this subject is called a "drop-in." Both dropouts and dropins pose problems because the differences in responses between the two groups are diluted. Friedman, Furberg, and DeMets (1985, p. 94) recommend that noncompliers should remain in their assigned groups and be included in the analysis because eliminating subjects or changing their groups would bias the study findings. However, the reduced o' means that the sample size must be increased or the researcher will have to settle for a less powerful study. A simple adjustment model by Lachin (1981) is to adjust the sample size for a dropout rate of proportion R. The unadjusted sample size N should be multiplied by the factor $\frac{1}{(1-R)^2}$. For example, if $R = .10$, the unadjusted sample size N should be multiplied by 1.23, or increased by 23%. In our previous example, increasing the sample (960) by 23% would result in an adjusted sample of 1181. Clearly, noncompliance affects the estimate of sample size and needs to be accounted for in the planning of the clinical trial. Also, efforts to keep dropins and dropouts to a minimum should be built into the design.

Sample Size for Continuous Response Variables

The conceptual issues of the previous discussion also apply to the calculation of continuous response variables, such as pulmonary function tests, blood pressure, cholesterol levels, weight, days of hospitalization, scores or psychometric and attitude scales, serum levels, and many others. Friedman, Furberg, and DeMets (1985) noted that these types of measurements can often be approximated by a normal distribution, or, when this is not the case, a transformation of values, such as logarithms, can approximate the normal distribution assumption.

For example, assume the response variable, X, is continuous with N_I and N_c subjects randomized to the intervention and control groups, respectively. Assume X has a normal distribution with mean u and variance σ^2. The true levels are not known but it is assumed that σ^2 can be estimated. Similarly, as before, to test the null and alternative two-sided hypotheses:

$$H_0 : \delta = u_c - u_I = 0$$

$$H_\alpha : \delta = u_c - u_I \neq 0$$

and the test statistic for estimated sample size is

$$Z = \frac{X_c - X_I}{\sigma \sqrt{1 / N_c + 1 / N_I}}$$

where a normal distribution is assumed and X_I and X_c denote the mean levels in the intervention and control groups. The same principles apply as before. If $\mid Z \mid > Z_\alpha$, then an investigator would reject H_0 at the α level of significance. From the above test statistic, this formula would be used to determine $2N$, the total sample size needed:

$$2N = \frac{4(Z_\alpha + Z_\beta)^2 \sigma^2}{\delta^2}$$

The previous principles apply as in the example with the dichotomous response variable. For other approaches to estimating sample sizes, consult Marks (1982a) and Friedman, Furberg, and DeMets (1985).

Analytic Considerations

Depending on which procedure was used for random assignment, there may be a need to give special attention to the methods used for statistical analysis of data in order to maximize the statistical power. Data analysis for clinical trials involves a great deal of time, energy, and response, which needs to be built into the design early in the planning phase. This section of the chapter will provide a brief discussion of some of the major issues in data analysis in clinical trials. For basic methods of statistical analysis, consult O'Brien and Lohr (1984).

Inclusion of Subjects for Analysis

Because of dropins and dropouts, the researcher must decide which subjects to include or exclude. Also, response variable data may be missing on some subjects or it may be revealed later that some subjects failed to meet the eligibility criteria for the study. *Exclusions* are those who are screened as potential subjects for a randomized study but fail to meet the inclusion criteria and so are excluded. Exclusions will not bias the randomization process but may influence interpretation of the results of the clinical trial. A follow-up of excluded people may help determine the generalizability of results. If the event rate in the control group is quite a bit lower than expected, the researcher may determine if most high-risk people were excluded.

Withdrawals are subjects who were in the clinical trial but are excluded from the analysis. Excluding withdrawals from the analysis may bias results because it undermines one of the purposes of randomization. This is an issue the researcher will have to address, also providing evidence to the scientific community that the results are unbiased. The usual reasons for excluding withdrawals from the analysis are nonadherence, missing data, occurrence of contemporary or competing events, and ineligibility. Clerical mistakes and laboratory or other diagnostic errors may occur, resulting in withdrawals. Certain design policies have been proposed to assist in preventing withdrawals and in the management of data analysis when it occurs. Subjects should not be enrolled in the trial until all the diagnostic tests have been confirmed and all entry criteria have been met. Once enrolled, no withdrawals are permitted and the analysis should include all subjects. Any policy on withdrawals should be made clear in the study protocol before the study begins. If withdrawal has to occur, it should be blinded, done early in the study, and not based on the response of the subject. Friedman, Furberg, and DeMets (1985, p. 247) warn that withdrawal from analysis because of noncompliance can lead to bias in that there may be an interaction between compliance and intervention: If noncompliance is greater in one group than another, then withdrawal of noncompliant subjects may lead to bias. The reasons for noncompliance in one group may not be the same as for noncompliance in the other group. The researcher needs to take note that, if compliance to an intervention is poor—that is, the intervention cannot be tolerated—widespread use of the intervention in a larger study population may not be feasible. Therefore, Friedman, Furberg, and DeMets (1985) and others suggest that no subjects be withdrawn due to compliance problems, but it is permissible to withdraw subjects from a trial because the data on them are of poor quality. Removing outliers is not recommended unless there is evidence to show that the data are erroneous. Measures to prevent loss to follow-up must be built into the design to ensure quality data.

Covariate adjustment may be used to minimize effects of group differences when randomization fails to produce comparable groups for prognostic or other factors such as age, ethnic group, or gender. Friedman, Furberg, and DeMets (1985) note that, if a covariate is discrete, or if a continuous variable is converted into intervals and made discrete, the analysis is stratified: that is, the subjects are subdivided into smaller, more homogeneous groups or strata and compared within each strata, then averaged to achieve a summary result for the response variable. If the response variable is discrete, the Mantel-Haenszel statistic is used, as shown in the example in Box 1.8. For a continuous response variable, the stratified analysis is called "analysis of covariance." Details on the use of analysis of covariance are found in Kerlinger (1986) and other basic statistical texts.

In most cases, changes in a response variable, such as reduction in cholesterol or blood pressure level, are highly correlated with compliance with the intervention. Therefore, adjusting for compliance is not recommended because it will bias the results.

For multicenter trials, as we pointed out earlier, randomization should be stratified by clinic and the analysis should incorporate the clinic as a stratification variable. Friedman, Furberg, and DeMets (1985, p. 255) suggest that randomization should also be blocked in order to achieve balance over time in the number of subjects randomized to each group.

Analysis of Multiple Response Variables

Some clinical trials use more than one response variable and a number of baseline variables and may have several statistical comparisons. If an investigator has 100 independent comparisons, 5 of them, on average, will be significantly different by chance alone, if a 0.05 level of significance is used. Therefore, response variables should be kept to a minimum.

The researcher may also consider analysis of subgroups to discover which groups of subjects respond best or worst to the intervention. Subgroup hypotheses should be defined in advance of the analysis. With small numbers of subjects, it will be difficult to detect significant differences. Post hoc analysis (often called "fishing") of subgroups is the weakest form of analysis and should not be used. Trends noted in the data should be used to generate hypotheses

---

Box 1.8. The Mantel-Haenszel Statistic to Analyze Strata

An investigator is comparing response rates on a dichotomous variable and divides the data into a number of strata using baseline characteristics. For each stratum i, a 2×2 contingency table is constructed as shown below.

A 2×2 Table for I^{th} Stratum

	Response		
	Yes	No	
Intervention	a_I	b_I	$a_I + b_I$
Control	c_I	d_I	$c_I + d_I$
Total	$a_I + c_I$	$b_I + d_I$	N_I

The elements a_I, b_I, c_I, and d_I represent the counts in the 4 cells and N_I is the number of subjects in the Ith stratum. Margin entries represent totals in each category. The value $(a_I + c_I) / N_I$ is the overall response rate for the Ith stratum. Within the Ith stratum, the rates $a_I / (a_I + b_I)$ with $c_I / (c_I + d_I)$ are compared. The standard chi-square test for 2×2 tables can be used to compare group differences in this stratum but the researcher wants to average the comparison over all strata. The statistic for combining several 2×2 tables over all strata is the Mantel-Haenszel (MH) statistic (Mantel & Haenszel, 1959). The MH statistic has a chi-square distribution with one degree of freedom. A value for MH greater than 3.84 is significant at the 0.05 level and a value greater than 6.63 at the 0.01 level.

---

for future clinical trials. For more information on analysis issues and statistical methods of analysis in clinical trials, consult Marks (1982b), Friedman, Furberg, and DeMets (1985), and Fleiss (1986).

Interpretation of Results

First, report complete statistics (exact t, p, and F values, degrees of freedom, and the sum of squares) in the findings section so the reader will be able to draw conclusions and understand how you arrived at your conclusions. Conclusions should be empirically based, that is, grounded in the data. Avoid making interpretations that go beyond the generalizability of the findings. Any biases that you are aware of in the study should be explained in terms of how they might affect any inferences made.

Be cautious in drawing conclusions about an intervention tested in a trial with an inadequate sample size. If a statistical test fails to reject a hypothesis, it cannot be assumed that the treatments are equivalent. In this case, the probability of a Type II error must be calculated before a valid conclusion is reached.

Reporting of correlation coefficients (r) needs to be placed into perspective. Often, r values are highly significant ($p < .0001$), but all this means is that the true correlation is not zero (Marks, 1982b). The value r yields more information in determining the relative value of the correlation.

Comparisons, such as subgroup analyses, made post hoc may contribute to incorrect conclusions. As discussed earlier, the chances of finding statistically significant levels in post hoc analysis are much higher than for a priori comparisons, even when no actual differences exist between the population means. Special statistical tests should be used for post hoc analysis, and the findings should be interpreted with caution. Trends noted in the data post hoc should be used to generate hypotheses for future trials. For more information on reporting and interpreting statistical findings of clinical trials, refer to Mosteller, Gilbert, and McPeek (1980).

Building Theories for Practice

Throughout this and other chapters, we have stressed the importance of formalizing the relationship between the theory and the research in order to test and build scientific theories for practice. An important part of interpreting the results is addressing the degree of empirical support the data have provided for the theoretical propositions of the clinical trial. And the next step is to suggest future work that will advance theory for the clinical domain of study, specifically:

(1) What revisions are suggested in the theoretical propositions as a result of the present study?
(2) What new theoretical propositions can be generated from the present study?
(3) Does the present study lend support to a broader theoretical framework or paradigm?

For more on this process, see Chapter 7 in Volume 1.

Box 1.9. Reducing Acute Confusional States in Elderly Patients with
        Hip Fractures

SOURCE: Williams, M. A., Campbell, E. B., Raynor, W. J., Mlynarczyk,
        S. M., & Ward, S. E. (1985). *Research in Nursing & Health, 8*,
        329-337.

The extent to which the incidence of postoperative acute confusional states
could be reduced in elderly (60 or >) patients with hip fractures was tested.
Before a quasi-experimental design could be instituted to test the effect of
interventions, it was necessary to develop a method of assessing risk for
confusion. Because the relative contribution of the many risk factors
implicated in confusion is not known, the first phase of this study focused
on the development of a quantitative method of risk assessment. Two
models were developed for predicting confusion. The sample used for
developing the predictive models became the comparison group in the
intervention phase. The admission prediction model contributed the
method for comparing probable confusion with actual confusion in both
the comparison (nonintervention) and the intervention groups. The second model served to identify factors that might be modified by certain
nursing interventions. Subjects were recruited from orthopedic units in
four acute care community hospitals for the nonintervention phase; three
of those hospitals we used in the intervention phase. The nonintervention
sample size was 170 and the intervention sample was 57. Inclusion criteria
were: age 60 or >, no validated history of mental impairment (DTs and
so on), and fracture by trauma. To keep the perioperative event similar,
persons were not included if their time from admission to surgery exceeded 2 days. Both samples were similar in characteristics. After adjustment for risk scores, a logistic regression model was fit in which both
groups were required to have the same slope (for the score function) but
were allowed to have different intercepts (i.e., level of confusion). A
significant difference between the intercepts implies that the incidence in
one group is lower than the incidence in the other group after adjustment
for the differences in their risk scores. The incidence of confusion was
reduced from 51.5% in the comparison group to 43.9%. Analysis that
controlled for risk factors in the two groups showed the drop in incidence
to be significant at p < .02. The most effective interventions appeared to
be those that provided orientation and clarification, corrected sensory
deficit, and increased continuity of care.

Summary

The main goal of Chapter 1 was to present the critical elements
involved in a successful clinical trial. Through successful clinical

trials, we can hasten our progress in determining effective nursing interventions and in building theories for clinical practice. Increasing the chances of a successful clinical trial are enhanced by the following:

- spending adequate time and resources in planning and designing the clinical protocol
- specifying the most critical response variable and explicating the main objective of the clinical trial in testable hypotheses
- randomizing subjects to the intervention and control groups
- developing a protocol for recruitment, selection, and retention of subjects
- deciding a priori how the statistical analysis will be performed and what measures will be taken to ensure quality data
- reporting complete statistics and basing the interpretations on the findings
- generating future hypotheses and addressing contributions made to theory building in the clinical domain of study.

Point-Counterpoint

(1) What factors related to a proposed clinical intervention trial might suggest that randomization would not be ethical? Friedman, Furberg, and DeMets (1985) suggest that, if a researcher thinks that randomization to an intervention is unethical, the clinical trial should not be conducted. Would this principle apply to the situation you just identified?

(2) Along this same line of thought, is there a situation you can think of where a "quasi-experimental" design is appropriate? Think of the criteria for experimental and quasi-experimental designs and consider the point made above by Friedman, Furberg, and DeMets (1985). Review the quasi-experimental study by Williams, Campbell, Raynor, Mlynarczyk, and Ward in Box 1.9. Could this study have been conducted using random assignment? What measures would you take to strengthen the design?

(3) Propose a number of interventions that could be appropriately tested in the form of randomized clinical trials in nursing. Develop a randomized clinical trial protocol for one of the identified interventions.

(4) Review three quasi-experimental studies published in the last two years in *Nursing Research*. Why were they conducted as quasi-experi-

mental studies? Could they have been conducted as randomized clinical trials? How would you design the studies?

Examples of Randomized
Clinical Trials in Medicine

Aspirin Myocardial Infarction Study Research Group. (1980). A randomized controlled trial of aspirin in persons recovered from myocardial infarction. *Journal of the American Medical Association, 242,* 2562-2571.

CASS Principal Investigators and Their Associates. Coronary Artery Surgery Study (CASS). A randomized trial of coronary artery bypass surgery, survival data. *Circulation, 68,* 939-950.

Multiple Risk Factor Intervention Trial Research Group, Multiple Risk Factor Interventional Trial. (1982). Risk factor changes and mortality results. *Journal of the American Medical Association, 248,* 1465-1477.

References

NOTE: Asterisked (*) entries denote experimental studies in nursing and references that may be of special interest or help to clinical researchers.

Alexy, B. (1985). Goal setting and health risk reduction. *Nursing Research, 33,* 9-14.*

Anderson, G. C., Gill, N. E., & Bodo, T. L. (1988, June). *Self-regulatory feeding and nonnutritive sucking: Effect of regular sleep after beginning bottlefeeding in preterm infants.* Paper presented at the biennial research conference of the Nurses Association of the American College of Obstetricians and Gynecologists, Toronto, Ontario, Canada.*

Anderson, G. R., & Glesnes-Anderson, V. A. (Eds.). (1987). *Health care ethics: A guide for decision makers.* Rockville, MD: Aspen.

Applebaum, P. S. (1987). *Informed consent: Legal theory and clinical practice.* New York: Oxford University Press.*

Barber, B. (1980). *Informed consent in medical therapy and research.* Brunswick, NJ: Rutgers University Press.*

Beauchamp, T. L. (Ed.). (1982). *Ethical issues in social science research.* Baltimore: Johns Hopkins University Press.

Beauchamp, T. L., & Rosenberg, A. (1981). *Hume and the problem of causation.* New York: Oxford University Press.

Beauchamp, T. L., & Walters, L. (Eds.). (1982). *Contemporary issues in bioethics* (2nd ed.). Belmont, CA: Wadsworth.*

Brody, H. (1982). *Ethical decisions in medicine* (2nd ed.). Boston: Little, Brown.

Bulpitt, C. J. (1983). *Randomized controlled clinical trials.* Hingham, MA/The Hague, the Netherlands: Martinus Nijhoff.*

Campbell, D. T., & Stanley, J. C. (1963). *Experimental and quasiexperimental designs for research.* Chicago: Rand McNally.

Code of Federal Regulations. (1983). *Protection of human subjects: 45CFR46* (revised as of March 8, 1983). Washington, DC: Department of Health and Human Services.

Cohen, J. (1977). *Statistical power analysis for the behavioral sciences.* New York: Academic Press.

Cook, T. D., & Campbell, D. T. (Eds.). (1979). *Quasi-experimentation: Design and analysis issues for field settings.* Chicago: Rand McNally.

Copp, G., Mailhot, C. B., Zalar, M., Slezak, L., & Copp, A. (1986). Covergowns and the control of operating room contamination. *Nursing Research, 35,* 263-267.*

Cottrell, B. H., & Shannahan, M. D. (1986). Effect of the birth chair on duration of second stage labor and maternal outcome. *Nursing Research, 35,* 364-367.*

Dickoff, J., & James, P. (1968). A theory of theories: A position paper. *Nursing Research, 17,* 197-203.

Dixon, J. (1984). Effect of nursing interventions on nutritional and performance status in cancer patients. *Nursing Research, 33,* 330-335.*

Doering, L., & Dracup, K. (1987). Comparisons of cardiac output in supine and lateral positions. *Nursing Research, 37,* 114-118.*

Ellenberg, A. S. (1984). Randomization designs in comparative clinical trials. *New England Journal of Medicine, 310,* 1404-1408.

Faden, R. R., & Beauchamp, T. L. (1986). *A history and theory of informed consent.* New York: Oxford University Press.

Finkel, M. J. (Ed.). (1976). *Factors influencing clinical research success.* Mount Kisco, NY: Futura.

Fleiss, J. L. (1986). *The design and analysis of clinical experiments.* New York: John Wiley.*

Fox, M. A. (1986). *The case for animal experimentation.* Berkeley: University of California Press.

Friedman, L. M., Furberg, C. D., & DeMets, D. L. (1985). *Fundamentals of clinical trials* (2nd ed.). Littleton, MA: PSG.

Frieman, J. A., Chalmers, T. C., Smith, H., & Kuebler, R. R. (1978). The importance of beta, the Type II error and sample size in the design and interpretation of the randomized control trial. *New England Journal of Medicine, 299,* 690-694.

Geden, E., Beck, N., Anderson, J., Kennish, & Mueller-Heinze, M. (1986). Effects of cognitive and pharmacologic strategies on analogued labor pain. *Nursing Research, 35,* 301-306.*

Geden, E., Beck, N., Hauge, G., & Pohlman, S. (1984). Self-report and psychophysiological effects of five pain-coping strategies. *Nursing Research, 33,* 260-265.*

Gill, N. E., Behnke, M., Conlon, M., & Anderson, G. C. (1988, September). *Nonnutritive sucking: Effect on behavioral state in preterm infants prefeeding.* Paper presented at the National Symposium of Nursing Research, San Francisco.

Gillett, P. A. (1988). Self-reported factors influencing exercise adherence in overweight women. *Nursing Research, 37,* 25-29.*

Goodwin, L. D. (1984). The use of power estimation in nursing research. *Nursing Research, 33,* 118-120.*

Gortner, S. (Ed.). (1987). *Nursing science methods: A reader.* San Francisco: Regents, University of California.

Hill, A. (1971). *Principles of medical statistics* (9th ed.). New York: Oxford University Press.

Jacobs, M. K., McCance, K. L., & Stewart, M. L. (1986). Leg volume changes with EPIC and posturing in dependent pregnancy edema. *Nursing Research, 35,* 86-89.*

Jones, J. H. (1981). *Bad blood: The Tuskegee syphilis experiment.* New York: Free Press.*

Keen, M. F. (1986). Comparison of intramuscular injection techniques to reduce site discomfort and lesions. *Nursing Research, 35,* 207-210.*

Keller, E., & Bzdek, V. M. (1986). Effects of therapeutic touch on tension headache pain. *Nursing Research, 35*, 101-105.*

Kerlinger, F. (1986). *Foundations of behavioral research* (3rd ed.). New York: Holt, Rinehart & Winston.

Koniak-Griffin, D., & Ludington-Hoe, S. M. (1988). Developmental and temperament outcomes of sensory stimulation in healthy infants. *Nursing Research, 37*, 70-76.*

Lachin, J. M. (1981). Introduction to sample size determination and power analysis for clinical trials. *Controlled Clinical Trials, 2*, 93-113.

Manderino, M. H., & Bzdek, V. M. (1984). Effects of modeling and information on reactions to pain: A childbirth preparation analogue. *Nursing Research, 33*, 9-14.*

Mantel, N., & Haenszel, W. (1959). Statistical aspects of the analysis of data from retrospective studies of disease. *Journal of the National Cancer Institute, 22*, 719-748.

Marks, R. (1982a). *Designing a research project*. Belmont, CA: Lifetime Learning.

Marks, R. (1982b). *Analyzing research data*. Belmont, CA: Lifetime Learning.

Meier, P. (1981). Stratification in the design of a clinical trial. *Controlled Clinical Trials, 1*, 355-361.

Meinert, C. L., & Tonascia, S. (1986). *Clinical trials: Design, conduct, and analysis*. New York: Oxford University Press.

Moody, L., Martin, D., & Notelovitz, M. (1989). *Clinical trial to improve health in aging women* (Grant proposal). Gainesville: University of Florida.

Moody, L., Wilson, M., Smyth, K., Schwartz, R., Tittle, M., & VanCott, M. (1988). Analysis of a decade of nursing practice research. *Nursing Research, 37*, 374-379.

Mosteller, F., Gilbert, J. P., & McPeek, B. (1980). Reporting standards and strategies for controlled trials. *Controlled Clinical Trials, 1*, 37-58.*

Oberst, M. T. (1979). Research ethics. Part II: The concept of risk in clinical studies. *Cancer Nursing, 2*, 481-482.

O'Brien, R. G., & Lohr, V. I. (1984). Power analysis for linear models: Time has come. In *Statistical User's Group International: Proceedings of the Ninth Annual Conference*. Cary, NC: Statistical Analysis Institute.

Pocock, S. J. (1979). Allocation of patients to treatment in clinical trials. *Biometrics, 35*, 183-197.

Scheetz, S. L. (1987). Randomized clinical trials. In S. Gortner (Ed.), *Nursing science methods: A reader* (pp. 133-141). San Francisco: Regents, University of California.

Silverman, W. A. (1985). *Human experimentation: A guided step into the unknown*. New York: Oxford University Press.

U.S. National Commission for the Protection of Human Subjects of Biomedical and Behavioral Research. *The Belmont report: Ethical principles and guidelines for the protection of human subjects of research*. Washington, DC: Government Printing Office.

Williams, M. A., Campbell, E. B., Raynor, W. J., Mlynarczyk, S. M., & Ward, S. E. (1985). Reducing acute confusional states in elderly patients with hip fractures. *Research in Nursing & Health, 8*, 329-337.

Wilson, H. (1989). *Research in nursing* (2nd ed.). Menlo Park, CA: Addison-Wesley.

2

Meta-Analysis:
Qualitative and Quantitative Methods

LINDA E. MOODY

> The use of statistics does not supplant analysis:
> it can only aid analysis.

Concern exists regarding how to hasten progress toward building a body of knowledge that can be used to address significant problems in nursing practice. Although there is an abundance of cross-sectional studies, that is, single, one-time studies with small samples, this type of study does little to add to an explanatory knowledge base for practice (Moody et al., 1988). Scientists have known for centuries that a single study will not resolve a major issue or that several studies of a problem with small samples will not resolve major or minor issues. The foundation of science is the cumulation of knowledge from the results of many studies, with adequate and representative sampling, over time. The process of knowledge accretion for any discipline includes these two phases:

(1) the cumulation of results across studies to establish facts or what is known, and
(2) the formation of theories to place the facts into a coherent and useful form.

The focus of this chapter will be on how findings across studies can be analyzed and summarized to establish facts and resolve important research issues through the use of qualitative and quantitative analyses (meta-analyses) of research.

Meta-Analysis Defined

Meta-analysis, or the averaging of results across studies, is a "new-discipline" (Sacks, Berrier, Reitman, Ancona-Berk, & Chalmers, 1987) that critically reviews and analyzes data pooled across several studies. In research, three types of analysis are often described: *primary analysis, secondary analysis, and meta-analysis.* Primary analysis is the original analysis of data from a single study while secondary analysis is a reanalysis of data, examining the same questions with different techniques or examining new questions from the original data set. *Meta-analysis* refers to "analysis of analyses" and is defined by Glass (1976, p. 3) in the following way:

> Meta-analysis . . . the statistical analysis of a large collection of analysis results from individual studies for the purpose of integrating the findings. It connotes a rigorous alternative to the casual, narrative discussions of research studies which typify our attempts to make sense of the rapidly expanding research literature.

The advantages, limitations, and procedures of meta-analysis and other methods of research analysis will be presented in this chapter. The main focus of the chapter will be on methods of meta-analysis: the first part of the process being a qualitative approach to synthesizing research and, then, the next phase, the quantitative approach to pooling research results. The use of various analytic approaches will be illustrated with exemplars from nursing research. Controversies surrounding meta-analysis will be presented and a set of standards for judging meta-analyses will be reviewed.

Review of Key Terms and Research Concepts

This chapter was prepared on the premise that the reader has an understanding of research designs and methods and basic statistical concepts and analytic procedures. If not, review Chapter 8 in Volume 1 and Chapter 1 of this volume to become familiar with the basic statistical concepts required to understand the process of meta-analysis. Key concepts and terms that you need to be familiar with are listed here: sampling methods, randomized clinical trials, experimental design, quasi-experimental, preexperimental, standard deviation, the normal curve, chi-square, t-test, probabilities, simple correlation (r), confidence intervals, effect size, and homogeneity/heterogeneity.

Methods of Research Analyses

How can identified lags in knowledge gain best be addressed? One way is through better literature reviews in preparation for conducting research, which was highlighted in Chapter 4, Volume 1. Other than the traditional literature reviews to analyze research, such as modified abstracting, there are quantitative approaches for analyzing and summarizing research results: vote counting, combined tests, such as p-values (integrating results), cluster approach, and other meta-analytic methods. Each of these methods uses a different approach depending on the data required for the analysis. Pitfalls of the traditional research review will be discussed, followed by a discussion of various qualitative methods and a detailed presentation of common quantitative approaches to meta-analyses. A comprehensive research analysis begins with the qualitative review, then, if there is an adequate number of experimental studies in the area, it culminates with a quantitative analysis.

The Traditional Research Review

The contribution of the literature review to knowledge building increases proportionately as research in a field expands. The growing importance and complexities involved in literature searches, and the limits of the human mind to sift through and comprehend a profusion of studies, restrict the quality of the outcomes of research reviews. There are several reasons why traditional literature reviews, which are often unsystematic and impressionistic, have provided such a weak foundation for research. Curlette and Cannella (1985, p. 293) explain the limitations of traditional research reviews:

(1) The rules for selecting the studies to be reviewed are rarely stated by the reviewer.

(2) The narrative summary typically does not include a systematic approach for resolving contradictory findings among the studies included in the review.

(3) The reviewer frequently applies some implicit rules to integrate the studies and draw conclusions.

(4) The reviewer's bias may creep into the summary in cases where methods or conclusions are in conflict with the reviewer's point of view.

Thus, in the traditional approach, the researcher may only include those studies that will support his or her study hypotheses or worldview and exclude studies that may provide opposing points of view. Another problem with this approach is the complexity involved in trying to analyze and synthesize results qualitatively without distorting the statistical findings. When we refer to the results of a study, it is not necessarily the conclusion drawn by the investigator, because that may be only slightly related to the study findings. The transformation that sometimes occurs between the results section and the discussion section of a published research report may be purely speculative. Therefore, reviewing the conclusions made by the author, which many researchers often do in a traditional review, without analyzing the study findings, can indeed provide misleading information.

Modified Abstracting

Another qualitative approach to literature review that has failed to contribute much to knowledge building is termed "modified abstracting" (Curlette & Ramig, 1979). In the modified abstracting approach, the reviewer presents a narrative précis of particular studies but makes no attempt to critique or integrate them. There is no systematic effort to select studies according to preestablished inclusion criteria. Modified abstracting, if precise, provides, at best, a summary of research in a particular area. It does not assist the researcher in resolving issues where there are conflicting findings or in integrating findings across studies. Many examples of modified abstracting can be found in the research literature but space limitations in journals permit the researcher to present only the most relevant research reviews.

A Systematic Approach to Research Analyses

If research in a particular area has been mostly descriptive and exploratory, then there are no options available other than a qualitative approach to literature review. But given this limitation, there are some standards that will ensure a more systematic approach to a qualitative literature review of research. Up to a certain point, these standards are the same as those that will be presented later in the chapter for quantitative research analyses. Steps in the research analysis process are depicted in Box 2.1.

Step 1. Delineating the Domain of Study

The researcher must first have a clear understanding of the domain of study. From this, the analyst then identifies the research hypotheses, study variables, or questions of interest across the studies that can be submitted to analysis.

Step 2. Defining Admissible Studies

Once the problem area has been defined, a rationale should be developed to specify the *inclusion criteria* for selecting studies to include in the review. This step is similar to deciding which subjects will be eligible for study participation. Studies are considered within the discipline of nursing and across other disciplines that may be studying the same research domain. For more information on this step, see the meta-analysis by Schwartz, Moody, Yarandi, and Anderson (1988).

Step 3. Locating Studies

The analyst engages in a comprehensive search for published and unpublished studies that meet the inclusion criteria. Several methods are available for locating studies:

(a) computerized searches, using several sources
(b) abstract service for theses and dissertations
(c) descendancy search (indexes that identify papers pertinent to a topic)
(d) ancestry search (citations in bibliographies of previously located literature)

Box 2.1. Steps in Qualitative or Quantitative Analysis

Step 1. Delineating the domain of study

Step 2. Defining admissible studies

Step 3. Locating studies

Step 4. Coding and classifying study variables

Step 5. Determining a common scale or metric

Step 6. Analyzing across studies

Step 7. Interpreting and reporting results

Step 8. Explicating theory and research outcomes

Step 9. Projecting future research needs

(e) formal and informal professional networks, such as ANA Council of Nurse Researchers, Sigma Theta Tau, and other professional research organizations within nursing and from other disciplines

(f) major publishers of primary research studies on the review topic

(g) major research institutions likely to be engaged in the topic of interest

(h) fugitive literature (retrieval of unpublished studies or studies published in obscure sources) in order to minimize sampling bias from selective reporting and publication bias

(i) senior investigators in the field of study who will help the researcher locate published and unpublished studies and studies in progress

Step 4. Coding and Classifying Study Variables

Both substantive (research domain and research questions) and methodological (sample, design, analyses) characteristics are delineated to describe the sample of studies. The coding system may be developed in the form of a precoded instrument that the researcher uses to analyze each study. Hedges and Olkin (1984) suggested that the following characteristics be assessed for each study: quality of research design, variation of treatment, type of outcome or response measures, and research procedures. An example of a coding instrument, the Nursing Practice Research Analysis Tool (NPRAT), is included in the Appendix of Volume 1. For other approaches to coding for meta-analysis, see Smith (1987) and Schwartz, Moody, Yarandi, and Anderson (1988). A coding instrument will assist the analyst in systematically evaluating each study according to the same standards. A summary table can then be constructed like the one shown

Box 2.2. An Example of Coding and Classifying Studies

Characteristics and Outcome Variables for Five Nonnutritive Sucking Studies

Study: Investigator	Sample Characteristics and Size; Method of Assignment	Method	Days of Hospitalization; (Cost)	Comparable Results	
				Weight Gain (in Gms)	Days to First Bottle
1. Measel & Anderson (1979)	Preterm infants GA = 28-32 wks. Birth weight = 1,000 Gms. e = 29, c = 30 Alternate sequential series	NNS during every tube feeding & for 5 min. afterwards, beginning with first gavage feeding	$\bar{X}e$ = 36.5, Se = 2.4, $\bar{X}c$ = 40.5, Sc = 23, p < .025	$\bar{X}e$ = 12.2 $\bar{X}c$ = 1.6 N.S.	$\bar{X}e$ = 14.4 Se = 1.6 $\bar{X}c$ = 17.8 Sc = 1.67 p < .05
2. Schwartz (1987)	Preterm infants GA = 32-34 wks. Birth weight = 1,200-2,000 Gms. e = 13, c = 12 Random assignment	NNS q 3 hrs. × 5 mins. beginning at birth & continued w/gavage feedings until infant was completely nourished by bottle	$\bar{X}e$ = 22.07, Se = 8.39, $\bar{X}c$ = 27.33, Sc = 11.58, t = 1.31, p = .102, $\bar{X}e$ = \$4929, Se = \$1715, $\bar{X}c$ = \$8698, Sc = \$6727, t = 1.95, p = .031	$\bar{X}e$ = 12.5 Se = 6.24 $\bar{X}c$ = 11.06 Sc = 4.72 t = .65 p = .261	$\bar{X}e$ = 11.05 Se = 4.74 $\bar{X}c$ = 12.5 Sc = 6.24 t = .465 p = .323
3. Field, Ignatoff, Stringer, Brennan, Greenberg, Widmayer, & Anderson (1982)	Preterm infants GA = < 35 wks. Birth weight = < 1,800 Gms. e = 30, c = 27 Random stratified for GA and birth weight	NNS during every tube feeding beginning with first gavage feeding	$\bar{X}e$ = 48, Se = 21, $\bar{X}c$ = 56, Sc = 18, p < .05, $\bar{X}e$ = \$16,800, Se = \$13,959, $\bar{X}c$ = \$20,394, Sc = \$11,339, p < .01	$\bar{X}e$ = 19.3 Se = 4.9 $\bar{X}c$ = 16.5 Sc = 5.5 p < .05	$\bar{X}e$ = 26 Se = 21 $\bar{X}c$ = 29 Sc = 18 p < .01
4. Caple (1982)	Preterm infants GA = 27-36 wks. Birth weight = > 1,300 Gms. e = 9, c = 10 Random assignment	NNS during every tube feeding & for 5 min. afterward or to satiety. Continuously fed infants were given a pacifier 3 hrs × 8 q min.	$\bar{X}e$ = 34.2, Se = 17.5, $\bar{X}c$ = 41.7, Sc = 26.0, p > .05		$\bar{X}e$ = 15.1 Se = 10.9 $\bar{X}c$ = 16.0 Sc = 11.4 p < .05
5. Bernbaum, Pereira, Watkins, & Perkins (1983)	Preterm infants GA = 32 wks. Birth weight ≤ 1,500 Gms. e = 15, c = 15 Infants were pair-matched, then assigned randomly	NNS during every tube feeding, beginning with first gavage feeding	$\bar{X}e$ = 51.9, Se = 8.2, $\bar{X}c$ = 58.7, Sc = 9.8, p > .05		$\bar{X}$ = 10.4 Se = 2.1 $\bar{X}c$ = 16.1 Sc = 5.1 p < .001

SOURCE: Reprinted with permission from: Schwartz, R., Moody, L., Yarandi, H., & Anderson, G. C. (1988). A meta-analysis of critical outcome variables in nonnutritive sucking in preterm infants. *Nursing Research, 36*, 292-295.
NOTE: e = experimental group; c = control group; GA = gestational age; NNS = nonnutritive sucking.

in Box 2.2 to assist in classifying and comparing studies. More than one coder should be prepared to analyze the research so that inter-observer agreement can be determined. This approach will assist in reducing selection bias and will improve the validity and reliability of the meta-analysis.

The discussion of Steps 5-9 here will be limited to the analyses of research that is nonexperimental and cannot be submitted to meta-analyses. Completion of Steps 5-9 for the quantitative research analyses of experimental studies will be addressed in the next section.

Step 5. Determining a Common Scale or Metric

For the research review, one of the most difficult tasks is to determine a common scale or metric that can be used to analyze findings across studies. For studies that do not lend themselves to quantitative analyses, qualitative indicators or categories that permit summarization of the study variables from the pooled research questions across the sample of studies need to be explicated, insofar as possible. In the qualitative or quantitative approach, the researcher has to demonstrate that indicators used are conceptually equivalent.

Step 6. Analyzing Across Studies

Summarizing across studies that do not permit quantitative analyses is arduous. Through the use of an analytic tool, such as the one in the Appendix in Volume 1, the analyst can identify common variables or research questions addressed by the studies and provide a qualitative summary of the most significant research outcomes. An example of a qualitative research summary is shown in Box 2.3. In this research analysis, the author was not able to proceed with a quantitative meta-analysis because exact statistics from the primary studies were not reported or were unavailable. This example illustrates the importance of researchers reporting exact p, t, F, and r as well as other important statistics, such as effect sizes, so that data can be analyzed across studies through meta-analytic methods. A great deal more will be said about this in the next section.

Step 7. Interpreting and Reporting Results

Similarly, providing an interpretation of results of pooled nonexperimental studies is based on the empirical evidence gained from the analysis. Summarizing qualitative information without losing

Box 2.3. An Example of a Qualitative Research Summary

Studies of Computer-Assisted Instruction in Nursing

Author Year	Education Level	CAI Content	Measurement Category	Research Design	Sample	Computer Language/ System	Additional Media	Methods Studied	Results
Bitzer & Boudreaux (1969); Bitzer & Bitzer (1973)	Diploma ADN	Maternity Nursing; Pharma- cology	Knowledge Application Attitude	Matched Random; & Intact Groups	N=22 [N>300]	PLATO	yes	CAI vs. class- discussion	NS
Boettcher Alderson Saccucci (1981)	BSN	Psycho- Pharma- cology	Knowledge Application	Pretest- Posttest Control Group	N=83 R	PLATO	no	CAI vs. PI	NS
Collart (1973)	BSN Junior class	Surgical Nursing	Knowledge Application	Survey Nonex- perimental	N=150 NR	?	no	CAI (tutorial)	—
Conklin (1983)	BSN (3rd year class)	Surgical Nursing	Knowledge Attitude	Pretest- Posttest Control Group	N=34 R	BASIC	yes	CAI vs. readings	S
Fishman (1984)	RN CE volunteers	Cancer Chemo- therapy	Knowledge (mastery; retention) Attitude	Pretest Posttest Control Group	N=64 R	BASIC	yes	CAVI vs. linear video vs. lecture	S

(Continued)

Box 2.3. An Example of a Qualitative Research Summary (Continued)

| | | | | | | | | Studies of Computer-Assisted Instruction in Nursing | |
Author Year	Education Level	CAI Content	Measurement Category	Research Design	Sample	Computer Language/ System	Additional Media	Methods Studied	Results
Huckabay Anderson Holm Lee (1979)	Graduate Nurse-Practitioner class	Hypertension	Knowledge Application Attitude	Pretest Posttest Control Group	N=31 NR (pretest)	?	no	CAI vs. Readings	NS
Kirchhoff Holzemer (1979)	Junior class	Surgical Nursing	Comprehension Application Attitude	Modified Posttest Only	N=100	PLATO	no	CAI vs. Written assignments	S
Morin (1983)	BSN (3rd & 4th year)	Nursing of Adults	Attitude Learning Style	Intact Group	N=41 Stratified	?	no	Learning Style vs. Attitude	NS (interaction)
Reynolds (1984)	BSN	Optional Course activities	Knowledge Application	Non-experimental	? NR	?	no	Sample course exams	No hard data
Timpke Janney (1981)	Basic nursing students	Dosage Calculation	Knowledge (mastery)	Non-experimental	N=92 NR	?	yes	CAI vs. part CAI vs. text	Frequent report only

SOURCE: Developed by Kearney, R. (1985) for NGR 7124: Theory Analysis and Critique. Gainesville: University of Florida.

important details is speculative and tedious. The reporting of the results of the summary should address this issue to assist the reader in knowing how much confidence to place in the research analyses.

Step 8. Explicating Theory and Research Outcomes

Use of a tool, such as the NPRAT (Moody et al., 1988), assists in identifying research outcomes and progress toward theory building. Addressing these outcomes in the form of a table will assist in identifying empirical support for middle-range practice theories or provide the basis for future theory testing.

Step 9. Projecting Future Research Needs

Again, from the information gained from using a tool to systematically analyze each study, the gaps in the research domain can be identified and summarized. From this, the analyst can specify which studies merit replication, speculate as to which areas are no longer fruitful for investigation, and provide recommendations for studies that will contribute new knowledge. This type of research synthesis and analysis may help provide vital data to influence clinical interventions, needed changes in health policy, or future funding for research in the area.

Meta-Analysis: The Quantitative Approach

The purposes of meta-analysis will be presented in this section, followed by a discussion of the historical development of meta-analysis and its potential uses in nursing. This will set the backdrop for our discussion of the actual process of conducting a meta-analysis and the use of the various statistical approaches.

Purposes of Meta-Analysis

Meta-analysis attempts to go beyond the traditional literature review by systematically analyzing and summarizing results from a cluster of studies in a specified domain of interest. We often hear the lament: "More research needs to be done in this area before we can apply the findings—after all, we are a practice discipline." And so concludes many a published nursing study. Yet, do we really need more research in an area or is it that we need to take another look at the data? Advocates of meta-analysis maintain that, before further research is conducted in an area, the "gold mines of information must first be excavated."

A meta-analysis should be considered if one or more of the following conditions are present:

(1) conflicting findings exist in an important area regarding effects of interventions on the dependent (response) variables

(2) analyzing results across experimental studies (especially clinical trials) would provide empirical support for a middle-range (practice-level) theory

(3) when remaining questions exist or new questions emerge about treatments or interventions that could be answered by statistically summarizing results across studies

(4) when controversy exists about the need for further research on an intervention

If conducted *properly*, meta-analysis transcends the traditional literature review in that it is systematic and the conclusions regarding the summary of findings are empirically based. If the literature review (which is a critical step in the research process) is approached haphazardly, or in a cursory manner, the researcher may jeopardize funding, fail to build a sound study design based on previous findings, or have the study rejected for publication because it was not theoretically sound. Thus the advantages of meta-analysis and its proper uses in knowledge building will be highlighted in the remainder of Chapter 2.

Historical Perspective

Although early meta-analytic procedures date back to the 1950s, appropriate statistical procedures were not available until the late 1970s to facilitate more valid analyses of results across studies. The developer of meta-analysis, Rosenthal, a social psychologist, traces his interest in meta-analytic methods back to the late 1950s when he questioned the effect of a study that suggested that the researcher's expectations might affect the results of the research. Since the early 1960s, Rosenthal taught a variety of meta-analytic procedures, although he did not call it that until his colleague Glass, in 1976, provided a prototype for what he called "meta-analysis." It was from this process that Glass summarized results across several studies and, from the pooled results, persuaded Rosenthal that the expectations of psychotherapists do affect outcomes: that is, therapists were most likely to help those patients they thought they could help.

Since the late 1970s, there have been hundreds of published and unpublished meta-analyses, mostly in social psychology, sociology, educational psychology, and, most recently, from clinical trials in medicine. In nursing, the number of meta-analyses is small but growing as the discipline conducts more clinical trials and experimental studies that lend themselves to meta-analyses. Examples of meta-analyses are provided throughout Chapter 2 to illustrate the process and use of analytic methods. Other examples are listed at the end of the chapter.

Rosenthal (1984) noted two obstacles to knowledge building in the social sciences: (a) the problem of poor cumulation (lack of orderly progress and development of science when compared with the older sciences such as physics and chemistry) and (b) the problem of small effects that only account for a trivial proportion of the variance—the effect is of no practical or clinical significance. In terms of building a body of knowledge based on past research, nursing faces the same obstacles. The appropriate use of meta-analyses will assist in our efforts toward knowledge cumulation.

The Traditional Versus the Meta-Analytic Approach

Rosenthal (1984) and his colleague Cooper designed an experiment to compare the traditional research review with meta-analysis. In their study, 32 graduate students and 9 faculty members were randomly divided into two groups and asked to summarize seven empirical studies that tested the hypothesis that females are more persistent at a task than males. The two groups used different summarization approaches for integrating the study results. The control group subjects used the traditional narrative approach, while subjects in the experimental group were instructed in meta-analysis, that is, combining p values from studies. After completing the reviews, they were asked whether the evidence supported the conclusion that females were more task persistent than males. Although the set of seven studies reviewed clearly showed a significant relationship between gender and task persistence, 73% of the control group, using the traditional review, concluded there was no relationship between gender and persistence, compared with 32% of the meta-analytic reviewers. The accumulated results of these studies showed that the null hypothesis of no relationship should be rejected ($p < .005$). Thus, with only brief instruction, the group using the quantitative approach with p values obtained a more accurate integration of the studies. Stated another way, the incidence of Type II errors (failing to reject null hypotheses that are false) may be far greater for the traditional literature review than for the meta-analytic procedure (Rosenthal, 1984, pp. 17-18).

Uses of Meta-Analysis

For pooling results of experimental studies, meta-analysis begins where the qualitative research analysis ends. Before proceeding to a discussion of the various statistical approaches to meta-analysis, we will review these topics: when to use meta-analysis and the assumptions and limitations of meta-analysis.

When to Use Meta-Analysis

The use of meta-analysis in research analysis and synthesis is limited, and, as Wolf (1986) points out, meta-analysis is not a "panacea" for the problem of knowledge cumulation methods. Meta-analysis is restricted to analysis of experimental studies and is appropriately applied for the following reasons:

(1) to resolve uncertainty in a domain of study when findings of research reports disagree
(2) to increase statistical power for primary end points and for subgroups
(3) to improve estimates of effect size
(4) to answer questions not posed when the original studies were conducted

As noted above by Sacks, Berrier, Reitman, Ancona-Berk, and Chalmers (1987, p. 450), meta-analysis is particularly useful in randomized clinical trials, because clinical trials often have sample sizes that are too small to detect clinically significant differences. This applies to the limited number of clinical trials in nursing, many of which have small samples.

How can we increase the use of meta-analysis in nursing to build our knowledge base and guide future research? One way is to clarify what is meant by the term "research results." Research results do not mean the conclusions drawn by the investigator, given that the author's conclusions may be only remotely related to the actual study findings. As you may have discovered from your own research reviews, the "metamorphosis" that often occurs between the results section and the conclusion section can lead a reviewer to unwarranted deductions. Reviewers who dwell too much on the conclusion section of a research report and only skim the findings section can easily be misled. Rosenthal points out another advantage of not jumping to the conclusion section and of taking time to carefully review the findings of studies (1984, p. 19): "Somewhere in the thicket of df there lurk one or more meaningful answers to meaningful questions that we had not the foresight to ask of our data." A precise review of the findings section may uncover new insights and important information. Thus what is meant by summarizing *research results* is the description of the relationship between any variable X and any variable Y in terms of these two factors:

(1) the *effect size*, which is the estimate of the magnitude of the relationship between variables X and Y, and
(2) the reliability or accuracy of the estimated effect size, usually provided in the form of a *confidence interval* placed around the *estimated effect size*.

Statistical tests of significance from a meta-analysis, and single studies for that matter, should be accompanied by estimated effect size and confidence intervals to provide indicators of the strength of the relationship. This tells the reader how much confidence to place in the results. We will discuss how to determine measures of effect size later in the chapter.

Assumptions and Limitations

What are the major assumptions and limitations of meta-analysis? When using meta-analysis, the researcher must consider these points regarding assumptions and limitations:

(1) representativeness of data from each study included in the analysis and the total sample included in the meta-analysis
(2) quality of data from each study
(3) independence of data from each study
(4) the specific assumptions usually associated with the *type of statistical method* used in the meta-analysis (t test, F, r, and so on)
(5) the specific assumptions and limitations of each original study

For more information on assumptions and limitations, see Wolf (1986).

Steps in Meta-Analysis

The meta-analysis consists of the steps presented earlier in Box 2.1. Steps 1-4 are the same for a qualitative or quantitative analysis. We begin our discussion of the meta-analytic process with Step 5.

Steps 1-4

These are the same as for the qualitative review.

Step 5. Determining a Common Scale or Metric

When reviewing studies for a meta-analysis, the analyst will likely face the problem of diverse research designs and reporting of varied significance results, such as t, F, r, chi-square, or some other statistic. To provide an index of the power of the analysis, the summary statistics must be converted to a simple common metric in order to pool and synthesize results. This allows the researcher to determine an effect size measure, which provides an index of the statistical strength of the findings.

The most common effect size measure is the Pearson product-moment correlation, r. Another method is converting to the effect size index d (Rosenthal, 1984; Wolf, 1986). Procedures for converting to r are shown in Table 2.1 andprocedures for converting to d are shown in Table 2.2. More will be presented on the calculation and interpretation of effect size measures after a discussion of the most frequently used combined statistical tests for analyzing across studies.

Step 6. Analyzing Across Studies

Combined tests. Combined methods are applied to the analysis of results of the same hypothesis from different studies in order to summarize an overall test of the hypothesis. Combined methods range from simple counting procedures to more complex summation methods that determine significance levels or raw or weighted test statistics, such as t test and z test statistics. Of the parametric tests, the most frequently used combined tests are the Fisher, Winer, and Stouffer. An early approach to meta-analysis was the vote counting

TABLE 2.1

Guidelines for Converting Various Test Statistics to r

Statistic to Be Converted	Formula for Transformation to r	Comment
t	$r = \sqrt{\dfrac{t^2}{t^2 + df}}$	
F	$r = \sqrt{\dfrac{F}{F + df(error)}}$	Use only for comparing two group means (i.e., numerator df = 1)
χ^2	$r = \dfrac{\sqrt{\chi^2}}{n}$	n = sample size Use only for 2 × 2 frequency tables (df = 1)
d	$r = \dfrac{d}{\sqrt{d^2 + 4}}$	

TABLE 2.2

Guidelines for Converting Various Test Statistics to d

Statistic to Be Converted	Formula for Transformation to d	Comment
t	$d = \dfrac{2t}{\sqrt{df}}$	
F	$d = \dfrac{2\sqrt{F}}{\sqrt{df(error)}}$	Use only for comparing two group means (i.e., numerator df = 1)
r	$d = \dfrac{2r}{\sqrt{1 - r^2}}$	

SOURCE: Reprinted with permission from Rosenthal (1984, p. 104).

TABLE 2.3

Advantages and Limitations of Nine Methods of Combining Probabilities

Method	Advantages	Limitations	Use When
1. Adding logs	Well established historically	Cumulates poorly; can support opposite conclusions	N of studies small (≤ 5)
2. Adding p's	Good power	Inapplicable when N of studies (or p's) large unless complex corrections are introduced	N of studies small (Σ p ≤ 1.0)
3. Adding t's	Unaffected by N of studies given minimum df per study	Inapplicable when t's based on very few df	Studies not based on too few df
4. Adding Z's	Routinely applicable; simple	Assumes unit variance when under some conditions Type I or Type II errors may be increased	Anytime
5. Adding weighted Z's	Routinely applicable, permits weighting	Assumes unit variance when under some conditions Type I or Type II errors may be increased	Whenever weighting desired
6. Testing mean p	Simple	N of studies should not be less than four	N of studies ≤ 4
7. Testing mean Z	No assumption of unit variance	Low power when N of studies small	N of studies ≤ 5
8. Counting	Simple and robust	Large N of studies needed; may be low in power	N of studies large
9. Blocking	Displays all means for inspection, thus facilitating search for *moderators* (variables altering the relationship between independent and dependent variables)	Laborious when N large; insufficient data may be available	N of studies not too large

SOURCE: Reprinted with permission from Rosenthal, R. (1984, p. 104).

method, which is no longer recommended because of its weak statistical power. The combined methods are discussed in this section with examples provided for the preferred combined tests. A summary of the most common combined tests is provided in Table 2.3, which describes the advantages, limitations, and recommended uses for each method. When using combined tests, it is recommended that the effect size as well as the overall probability level be reported (McGaw & Glass, 1980). The Stouffer, Winer, and combined tests will be illustrated in this section, with examples, because they are used most frequently.

Adding probabilities (p values method). This powerful approach, developed by Edgington (1972), integrates study results using the levels of significance or the probabilities associated with the test statistics (*p* values) from each of the original studies. It is based on the binomial or chi-square distributions. The test has good power and is best applied when the *N* of studies is small (< 5) and the sum of the *p* values is less than 1.0. The formula for adding probabilities is

$$P = \frac{\Sigma p^N}{N!}$$

The one-tailed *p* associated with each *t* is determined for each study. A sign preceding the *t* gives the direction of the results. A positive sign means that the difference is consistent with the bulk of the results; a negative sign means the difference is inconsistent. When the results are in the consistent direction, one-tail *p*'s are always less than .50. When the results are not consistent, *p* values are always greater than .50. When calculating *p*'s, it is customary also to provide the size of the effect in terms of the Pearson *r* or the *d*, and the standard normal deviate, *Z*, for each *p* value. Determination and interpretation of effect size will be discussed in the next section. Rosenthal (1984, p. 96) notes that when the sum of the *p* levels exceeds unity (> 1), the overall *p* obtained will be too conservative unless corrections are made.

Cluster approach. Proposed by Light and Smith (1971), the literature is reviewed, studies relevant to the problem of interest are identified, and studies that meet specific selection criteria are included. The criteria are

(1) subject selection
(2) measurement of variables

(3) instrumentation

(4) research design

The original data used for the reported statistical analysis in each side must then be obtained and analyzed. Using the original data, clusters are defined based on the research question under consideration. A cluster is a natural unit of analysis that the reviewer identifies in the selected studies, such as schools, classrooms, groups, or subgroups within groups. The clusters are analyzed for differences between them and within them. The differences in effects among clusters are analyzed as well as the sources of the differences. One problem with this approach is that the original data must be accessible. This test is not used often because of the difficulties involved in accessing original data across studies.

Stouffer Combined Test (adding Zs). Developed by Stouffer et al. (Wolf, 1986), this test converts p values to Z's and the Z's are then summed. The formula for the Stouffer Combined Test is

$$Z_c = \frac{\Sigma Z}{\sqrt{N}}$$

The denominator is the square root of the number of tests combined. As Wolf notes (1986), this test is based on the sum of normal deviates being itself a normal deviate, with the variance equal to the number of observations summed. The Stouffer Test is easy to calculate and is slightly more powerful than the Winer Combined Test. An example of the Stouffer procedure is provided in Box 2.4.

Fisher Combined Test (adding logs). Also referred to as "adding logs," this test is well established historically. It is best used when the N of studies is < 5 and all the studies test a common hypothesis. The natural logarithms of the probabilities are calculated, multiplied by –2, and then summed, to provide a χ^2 statistic with the degrees of freedom equal to two times the number of tests combined ($2n$). The formula for the Fisher Combined Test is shown here:

$$\chi^2 = -2\,\Sigma \log_c p$$

According to Wolf (1986, p. 19), the chi-square statistic obtained in the above equation has a sampling distribution that is approximated by the chi-square distribution, with degrees of freedom equal to $2n$, where n is the number of tests combined, and p is a one-tailed

---

Box 2.4. Use of the Stouffer and Winer Combined Tests

Schwartz, Moody, Yarandi, and Anderson (1988) conducted a meta-analysis to synthesize the existing body of nonnutritive sucking (NNS) research and assess the effects of NNS on clinical outcomes of preterm infants. Outcome variables for the meta-analysis were: days of hospitalization, hospital costs, days to first bottle feeding, and weight gain. In order to obtain an overall summary test of the hypothesis, the t Test statistic and the one-tailed significance level were calculated for each study, as shown below. The Stouffer and Winer Combined Tests were then applied, as illustrated below, to test two null hypotheses: (1) there will be no significant difference in days to first bottle feeding, and (2) there will be no significant difference in days of hospitalization.

Results of Test Statistics: Days to First Bottle Feeding and
Days of Hospitalization

Study	Pooled Standard Deviation	df	t	One-Tailed Significance Level	Z
Days to First Bottle Feeding					
1	1.64	57	7.96	.00005	4.0
2	5.51	23	0.657	.259	0.70
3	19.64	55	0.576	.285	0.65
4	11.17	17	0.175	.432	0.02
5	3.90	28	4.00	.0002	3.10
Days of Hospitalization					
1	2.35	57	6.53	.00005	4.0
2	10.04	23	1.31	.102	1.17
3	19.64	55	1.54	.065	1.51
4	22.41	17	0.73	.238	0.72
5	9.04	28	2.06	.024	1.85

Stouffer Combined Test. Using the formula for the Stouffer Combined Test for the data in the above table, Z_c was calculated for the dependent variables, days to first bottle feeding and days of hospitalization, and was 3.78 and 4.13, respectively. The probability of obtaining these values of Z_c is less than .05.

Winer Combined Test. Using the formula for the Winer Combined Test and the same data in the above table, Z_c for the dependent variables, days to first bottle feeding and days of hospitalization, was 5.76 and 2.26, respectively. Both Z values were statistically significant at the .05 level.

Both combined tests results provided evidence that NNS intervention was effective in reducing days to first bottle feeding and days of hospitalization in preterm infants. It should be noted that the Winer and Stouffer Combined Tests are more powerful if the number of studies is greater than 10. Effect size will be discussed in the next section.

probability associated with each test. The use of the Fisher Combined Test is demonstrated in Box 2.5 and compared with the use of the Stouffer and Winer Combined Tests.

Vote counting. One of the first methods of meta-analysis was the vote counting method. In this approach, the reviewer examines the relationship between the independent and dependent variables, tallying the number of studies within selected outcome categories, such as these:

(1) statistically significant results in a positive direction
(2) statistically significant results in a negative direction
(3) lack of significant results in either direction

The category containing the largest number of studies is assumed to represent the direction of the true relationship (Light & Smith, 1971). A limitation of the vote counting method exists when the mean statistical power is < .5 and there is a true effect. Therefore, increasing the number of studies included in the review increases the probability of falsely concluding that an effect does not exist. For this reason, and because improved statistical methods now exist, vote counting is no longer recommended. As illustrated earlier in Box 2.3, a few years back, vote counting might have been used to analyze these studies but the probability for error with this method is now recognized.

Winer Combined Test (adding t's). In 1971, Winer introduced a procedure for combining independent tests that derives from the sampling distribution of independent t statistics. The t statistics associated with each test are summed and divided by the square root of the sum of the degrees of freedom (df) associated with each t after each df has been divided by df – 2. The Winer Combined Test formula is

$$Z_c = \frac{\Sigma t}{|\, df / (\, df - 2\,)\,|}$$

The Winer procedure is based on df/(df – 2) being the variance of a t distribution, which is approximately normally distributed. The Winer method is not recommended for very small samples where the df are few. An example of the use of the Winer method is shown in Box 2.4 from the study by Schwartz, Moody, Yarandi, and Anderson.

Box 2.5. Comparing the Stouffer, Winer and Fisher Tests Effects of Exercise on Self-Esteem Across Four Studies[a]

Study	t	df	One-tailed p	Z	$-2 \Sigma \log_e p$
A	2.72**	80	.004	2.65	11.04
B	−1.95	60	.97	−1.88	.06
C	2.03*	200	.024	1.98	7.46
D	1.56	20	.06	1.52	5.63

SOURCE: Wolf, F. (1986). *Meta-analysis: Quantitative methods for research synthesis* (pp. 18-23). Beverly Hills, CA: Sage.
a. A minus sign preceding the t indicates the direction of the result. In the example, findings from Study B were inconsistent with the majority of the results.
*p < .01, two-tailed test

This example illustrates the use of three combined tests: the Fisher, Stouffer, and Winer tests—in testing the hypothesis across four studies that exercise enhances self-esteem. Each study used a different method for testing self-esteem. The table above shows the results from each study as well as the pooled results for each combined test. The results indicated significantly greater self-esteem on the average for the experimental subjects in studies A and C, but in studies B and D, self-esteem was nonsignificantly higher for the control group. Disparate results from several studies may be resolved through meta-analysis, to address the remaining question: Does exercise improve self-esteem? Applying the formulas for the Fisher, Winer, and Stouffer procedures (see discussion in Chapter 2 for formulas), the results are as follows:

1. Fisher Combined Test: $X^2 = 24.19$, with 8 df, $p < .01$
   (Adding Logs)
2. Winer procedure: $Z_c = 2.10$, the probability of obtaining this p value is
   (Summing ts) $p (\geq 2.10)$, < .018, one-tailed
3. Stouffer procedure: $Z_c = 2.13$, the probability of obtaining this value or
   (Summing Zs)   larger is $p (Z \geq 2.13) < .017$, one-tailed.

In using the procedures, the one-tailed hypothesis tests are used because of the directional nature of the hypothesis resulting from the known direction of the majority of the results of each study.

In this example, analogous results are obtained with each procedure, indicating that the null hypothesis of no significant effect common to each of the studies should be rejected when the scope of the inference concerns the combined populations (Wolf, 1986, p. 23).

Comparing the Fisher, Stouffer, and Winer Tests. Deciding which tests to use depends in large part on what data are available from the sample of studies. In the Schwartz, Moody, Yarandi, and Anderson (1988) study, it was not possible to use the Fisher Test, because exact *p* values were not available for all studies. Wolf (1986) provides an illustration of the comparative use of these three methods to test the hypothesis across four studies that exercise improves self-esteem (Box 2.5). Thus the results of the three methods in this example are comparable. The analyst may also select a specific test due to its ease of calculation, such as the Stouffer Test, which is straightforward. If all the independent studies are reported as *t*'s, then it is easy to use the Winer procedure. The Fisher procedure is recognized as being the most asymptotically efficient of the combined tests (Littrell & Folks, 1973).

Effect Size

The combined tests described in the previous section provide a summary index of the statistical significance of the results pertaining to a hypothesis but do not yield information about the strength of the relationship. Therefore, indexes of the effect size should accompany the combined tests. Effect size is defined by Cohen (1977, pp. 9-10) in this way:

> ... "the degree to which the phenomenon is present in the population," or "the degree to which the null hypothesis is false." Whatever the manner of representation of a phenomenon in a particular research in the present treatment, the null hypothesis always means that the effect size is zero.

Thus effect size measures the research results on a common scale or metric. For example, as presented earlier in Table 2.3, Cohen's *d* is the difference between the means of the experimental group and the control group divided by a standard deviation. If an overall standardized effect size of one were obtained, this would imply that the average experimental subject scored one standard deviation above the average control subject. An example of calculation of effect size is depicted in Box 2.6.

Interpreting effect sizes. Proper interpretation of the effect size is important in that it provides insight into the strength of the statistical significance finding. Wolf (1986, p. 27) describes the procedure of constructing a 95% or 99% confidence interval around the average

---

Box 2.6. Calculation of Effect Size

In the study described in Box 2.5 by Schwartz et al., effect size was calculated on all outcome variables where the necessary information was available, using the formula

$$\text{Effect Size} = \bar{d} = \frac{|X_e - X_c|}{S_p}$$

where X_c is the mean for the control group, X_e is the mean for the experimental group, and S_p is the pooled standard deviation. The Winer and Stouffer Combined Tests provided a test of significance for the collection of studies, and the effect size determined the strength of the relationship between the groups. The table below shows the results of effect sizes between the experimental and control groups of each study and the overall average regarding days to first bottle feeding and days of hospitalization.

Effect Size: Days to First Bottle Feeding and Days of Hospitalization

Study	Group Mean C	E	$\bar{d}$	U3 (%)
	Days to First Bottle Feeding			
1	17.8	14.4	2.07	98.1
2	12.5	11.1	0.26	60.3
3	29.0	26.0	0.15	56.0
4	16.0	15.1	0.08	53.2
5	16.1	10.4	1.46	92.8
Average			$\bar{d} =$ 0.80	78.8
	Days of Hospitalization			
1	40.5	36.5	1.70	95.5
2	27.3	22.07	0.52	69.6
3	56.0	48.0	0.41	95.6
4	41.7	34.2	0.33	63.3
5	58.7	51.9	0.75	77.3
Average			$\bar{d} =$ 0.74	77.0

NOTE: C = control, E = experimental.

The results indicated that the average experimental subject across studies had the first bottle feeding .80 standard deviation units earlier than the average control subject. Or, put another way, the percentile of nonoverlap, U_3, suggests that the average experimental subject received the first bottle feeding earlier than 78.8% of subjects in the control group. To test the significance of the mean effect size, the t statistic was calculated and found to be significant at the .06 level, $t = 1.97$.

Also shown in the above table is effect size results using days of hospitalization. The average effect size indicated that experimental subjects for the combined studies were discharged from the hospital .74 standard deviation units earlier than the average control subject. The information on U_3 nonoverlap suggests that the average experimental subject was discharged from the hospital earlier than 77% of the control-group subjects. The calculated t Test for mean effect size was 2.9, significant at the .02 level.

TABLE 2.4

Interpreting Magnitude Effect Size

$d =$	Magnitude of Effect Size
.2–.49	Small effect
.5–.79	Medium effect
.8 or >	Large effect

effect size to examine whether it encompasses zero. The standard deviation associated with the average effect size across studies is reported to indicate the variability associated with it. In the example in Box 2.6, the average experimental subject across studies had the first bottle-feeding .80 standard deviation units earlier than the average control subject. Another way to interpret this finding is to say that the percentile of nonoverlap, U_3, suggests that the average experimental subject received the first bottle-feeding earlier than 78.8% of subjects in the control group. Thus, you may ask, how significant is this finding in view of the fact that the results of the Winer and Stouffer Combined Tests also showed statistically significant results across studies? To test the significance of the mean effect size, .80, the t statistic was calculated and found to be significant at the .06 level, $t = 1.97$.

Cohen (1977) provides standards for interpreting the magnitude of the effect size when d is used (Table 2.4). Cohen warns that these standards are still being developed and refined. Because effect sizes, when reported as standard deviation units, are not easily interpreted, Cohen (1977) used the normal curve table for translating the effect size d into measures of nonoverlap. Using this approach, the average effect size is transformed into a graphic representation of the effect on the degree of overlap between the control and experimental groups. For example, in the Schwartz, Moody, Yarandi, and Anderson (1988) meta-analysis (Box 2.6) of the variable "days of hospitalization," the average effect size indicated that experimental subjects for the combined studies were discharged from the hospital .74 standard deviation units earlier than the average controlling subject. The information on U_3 suggests that the average experimental subject was discharged from the hospital earlier than 77% of the control group subjects. The calculated t test for the mean effect size was 2.9, significant at the .02 level.

Another interpretation of effect size is that a .50 standard deviation improvement in achievement scores is accepted as a conventional measure of practical significance (Rossi & Wright, 1977). Tallmadge (1977) reported that a .25 or > standard deviation improvement is considered educationally significant. As more meta-analyses are conducted in nursing, effect sizes will become standardized and less difficult to interpret.

Confidence intervals. Use of confidence intervals to interpret effect size may also provide insight as to the importance of the findings, as Wolf (1986) and Rosenthal (1984) recommended. Referring again to the Schwartz, Moody, Yarandi, and Anderson study (1988) in Box 2.6, analyses of the outcome variable "hospital costs" were constructed for a single study (Study 2) with a sample size of 25. The confidence interval ranged from –$10,560 to $44,160. The range, unrealistic due to the effect of the small sample size, yielded no useful information. But when Study 2 and Study 3 data were combined, increasing the sample size to 82, construction of the confidence interval resulted in a range of $2,525 to $23,897. This example illustrates that, as the size of the confidence interval narrows, there is less likelihood of error in the estimation. For more detailed information about interpretations of effect size, refer to Wolf (1986) and Rosenthal (1984).

Mediating effects. Another important consideration in the meta-analysis is the examination of whether third variables are mediators of the effect under study in the primary research hypothesis. For example, we may want to know which, if any, demographic variables mediated the relation between selected variables. Wolf (1986) provides an example of 180 fictional studies of which 60 were conducted with females and 120 included males. Suppose there was reason to suspect that gender mediated the relation between personal income and self-esteem. Analyzing effect size by gender, the results showed that average effect size for females was .14 and for males .46. The effect size for each of these 180 samples could then be correlated with the gender of the samples. Assume this resulted in a correlation of .38 ($p < .01$, $n = 180$). This would indicate that male samples yielded stronger effect sizes than female samples or the relation between personal income and self-esteem tended to be stronger for males than for females. This example also illustrates that subgroup analysis might yield important information. Additionally, multiple linear regression methods may be used to regress effect sizes on a number of potential mediating variables (Hedges & Olkin, 1985).

If the average *d* rather than the average *r* is used as the effect size indicator across studies, a similar approach is used to assess mediator variables. Using the above example, d for females and males, respectively, is determined, and the d for each sample is correlated with gender, with females coded 0 and males 1. Then, the differences between $\bar{d}$'s for males and females are tested statistically using the methods proposed by Hedges (1982).

Weighting studies. Many would argue that not all studies in a meta-analysis should be given equal weight because some studies may have small, unrepresentative samples while others may have used well-controlled randomized designs with adequate samples. To correct for variation in quality, some meta-analysts have recommended weighting each of the standard normal deviates (Zs) used for the Stouffer Combined Test by the size of the sample on which it was based (Mosteller & Bush, 1954). This can be done using the formula

$$\text{weighted } Z_c = \frac{\Sigma \, df \, Z}{\sqrt{\Sigma \, df^2}}$$

Z is the standard normal deviate associated with the one-tailed p value for each statistic synthesized and df = the degree of freedom associated with the statistic. In the Schwartz, Moody, Yarandi, and Anderson (1988) study, using this formula for the variable "days to first bottle-feeding," the results would be as follows:

$$\text{weighted } Z_c = \frac{(57)(4) + (23)(.7) + (55)(.65) + (17)(.02) + (28)(3.1)}{(57)^2 + (23)^2 + (55)^2 + (17)^2 + (28)^2}$$

$$\text{weighted } Z_c = \frac{366.99}{88.75} = 4.14$$

The probability of obtaining this value of weighted Z_c or larger is $p(Z \geq 4.14) < .0001$, one-tailed. When studies are weighted using this method, it is recommended that both weighted and unweighted Zs be reported. The difference in the weighted, 4.14, and the unweighted Z, 5.76, in the Schwartz et al. study in this case does not alter the conclusion but it is obvious that the weighted method adjusts for sample sizes for each corresponding Z score.

As Wolf (1986, p. 40) notes, the advantage of this method is clear. For example, studies with small samples that contain results inconsistent with most other studies could exert an unwarranted influence on the pooled results if unweighted Zs are used.

Unbiased estimate of effect size. A weighted estimator of effect size was developed by Hedges (1982) that is more asymptotic and accurate when sample sizes in the experimental and control group are greater than 10 and effect sizes (d) are less than 1.5, which is usually the case. Wolf (1986, p. 41) provides this following formula for calculating the weighted $\bar{d}$

$$\bar{d} = \frac{\Sigma\, wd}{\Sigma\, w}$$

where d is the unweighted effect size and w is the reciprocal of the estimated variance of d in each of the studies to be aggregated in the meta-analysis. To calculate w when the experimental and control group sample sizes are almost equal and greater than 10, the following formula is used (Rosenthal & Rubin, 1982):

$$w = \frac{2\, N}{8 + d^{2}}$$

In the above formula, d is the unweighted effect size and N is the total sample size in the study for both groups. Using this formula for the Schwartz, Moody, Yarandi, and Anderson (1988) study for the variable "days to first bottle-feeding," results are depicted in Box 2.7. As illustrated in Box 2.7, this procedure provides a way of checking for bias of the effect size.

Tests of homogeneity. An important theoretical consideration underlying meta-analysis is whether the pooled studies are homogeneous and are representative of the population effect size (Wolf, 1986, p. 42). If the population is homogeneous, then it is more likely that a common hypothesis is being tested. If the estimates are heterogeneous, then it is questionable whether the studies share a common hypothesis.

How can homogeneity be assessed? A number of statistical tests have been proposed by Rosenthal (1984) to assess for homogeneity/heterogeneity of the standard normal deviates Z corresponding to the one-tailed p values from the combined studies. It may be necessary to use extended tables of the t distribution (Rosenthal & Rosnow, 1984). The formula is

Box 2.7. Calculation of Unbiased Estimate of Effect Size

Study	N	d	w
1	59	2.07	9.61
2	25	0.26	6.20
3	57	0.15	14.21
4	19	0.08	4.74
5	30	1.46	5.92

SOURCE: Data are from the Schwartz, Moody, Yarandi, and Anderson (1988) study.
NOTE: Unbiased Estimate of Effect Size = .80. Referring to the results of the unweighted estimate of effect size for the variable, days to first bottle feeding (Box 2.6), note that it is also .80, the same as the unbiased estimate of effect size. This example illustrates a method of checking for bias. Ideally, both results should be reported.

$$Z = \frac{Z_1 - Z_2}{\sqrt{2}}$$

Using the data from Box 2.4 for the variable "days of hospitalization," we use the above formula to test whether Study 1 is significantly different than Study 4, which had a much smaller sample size than Study 1. The formula yields the following results, $Z = 2.82$, which has a p value of .03. Thus this finding warrants a search for a plausible explanation as to why the two studies are significantly different and for a rationale for including Study 4 in the sample. This is why analysis of the substantive and methodological characteristics are imperative in the coding and classifying of studies.

To further test this, we use another approach, the Omnibus Test, also called the Diffuse Test, to examine the entire collection of studies in the meta-analysis. The following equation (Wolf, 1986, p. 45) is used for the Omnibus Test

$$\chi^2 = \Sigma (Z - \overline{Z})^2$$

Using the same variable, days of hospitalization, from the Schwartz, Moody, Yarandi, and Anderson (1987) study, homogeneity is examined with the Omnibus Test. The resultant χ^2 value of 6.48, with 4 df, is nonsignificant. This indicates that there is sufficient homogeneity among the studies to warrant their inclusion. For more information on assessing homogeneity, refer to Wolf (1986), Rosenthal and Rubin (1982), and Abraham and Schultz (1983).

Nonparametric Methods and Effect Size

Methods exist for pooling data across studies that measure variables on ordinal or dichotomous scales. In addition, use of a nonparametric indicator of effect size is appropriate when the data are skewed or not normally distributed. One solution is to use the median as the measure of central tendency to describe effect size. Rosenthal (1984) believes that use of medians in meta-analysis provides results that usually favor Type II errors, that is, results that favor the null hypothesis. Wolf (1986, p. 50) explains that the nonparametric effect size D for each study may be obtained from the formula

$$D = \varphi^{-1}(p)$$

where D is a standard normal deviate, φ^{-1} is the inverse of the cumulative standard normal distribution function, and p is the proportion of the control group subjects whose values on the dependent variable are less than the median value for the experimental group. For additional information on the use of nonparametric tests and calculating effect sizes for small samples, see Kraemer and Andrews (1982).

Step 7. Interpreting and Reporting Results

Providing the reader with a clear and explicit summary of the research results and an interpretation of how much confidence can be placed in the analysis is of paramount importance. As we discussed in Step 6, the analyst must provide adequate statistical information that will permit the reader to interpret the findings and to know how much confidence can be placed in the analysis. As discussed later in the "Standards for Meta-Analysis" section, the analyst is obliged to present an estimation of the validity and reliability of the results, a full discussion of the sampling process, and identified limitations of the review. Refer to the Schwartz, Moody, Yarandi, and Anderson (1988) article for an example of such a discussion.

Step 8. Explicating Theory and Research Outcomes

If the analyst has used a coding tool, such as the NPRAT, then developing this section of the report is greatly facilitated. The research outcomes should be summarized as discussed previously for the qualitative review. Advances in theory development and rec-ommendations for future theory testing are identified. It may be possible in some meta-analyses, in which there is existing empirical support and the effect size is large, that middle-range theories for practice can be supported or formulated for further testing. For an example of how this can be accomplished, see Box 2.8.

Step 9. Projecting Future Research Needs

This step is the same as discussed previously for the qualita-tive analysis. A quantitative analysis, accompanied by information gleaned from the qualitative analysis, may provide more compelling data for influencing health policy or increasing funding for clinical intervention studies.

Sources of Bias

A number of methods exist to examine and reduce bias in the meta-analysis process. Some of the contributing factors to biased analyses are these (Wolf, 1986, p. 37):

(1) journals' biases for publishing positive, but not negative, results
(2) weighing results of all studies equally even though there are obvious qualitative differences
(3) including multiple tests of a hypothesis from a single study
(4) failure to ensure high reliability among raters in the coding of study characteristics

While many of these issues have been discussed in "Step 6, Analyz-ing Across Studies," key points will be highlighted in the next section on standards for meta-analysis.

Standards for Meta-Analysis

What criteria can be used to judge the merits of a meta-analysis in order to know how much confidence to place in the research out-comes? A number of researchers have addressed this topic—Smith (1987), Sacks, Berrier, Reitman, Ancona-Berk, and Chalmers (1987), and Curlette and Cannella (1985), to mention a few. Sacks and col-

---

Box 2.8. Nursing Interventions and Patient Outcomes: A Meta-Analysis
of Studies

SOURCE: Heater, B., Becker, A. and Olson, R. (1988). *Nursing Research, 37,*
303-307.

This meta-analysis sought to determine the contribution that research-based nursing practices make to health care by comparing patient outcomes from experimental nursing interventions with patient outcomes from routine, procedural nursing care. All published and unpublished experimental studies from 1977 through 1984 using independent nursing interventions were evaluated to compute an estimate of the effect size for the patient outcomes. All studies were conducted by nurses. Independent nursing interventions were defined as actions by professional nurses not requiring a physician's order. The aim of the nursing actions or interventions is promotion of health or prevention of illness. Patient outcomes were defined as the effects of interventions provided by a nurse that produced measurable responses in relation to identified criteria. Using content analysis, four types of outcomes were identified: behavioral, knowledge, physiological, and psychosocial.

The major finding was that research-based nursing practice can offer patients better outcomes than routine, procedural nursing care. A mean ES of .59 was found which is associated with U_3 of 72.2 and $r = .282$, meaning that the average subject in an experimental group had better outcomes than 72% of the subjects who received routine care. An r of .282 is associated with a 28% improvement in patient outcomes. In other words, 72% can have better outcomes and the outcomes are 28% better.

Patient Implications: Benefits resulting from 28% better outcomes for 72% of the patients when research-based nursing interventions are used strongly suggest that it is wasteful for professional nurses to perform nonnursing tasks.

How can these data be used to argue against the AMA's proposal to create a new health care worker, the RCT?

---

leagues (1987) reviewed 86 reports of randomized controlled trials and evaluated the quality of these meta-analyses. Their evaluation was based on 23 items in six major areas: study design, combinability, control of bias, statistical analysis, sensitivity analysis, and application of results. From the work of Sacks et al. (1987, pp. 451-453) and other researchers, the following standards can be applied in judging whether a meta-analysis was rigorous and conducted scientifically.

A. Study Design

(1) Protocol. The questions to be answered, the criteria for inclusion in the study, and the methods to be used should be established beforehand and made explicit. A planned protocol for conducting the meta-analysis will assist in a more rigorous and systematic analysis.

(2) Literature search. Details of the search procedures should be provided. The search should include as many relevant sources as possible, published and unpublished. Kraemer and Andrews (1982) note that published research tends to be biased toward studies with positive findings. It is speculated that many researchers abandon studies if they believe the outcome will be nonsignificant and file the results away somewhere in the office. Rosenthal (1984) refers to this as the "file drawer problem." Thus the fact that studies with significant findings are more likely to be published increases the probability of a Type I publication bias error in identifying more positive results than is really the case were it is possible to include all studies.

Rosenthal (1984) addressed this problem by recommending that the meta-analyst determine the number of studies confirming the null hypothesis that would be needed to reverse a conclusion that a significant relationship exists. Cooper (1979) referred to this as the Fail Safe N (N_{fs}) for the number of studies needed in the meta-analysis to reverse the overall probability obtained from the combined test to a value higher than the established critical value for statistical significance, .05 or .01. Wolf (1986, p. 38) provides the following formulas for computing N_{fs}, for the .05 and .01 levels:

$$N_{fs}\,.05 = \left\{ \frac{\Sigma\,Z^2}{1.645} \right\} - N$$

$$N_{fs}\,.01 = \left\{ \frac{\Sigma\,Z^2}{2.33} \right\} - N$$

Here $\Sigma\,Z$ is the sum of individual Z scores and N is the number of studies combined using the Stouffer combined significance procedure. The Fail Safe N can then be assessed by senior researchers in the field to determine the likelihood that these unpublished studies in the research domain exist that show no effect. For more information on this process, see Orwin (1983) and Wolf (1986).

(3) Studies analyzed and studies rejected. The meta-analyst should keep an account of all studies included and excluded in the meta-analysis. Criteria for including and excluding studies should be made explicit.

(4) Treatment assignment. Sacks, Berrier, Reitman, Ancona-Berk, and Chalmers (1987) note that the most important question bearing on validity of the pooled data is the method of treatment assignment in each primary study because results of trials using historical controls are more likely to favor the new treatment than results of the same therapy tested in randomized controlled trials. Thus the method of treatment assignment is important and should be noted.

(5) Ranges of subject characteristics, diagnoses, and treatments. The reader will be able to judge the validity and generalizability of a meta-analysis if the researcher provides data on the subjects (relevant demographic variables), diagnoses (including stages of severity of disease), range of therapies, and end points from the original studies.

(6) Combinability. Another major issue in pooling data is whether the results of the separate studies are such that they can be combined to produce valid outcomes. The studies must address common hypotheses and be conceptually and methodologically equivalent to warrant pooling across studies. This issue needs to be addressed clearly and in sufficient detail to convince the reader that the results of the meta-analysis are useful and clinically relevant.

(7) Criteria. The researcher should address which criteria were used to decide that studies analyzed were comparable to be pooled and note any differences in the primary study that might affect the conclusions.

(8) Measurement. As Sacks, Berrier, Reitman, Ancona-Berk, and Chalmers (1987) noted, related to the issue of combinability is the issue of statistical homogeneity or heterogeneity. Two possible models of combining estimates are recognized for meta-analysis. These models were demonstrated earlier in the chapter. In the first model, the within-study variability model, each study is considered to be a sample from the same population and provides an estimate of a single, underlying true rate, and differences are due to experimental error. In the second model, the between-study variability model, each study is considered to be from a different population, the rate varies from study to study, and differences are due to experimental error and to differences in the populations. Methods exist to deter-

mine which model is appropriate (Wolf, 1986). If the between-study variability model applies, the analyst should apply tests for homogeneity to help decide the degree of caution needed in interpreting the pooled results (Sacks, Berrier, Reitman, Ancona-Berk, & Chalmers, 1987, p. 152).

B. Control and Measurement of Potential Bias

(1) Selection bias. Sacks, Berrier, Reitman, Ancona-Berk, and Chalmers recommended that the inclusion of studies should be based on an examination of the study methods and not based on whether the study outcomes were statistically significant.

(2) Data extraction bias. In any data gathering process that requires interpretation and judgment calls, reviewers may disagree. This type of bias can be controlled by training more than one coder or interpreter, who is blinded to the various treatment groups, to extract the data, and then measuring interobserver agreement. This process is illustrated in the study by Schwartz, Moody, Yarandi, and Anderson (1988).

(3) Source of support. The source of funding should be noted to assist in determining whether a conflict of interest or vested interest may have influenced study outcomes. This helps to determine how much credence to give to the results.

C. Statistical Analysis

(1) Statistical methods. A standard method of statistical pooling should be used. Analysts should specify why certain methods were used. Many authors recommend the use of more than one method to provide multiple indicators for interpretation, which will increase the validity and reliability and strengthen the statistical findings.

(2) Statistical errors. The potential for Type I error (concluding that there is difference when none exists) and Type II error (concluding that there is no difference when there is) should be addressed.

(3) Confidence intervals. As discussed in Step 6, a more useful statistic for the reader is an estimate with confidence intervals of the difference between the success rates of the interventions being compared rather than only having the results of significance tests.

(4) Subgroup analyses. A major purpose of meta-analysis is to increase the statistical power of subgroup analyses. The analyst should specify why subgroups were or were not analyzed.

D. Sensitivity Analysis

Sacks, Berrier, Reitman, Ancona-Berk, and Chalmers (1987) explain that, depending on the statistic chosen, the same set of data can be combined to yield different conclusions. Likewise, the results may vary depending on the overall quality of the primary trials and on whether certain trials, subgroups, or other variables have been excluded or changed.

(1) Quality assessment. The analyst should provide an overall summary of the quality of the studies that were combined to assist the reader in formulating conclusions. Items to be addressed are the sampling procedures, measurement of subject compliance, blinding process of subjects and observers, statistical analyses, and management of subjects who withdrew.

(2) Varying methods. Sacks, Berrier, Reitman, Ancona-Berk, and Chalmers (1987) note that each meta-analysis should include an analysis of how the results vary, through the use of different assumptions, tests, and criteria.

(3) Publication bias. The analyst should note how unpublished studies were retrieved and how negative studies were addressed. Refer to the earlier discussion of a method for calculating the number of unpublished negative studies required to refute the published evidence. This procedure provides a useful measure of the strength of the published evidence.

E. Application of Results

(1) Caveats. Once the study results are available, the analyst should put them into perspective for the reader based on the above considerations. For example, is the experimental therapy now established as more effective than the old treatment for all subjects or for certain subgroups? Should the conclusions only be suggestions for future study? What implications the research results have for health policy also need to be addressed. The contribution toward theory building should be stated and recommendations provided for theory refinement or theory testing.

(2) Economic impact. In an era of fiscal parsimony in health care, the economic impact of adopting new methods for treatment need to be addressed. The use of research results from meta-analysis can be a compelling tool for addressing the need for future research or the effects of a new intervention on health policy.

Summary

The need for improved methods for qualitative and quantitative research reviews has been a major focus of this chapter. As with any procedure, meta-analysis must be used appropriately to yield a plausible analysis of the results of pooled studies within a research domain. Many of the advantages of meta-analysis have been addressed throughout the chapter and are briefly summarized here:

(1) It is an effective method for synthesizing and analyzing a domain of research, permitting the use of statistical methods to reach empirically based conclusions.

(2) It assists in resolving important issues in a field where there are many studies with conflicting findings.

(3) It assists in highlighting gaps in a field of research and in protecting future research.

(4) It may serve as an analytic tool for influencing health policy and funding for future research.

(5) It assists in explication of explanatory or predictive-level theories.

As nursing expands the use of randomized clinical trials to test nursing interventions in specific research domains, there will be more studies available that permit researchers to take advantage of this powerful method of research synthesis and analysis. Through appropriate use of qualitative and quantitative meta-analyses, we can accelerate our progress in knowledge building for nursing practice.

Point-Counterpoint

(1) Select one of the meta-analyses in nursing listed at the end of this chapter. Using the "standards for meta-analysis" included in this chapter, critique the meta-analysis accordingly.

(2) In your own particular area of research interest, is there a domain in which a number of experimental studies exist to permit the use of meta-analysis?

(3) If the answer to the above question is no, explain how you would proceed with a systematic qualitative review of the literature. Construct a coding scheme and a summary table similar to the ones included in this chapter.

(4) Discuss why it is important to address the issue of homogeneity/heterogeneity in a meta-analysis?

(5) Critique the article by Wachter, "Disturbed by Meta-Analysis?" (see References). Discuss the "four charges" made against meta-analysis and how these problems can be avoided or attenuated.

Examples of Meta-Analytic Studies

Nursing

Broome, M., Lillis, P., & Collete-Smith, M. (1989). Pain interventions with children: A meta-analysis of research. *Nursing Research, 38,* 154-158.

Devine, E., & Cook, T. (1983). A meta-analytic analysis of effects of psychoeducational interventions on length of postsurgical hospital stay. *Nursing Research, 32,* 267-274.

Hathaway, D. (1986). Effect of preoperative instruction on postoperative outcomes: A meta-analysis. *Nursing Research, 35,* 269-275.

Heater, B., Becker, A., & Olson, R. (1988). Nursing interventions and patient outcomes: A meta-analysis of studies. *Nursing Research, 37,* 303-307.

Hyman, R., Feldman, H., Harris, R., Levin, R., & Malloy, G. (1989). The effects of relaxation training on clinical symptoms: A meta-analysis. *Nursing Research, 38,* 216-220.

Schwartz, R., Moody, L., Yarandi, H., & Anderson, G. C. (1988). A meta-analysis of critical outcome variables in nonnutritive sucking in preterm infants. *Nursing Research, 36,* 292-295.

Other Disciplines

Beecher, H. K. (1955). The powerful placebo. *Journal of the American Medical Association, 159,* 1602-1606.

Elashoff, J. D. (1978). Combining results of clinical trials. *Gastroenterology, 75,* 1170-1172.

Goldman, L., & Feinstein, A. R. (1979). Anticoagulants and myocardial infarction: The problems of pooling, drowning, and floating. *Annals of Internal Medicine, 90,* 92-94.

Levitt, S. H., & McHugh, R. B. (1977). Radiotherapy in the postoperative treatment of operable cancer of the breast. Part I. Critique of the clinical and biometric aspects of the trials. *Cancer, 39,* 924-932.

Louis, T. A., Fineberg, H. V., & Mosteller, F. (1985). Findings for public health from meta-analyses. *Annual Review of Public Health, 6,* 1-20.

Yusuf, S., Peto, R., Lewis, J., Collins, R., & Sleight, P. (1985). Beta blockade during and after myocardial infarction: An overview of the randomized trials. *Progress in Cardiovascular Disease, 27,* 335-371.

References

Abraham, I. L., & Schultz, S. (1983). Univariate statistical model for meta-analysis. *Nursing Research, 32,* 312-315.

Brooten, D., Kumar, S., Brown, L., Butts, P., Finkler, S., Sachs, S., Gibbons, A., & Papadopoulos, J. (1986). A randomized clinical trial of early hospital discharge and home follow-up of very-low-birth-weight infants. *New England Journal of Medicine, 315,* 924-938.

Cohen, J. (1977). *Statistical power analysis for the behavioral sciences* (rev ed.). New York: Academic Press.

Cooper, H. (1979). Statistically combining independent studies: A meta-analysis of sex differences in conformity research. *Journal of Personality and Social Psychology, 37,* 131-145.

Curlette, W. L., & Cannella, K. S. (1985). Going beyond the narrative summarization of research findings: The meta-analysis approach. *Research in Nursing and Health, 8,* 293-301.

Curlette, W., & Ramig, C. (1979). An overview of meta-analysis. *Georgia Journal of Reading, 4,* 36-39.

Devine, E., & Cook, T. (1983). A meta-analytic analysis of effects of psychoeducational interventions on length of postsurgical hospital stay. *Nursing Research, 32,* 267-274.

Edgington, E. S. (1972). An additive method for combining probability values from independent experiments. *Journal of Psychology, 82,* 85-89.

Fiske, D. W. (1983). The meta-analytic revolution in outcome research. *Journal of Consulting and Clinical Psychology, 51,* 65-70.

Glass, G. V. (1976). Primary, secondary, and meta-analysis of research. *Educational Researcher, 5,* 3-8.

Glass, G., McGaw, B., & Smith, M. (1982). *Meta-analysis: Cumulating research findings across studies.* Beverly Hills, CA: Sage.

Hathaway, D. (1986). Effect of preoperative instruction on postoperative outcomes: A meta-analysis. *Nursing Research, 35,* 269-275.

Hedges, L. (1982). Estimation of effect size from a series of independent experimenters. *Psychological Bulletin, 92,* 490-499.

Hedges, L., & Olkin, I. (1985). *Statistical methods for meta-analysis.* Orlando, FL: Academic Press.

Hunter, J. E., Schmidt, F. L., & Jackson, G. B. (1982). *Meta-analysis: Cumulating research findings across studies.* Beverly Hills, CA: Sage.

Jones, L. C. (1985). *Conducting meta-analytic procedures for social research.* Beverly Hills, CA: Sage.

Kraemer, H., & Andrews, G. (1982). A nonparametric technique for meta-analysis effect size calculation. *Psychological Bulletin, 91,* 404-412.

Light, R., & Smith, P. (1971). Accumulating evidence: Procedures for resolving contradictions among different research studies. *Harvard Educational Review, 41,* 429-471.

Littrell, R. C., & Folks, J. L. (1973). Asymptotic optimality of Fisher's method of combining independent tests II. *Journal of the American Statistical Association, 68,* 193-194.

McGaw, B., & Glass, G. (1980). Choice of the metric for effect size in meta-analysis. *American Educational Research Journal, 17,* 225-227.

Moody, L., Wilson, M., Smyth, K., Schwartz, R., Tittle, M., & VanCott, M. (1988). Analysis of a decade of nursing practice research. *Nursing Research, 37,* 374-379.

Mosteller, F. M., & Bush, R. R. (1954). Selected quantitative techniques. In G. Lindzey (Ed.), *Handbook of social psychology* (Vol. 1). Cambridge, MA: Addison-Wesley.

Orwin, R. G. (1983). A fail-safe N for effect size. *Journal of Educational Statistics, 8,* 157-159.

Rosenthal, R. (1984). *Meta-analytic procedures for social research.* Beverly Hills, CA: Sage.

Rosenthal, R., & Rubin, D. (1982). Comparing effect sizes of independent studies. *Psychological Bulletin, 92,* 500-504.

Rossi, P., & Wright, S. (1977). Evaluation research: An assessment of theory, practice and politics. *Evaluation Quarterly, 1,* 5-52.

Sacks, H. S., Berrier, J., Reitman, D., Ancona-Berk, V. A., & Chalmers, T. C. (1987). Meta-analyses of randomized controlled trials. *New England Journal of Medicine, 316,* 450-455.

Schwartz, R., Moody, L., Yarandi, H., & Anderson, G. C. (1988). A meta-analysis of critical outcome variables in nonnutritive sucking in preterm infants. *Nursing Research, 36,* 292-295.

Smith, M. C. (1987). Meta-analysis: Conceptual issues. In S. Gortner (Ed.), *Nursing science methods: A reader* (pp. 59-76). San Francisco: University of California.

Smith, M. C., & Naftel, D. C. (1984). Meta-analysis: A perspective for research synthesis. *Image, 16,* 9-13.

Tallmadge, G. K. (1977). *The Joint Dissemination Review Panel ideabook.* Washington, DC: National Institute of Education and U.S. Office of Education.

Wachter, K. (1988). Disturbed by meta-analysis? *Science, 241,* 1407-1408.

Winer, B. J. (1971). *Statistical principals in experimental design* (2nd ed.). New York: McGraw-Hill.

Wolf, F. M. (1986). *Meta-analysis: Quantitative methods for research synthesis.* Beverly Hills, CA: Sage.

3

Causal Modeling

SANDRA L. FERKETICH AND JOYCE A. VERRAN

> ... model testing can only be evaluated within the context of
> adequate theory development.

The Nature of Causation

One of the most controversial topics in the philosophy of science involves the nature of causation. A review of the different philosophical stances is beyond the scope of this chapter. In general, however, a causal relationship may be viewed as a connection between an antecedent phenomenon (cause) and a consequence (effect) such that if the antecedent occurs then the consequence also occurs. There are three basic criteria necessary for making causal statements. The first criterion is temporal ordering. This means that the causal agent must occur prior to the effect. For some phenomena, the time between cause and effect may be very short, appearing almost instantaneous; and for other phenomena, the delay between cause and effect is so long that the association is difficult to interpret. The second criterion is covariation of the cause and effect. In other words, there is a systematic relationship between the phenomena that can be observed and measured. The third criterion for making causal statements is that the possible causal effects of other phenomena on the consequence have been accounted for or controlled.

The Need for Causal Modeling

Under constraints derived from the three criteria for causation, experimental designs allow an examination of whether a specific cause results in a specific effect. One of the established constraints for examining causation is the ability to manipulate the causative agent, which assures that there will be variation in the cause. This is not, of course, always possible or even desirable in certain areas of research. Experimental designs cannot be implemented when causal inferences are to be made with naturally occurring events that cannot be manipulated by a researcher. Nor can they be used in situations where there may be multiple causes and effects that are difficult to isolate in one experimental setting.

Because of the need to study cause-and-effect relationships in a variety of situations, not all necessarily amenable to experimental designs, multiple ways have been proposed to study causation without experimentation. *Causal modeling* is the unifying term for a number of statistical analysis approaches that have been devised for this purpose. The commonality that underlies the various sets of procedures is the evaluation of the validity of causal hypotheses by examining the fit between a theoretical model and empirical data. When a theoretical model is shown to have a good fit with the data, the model has been confirmed and the causal hypotheses have been supported. In summary, experimental designs allow the direct examination of a cause-and-effect relationship under controlled circumstances, while causal modeling permits plausible inferences to be made about causation with naturally occurring events.

Causal modeling permits examination of a simple or complex system of causal agents that may effect a change; but this is only possible given a fairly defined set of underlying assumptions. These assumptions, or conditions, may be divided into two distinct areas. The first area relates to the conditions that specify the manner in which the theory underlying the model is organized. The second refers to the assumptions that support the analysis technique used to test the specified model. The underlying assumptions about both areas will be discussed in the next sections of this chapter.

Theory Development for Causal Modeling

A causal model is a set or sets of interrelated hypotheses that attempt to explain the occurrence of phenomena. The basic components of the model include the variables that act as causes and effects and the hypothesized associations between these causes and effects. The quality of the model structure and the subsequent model testing can only be evaluated within the context of adequate theory development. The following subsections emphasize the need for adequate theory before the researcher attempts to develop and test a causal model. Only when the researcher has a well-supported theory with appropriate causal connections and temporal ordering among variables can the analysis techniques to test the model be applied. It is the formal statement of the theory underlying the causal model that actually allows inferences about cause-and-effect relationships.

Specifying the Formal Statement of Theory

A theory that is appropriate for causal modeling must be supported by a sound theoretical rationale available from the literature and/or previous research. Consideration needs to be given to the form of the theory with respect to its elaborateness, its complexity, and its boundaries (James, Mulaik, & Brett, 1982).

Elaborateness of the theory. The term *elaborateness* refers to the number of effects that are included in a theory. A theory with one effect would be considered nonelaborate. In a causal model, effects can be intermediate results or final outcomes. Causal modeling can be used with both elaborate and nonelaborate theories. However, most researchers attempt to derive a model that is both parsimonious and powerful in terms of its explanatory power. In considering elaborateness, a key issue is whether all relevant causes of each effect are included in the theory.

Of course, the issue of what are relevant causes comes to mind at this point. The definition of *relevant* is not easy to provide. Certain conditions must be considered, the first of which is that the inclusion of the cause must be sound within the framework of the posed model. The inclusion of any particular causal agent is less open to question when adequate theory is behind its selection. In other words, relevancy also relates to whether the causal variable makes theoretical sense within the system of cause-and-effect relationships. A second consideration is that, when examining the system of causal agents for one variable, errors in testing the model are more likely when a cause that is related to other causes is not included. The implications of failure to include a related variable are that the other variables may assume unwarranted importance in the system of prediction. A third consideration is that the causal agent consistently exerts a substantive effect, that is, there must be a consistent pairing of the two variables at a magnitude that has theoretical significance. In models that are not designed to be elaborate, only the most powerful causal agents are selected from the total set of causal agents. This would maximize the predictive power of the most parsimonious model. Inclusion of all relevant causes in a model is a critical factor in causal modeling because, by including all relevant causes, the theorist is addressing one of the major criteria for making causal statements: that all other possible effects have been accounted for or controlled. In an experimental design, this criterion is met by such techniques as random assignment and sample selection. In causal modeling, the researcher can only satisfy the criterion by dependence on previously developed theory that indicates the relevant causes of each major outcome variable important to the model.

The reader may question such dependence on previous theory. After all, if all theoretical specification has been completed, why bother doing it again? However, unless the model is a replication of previous work, all of the work has not been done. The basis of each causal link may have originated from a series of small studies that defined the causes of one or more of the variables included in the model. The model-building process, in this case, starts with the synthesis of the literature into a unified whole.

Complexity of the theory. In addition to elaborateness, models may also be examined in relation to their complexity. While elaborateness deals primarily with the number of causal connections, complexity addresses both the level of abstraction of the individual variables in the model and the subsequent causal connections. A very complex model would be one in which causal linkages are made between abstract variables without the inclusion of intervening causes and effects. In this type of model, the causal linkages may be supported by discussing the actions of intervening variables, but these variables are not formally explicated in the model. Of course, these mediating variables may be included as part of the formal model. In this case, the inclusion of mediating variables makes the theory more elaborate but less complex.

As Cook and Campbell (1979) discuss, the value of any given model is not a function of the degree of complexity. Both complex and noncomplex models can be supported through literature and previous empirical work. It is this support that adds value to a model, rather than the complex nature of the variables and their causal connections. However, it should be noted that, with highly complex models, linkages are more vulnerable to misspecification.

Because the relationships, by definition, are contingent upon many unspecified intervening variables, they are more prone to error. Therefore, it is of benefit to examine a theory for its level of complexity and the fallibility of the causal linkages.

Boundaries. In the context of causal modeling, *boundaries* refers to the parameters or subgroups for which the model is appropriate. It is imperative that the theoretician clearly specify the range of possibilities over which the model is expected to apply. For example, if a model is proposed such that it is expected to have different causal relationships for men than for women, one of the boundaries for the model is male gender. If a theory is proposed that sets boundaries so that a variable representing a subgroup moderates the effect of the proposed linkages, then the model has been misspecified. Under this circumstance, the results of testing will be biased. In order to solve this problem of inappropriate boundaries, the researcher can specify a different model for each of the subgroups or include more complex terms in the model.

Another aspect of specifying boundaries has to do with setting a time frame within which the theory functions. The specified relationships should be stable across a reasonable period of time. If stability is only within a very short period of time, the generalizability of the model becomes correspondingly limited. The relationships in a stable model remain the same during several time periods.

In a longitudinal study, the same rule for model stability is required for each measurement time. This increases the complexity of the task of model building because the relationships among variables might not be the same at each time period. With a change in time, there may be a corresponding disorganization of the relationships in the model. The efficacy of the model will in part be dependent upon assessing the relationships when organization reoccurs. In other words, part of the theoretical framework in a longitudinal design must include the specific times at which measurement will take place.

Summary. This section has examined the areas that need to be considered when specifying a theory to be used in a causal model. The major issue in developing such a theory is the need to have firm support for the causal relationships that will be tested with nonexperimental data. The researcher who assumes that the causal modeling approach provides an easy way to show cause and effect without the stringent assumptions of the experimental design has seriously overestimated the power of the analytic technique. To reiterate, the causal modeling technique is only as good as the theory that drives the model. Although the analysis for causal modeling is complex and in some respects sophisticated, the procedures are systematic and repetitive. It is the theoretical development of the model that constitutes the science of causal modeling.

Model Representation

Although models can be representations of many sorts, from a simple paper model of an airplane to a refined wind tunnel simulator, all models represent real phenomena. For instance, the paper model of an airplane is a physical model while the wind tunnel simulator could be modeled with mathematical formulas. It is also possible to have verbal models or diagrammatic models. In causal modeling, verbal models, diagrammatic (pictorial) models, and mathematical models are used sequentially to test theory.

The verbal model is a statement or set of statements that describe the concepts and relations that constitute the model. In the previous section of this chapter, the need for a strong theoretical base for a causal modeling approach was delineated. The resultant theory is formalized into a set of verbal definitions and propositions about causal relationships. The purpose of this section is to delineate the conventions for displaying a causal model in a pictorial format. Additionally, other pertinent issues of model representation, such as causal ordering and direction, will be examined. The conventions are important because they provide the standards by which the content of the models can be easily communicated to others.

Pictorial Formulation and Conventions

Although there are many ways to pictorially represent a causal model, we will summarize the conventions associated with the path analytic technique. At this point, it is not necessary to understand path analysis to learn the conventions used in depicting path diagrams.

Staging of variables. Figure 3.1 illustrates a very simple four-variable causal model. In this type of convention, the placement of the variables on the page indicates temporal ordering. The variables to the left of the page are thought to occur before those to the right. Simultaneously occurring variables are placed in the same vertical block. These blocks are often called "stages" in the model. In Figure 3.1, x_1 and x_2 are in stage 1 and are posited to occur at the same time.

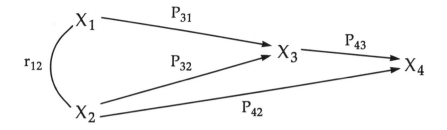

Figure 3.1. A Four-Variable Causal Model

Relationship coefficients. Each of the relationships indicated in a pictorial model is identified by a specific coefficient that indicates the type of relationship and the variables involved. Two types of relationship are usual: simple bivariate correlations and causal effects. The bivariate correlation is indicated by the usual notation of r. The subscripts indicate the variables involved in the relationship, usually with the lowest numbered variable listed first. Causal relationships are indicated by *path coefficients* (p), which indicate the direct effect of the antecedent variable on the outcome variable. The subscripts, again, indicate the variables involved in the relationship. With path coefficients, however, the first subscript indicates the outcome or effect, while the second represents the antecedent or cause.

Relationships among variables. The lines connecting any two variables indicate relationships between the variables. A curved line with no arrowhead or with bidirectional arrows indicates a bivariate correlation. In this case, the variables covary but no temporal ordering is posited. Line r_{12} is an illustration of this type of bivariate, but noncausal, relationship in stage 1 of the model depicted in Figure 3.1. Usually, in a causal model, bivariate correlations are only examined within the same time stage rather than across stages.

Straight unidirectional arrows are used to depict a directional causal relationship between variables. The arrow leads from the antecedent variable to the outcome variable. Line p_{31}, in Figure 3.1, indicates such a causal link. In this case, X_1 is posited as a direct cause of X_3.

It is possible to have variables linked by two arrows as is shown in Figure 3.2. These arrows may be straight or curved with single arrowheads. In either case, the arrows indicate that there is reciprocal

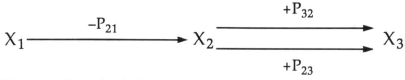

Figure 3.2. Example of a Nonrecursive Causal Model

causation between the two variables. We will further discuss reciprocal, or nonrecursive, models in the section on causal direction.

Only those variables that are connected with arrows are proposed as a cause-and-effect relationship. Absent linkages between variables indicate no association, or no cause-and-effect relationship. At a later point in this chapter, testing of both hypothesized and non-hypothesized linkages will be discussed.

In causal models, the relational statements between variables have an additional notation that describes the type of effect exerted by the antecedent variables. Figure 3.2 shows a model with type of effect noted. The theory on which the model was based was sufficiently explicit to posit not only the causal direction but whether the type of effect of each variable was positive (direct) or negative (inverse).

One other aspect of model links needs to be addressed at this point. This involves direct, as opposed to indirect, causal effects. An indirect causal relationship is one in which the effect of a given antecedent variable on an outcome variable is experienced through an intervening variable. In Figure 3.1, there are two indirect causal relationships indicated, the relationship of X_1 on X_4 through X_3 and the relationship of X_2 on X_4 again through X_3. Note that X_2 also has a direct causal effect on X_4 as indicated by the arrow p_{42}. There is no specific convention for indicating indirect causal links. They are inferred through an analysis of the depicted direct causal relationships.

In some theories, *mediating variables* play an important role and, therefore, need to be designated specifically in pictorial diagrams of causation. A classic example of such theories is the relationship of social support on the effect of stress on outcome variables. In this case, social support mediates the effect of stress but does not necessarily have a direct influence on either stress or the outcome. Such a relationship may be indicated by a dotted unidirectional arrow leading to the direct link between stress and the outcome. Figure 3.3 shows such a relationship.

Naming of variables. The variables in a pictorial representation of a causal model are also named by a series of conventions. Endogenous

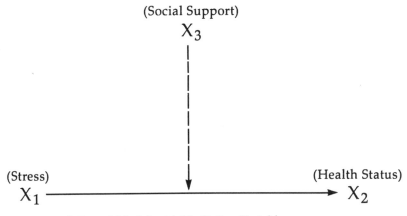

Figure 3.3. A Causal Model with Mediating Variable

variables are those that are explained by other variables in the model. In Figure 3.1, there are two endogenous variables, X_3 and X_4. Exogenous variables are those that act as a cause but have no causal antecedents in the model. In other words, the occurrence of exogenous variables is not explained by the theory. In Figure 3.1, there are also two exogenous variables, X_1 and X_2.

In presenting the previous material on relationships and variables, we have been primarily referring to manifest variables. A *manifest variable* is a measured or observed variable. A *latent variable* is an abstract construct that is not directly observed or measured. Usually, a latent variable is indexed by several manifest variables. Figure 3.4 illustrates the simplest way of depicting a latent variable. In Figure 3.4, the circle indicates the latent variable and the squares indicate manifest variables that are measures or effects of the latent variable. For the time being, do not be concerned about the temporal ordering and direction of the arrows in Figure 3.4. These are conventions of a latent variable model that will be described more fully at a later point.

Causal order. It was mentioned that the location of a variable within the diagrammatic representation indicates its temporal ordering. Those variables that are located more to the left are theorized to occur prior to those on the right.

The temporal ordering of variables in a causal model is theory based and must be justified in the verbal model accompanying the diagram. The time intervals between the occurrence of variables are not necessarily specified. For some theories, the span of time be-

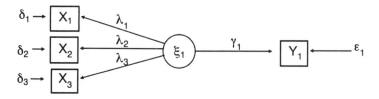

Figure 3.4. Diagram of a Latent Variable

tween cause and effect is very narrow and the occurrence appears to be simultaneous. In positing the theory for a causal model, it is usually not necessary to propose the exact time interval between stages of the model. It is sufficient, with most models, to explain the basic ordering of variables in the model. With the measurement of these variables, however, the investigator may need to support the length of temporal intervals in order to plan the appropriate times for data collection.

One special aspect of temporal ordering of variables is concerned with the testing of alternative models that propose different sequencing of the same variables. It is not possible to discern different causal order based solely on analysis; but it is possible to test different models when the theoretical base offers conflicting temporal sequencing. This is only possible, however, when the models have been specified a priori and the data are used to determine the model of best fit (Billings & Wroten, 1978; Griffin, 1977).

Causal direction. Causal models may be asymmetrical or symmetrical in terms of the direction of causal flow. An asymmetrical model is one in which the causal flow moves solely in one direction. Usually the direction is indicated in a diagrammatic model from left to right. The arrows are all unidirectional and point in the same direction. This type of model is called a "recursive model." Recursive models are somewhat easier to analyze and, therefore, have been more popular in the literature. The drawbacks to the model have caused some problems in posing theoretical solutions to the study of phenomena. For many phenomena, variable X not only has an effect on variable Y but variable Y has an effect on variable X. Effects, therefore, in the symmetrical (nonrecursive) model do not flow only in one direction. The reciprocal nature of the effect is not only intuitively appealing but is sound in terms of the theoretical structure of some phenomena. Nonrecursive models require special analytic techniques, which are discussed later in the chapter. Figure 3.1 was an illustration of a recursive model, while Figure 3.2 was an illustration of a nonrecursive model. Models may have elements of both recursive and nonrecursive relationships. If any part of the model is nonrecursive, however, the model is generally termed "nonrecursive."

Summary. In this section, we have discussed the requirements for depicting a causal model diagrammatically. When the pictorial representation is sufficiently clear, the researcher is able to move from this type of model to the mathematical model. The next section will discuss the translation of the pictorial model into the mathematical equations that form the basis of the statistical analysis.

Mathematical Formulation

The model shown pictorially in Figure 3.1 may be termed a "linear structural model." *Linear structural models,* or, simply, structural models, are usually a series of equations, containing manifest variables, which specify a set of cause-and-effect relations. *Covariance structure models,* or latent variable models, are linear structural models, the equations of which contain one or more latent variables. Latent variable models have been proposed as solutions to problems encountered with structural modeling when there is significant measurement error with operational indices or when there are dependencies among measures. Thus covariance structure modeling is a more complex form of structural modeling in which a measurement model and a causal model are both analyzed.

A *structural equation* is a mathematical formulation of a cause-and-effect relationship assuming that the causal agents are unique determinants of the effect (dependent variable). Thus, in a true structural equation, there is no error term (Turner & Stevens, 1971). However, errors in measurement and errors in response do occur and equations for the model are usually formulated to describe these effects on the dependent variable. For the purposes of this chapter, we will refer to those equations that contain an error term and describe a cause-and-effect relationship as "functional equations." The functional equation takes the form of a regression equation, as follows:

$$Y = a + b_1 X_1 + \ldots + b_n X_n + e_l$$

where Y indicates the effect of several causal variables, denoted by X_1 to X_n. Each of the causal variables is weighted (denoted by b_1 to

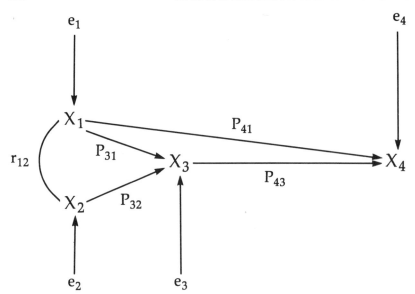

Figure 3.5. Four-Variable Causal Model with Full Path Notation

b_n) according to its relative impact on Y. In the functional equation, e represents the portion of the variance in Y that is unexplained by the antecedent variables. The α is a constant term that equalizes variable values on each side of the equation.

The causal relationships in a causal model may be written in mathematical terms by using the functional equations described above. In this chapter, we will describe in detail the use of path analysis as the method for analyzing causal models. Although there are other methods of analysis, the researcher who understands one method can extend that knowledge to include other analytic techniques. It is logical, therefore, to begin writing equations using the notation appropriate for path analysis. Figure 3.5 shows a four-variable model with full path notation consistent with previous definitions in the chapter.

Once the notation has been included, the next step is to construct the set of functional equations that describe the model. Some authors (see, for example, Stember, 1986) construct a set of what are known as "simultaneous equations." When simultaneous equations are used, there is an equation for each variable in the model. Equations are ordered from exogenous variables to final outcome variables. A set of functional equations, as we are using it in this chapter, only contains equations for each endogenous variable in the model.

The rules (based on Turner, 1971) that apply when writing equations are these:

(1) When writing functional equations, there will be exactly p functional equations for p endogenous variables.

(2) When writing simultaneous equations, there will be exactly p functional equations for the p endogenous and exogenous variables included in the model.

(3) Each functional equation is unique.

(4) The variable at the head of the arrow, the outcome variable, is a function of the variable(s) and/or error term at the tail(s) of the same arrow(s).

(5) A variable not connected to the outcome variable may have an indirect effect but is not included in the functional equation.

(6) Equations are considered to be in standard score form, therefore, a constant is not included.

Using these rules, we know that exactly two functional equations will be needed for the model in Figure 3.5. The form of the equations is as follows:

$$X_3 = p_{31}X_1 + p_{32}X_2 + e_3$$

$$X_4 = p_{43}X_3 + p_{41}X_1 + e_4$$

When simultaneous equations are stated, we know that there are exactly four equations written as follows:

$$X_1 = e_1$$

$$X_2 = e_2$$

$$X_3 = p_{31}X_1 + p_{32}X_2 + e_3$$

$$X_4 = p_{43}X_3 + p_{41}X_1 + e_4$$

Summary. The final type of model that can be obtained when using a causal modeling approach is a mathematical model. Equations are developed based upon the hypothesized causal relationships in the pictorial diagram. This section has developed these mathematical formulations using the notation of path analysis. Using the information from this section, analytical methods to test the model will be examined.

Model Testing

Operationalization

The choice of measures for the variables included in the model is an important aspect of providing an adequate test of theory. Measurement error in the independent variables can lead to severe bias in parameter estimation (Cohen & Cohen, 1983). In a manifest variable causal model, it is important that this bias be minimized through the use of well-developed and tested instruments to index each concept. In other words, instrument reliability should be sufficiently high to preclude problems with attenuation in bivariate correlational relationships. (For a discussion of attenuation, see Murdaugh, 1981.) Although there is no firm definition of "sufficiently high reliability," James, Mulaik, and Brett (1982) note that a reliability of .70 is not sufficient to minimize parameter and estimation bias. Nunnally (1978) indicates that developed instruments should have reliabilities of .80 or above. Therefore, in operationalizing manifest variables in a causal model, instrument reliabilities should be high and certainly no less than .80.

The developers of analytic techniques for latent variable models claim that the method is capable of accounting for measurement error. Therefore, the requirement for high reliabilities is less stringent in latent variable models. Nevertheless, the prudent researcher selects the best instruments available to index concepts. No analysis method can be expected to solve all problems with measurement error.

A second aspect to be considered when operationalizing variables for a causal model is instrument validity. As Bohrnstedt and Carter (1971) note, there will be significant bias in parameter estimation if instrument validity is questionable. There is little chance that the model test will be adequate when validity of the indices is suspect; therefore, attention to the quality of instruments is crucial.

Issues in Data Collection

Data for causal modeling is collected with descriptive, or nonexperimental, designs. The same threats to the legitimacy of the data hold in the causal model as in survey research or any other descriptive type of research. These designs require as rigorous data collection protocols as any experimental study; therefore, it is imperative that the investigator develop a sound research design when collecting data to be tested in a causal model.

Of major concern in causal modeling designs is the size of the sample used to test the theoretical model. Technically, the sample size needed to invert a matrix and perform the necessary calculations for parameter estimation is $k + 1$, where k equals the number of parameters being estimated. Although a solution may be obtained, the stability of the estimated parameters is seriously in doubt. In other words, to reduce such instability and the artificial inflation of the explained variance due to small sample size, larger samples are required. Some researchers use a simple rule of thumb, 10 subjects per variable plus 50 subjects, to estimate the sample required for the analytic procedures (Thorndike, 1978). Power analysis can also be used to determine sample size in a causal model (Cohen, 1988). When using the power of the statistical test to determine sample size, each individual equation is considered as a separate test. Because one of the factors used to determine power in multiple regression is the number of variables in the equation, calculations for sample size could vary depending on the complexity of the equation used. For a conservative estimate of sample size, the equation with the greatest number of variables is used. For example, in Figure 3.6, the equation describing X_4 has three independent variables. The equation describing X_3, however, has only two independent variables. For the most conservative estimate of sample size necessary to test the various equations in this model, the equation for X_4 should be used.

Testing Fit Between Data and Theoretical Formulations

The purpose of this section is to present a path analytic method to test causal models. The assumptions that underlie the procedure of path analysis are these:

(1) The relations indicated in the model are linear, additive, and causal.
(2) Each set of residuals is not correlated with the variables that precede it in the model nor are the sets correlated among themselves.
(3) The model being tested is recursive.
(4) The variables in the model are measured without error.

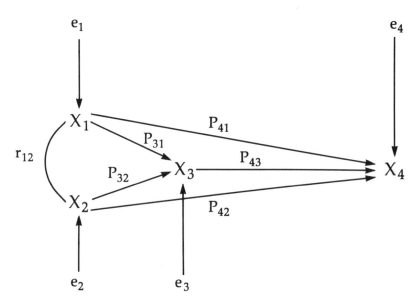

Figure 3.6. A Just-Identified Causal Model

Given these assumptions, the method of path analysis reduces to the solution of one or more multiple linear regression analyses. Therefore, the statistical analysis method proposed in this section involves multiple regression in a basic two-step process to examine a causal model. The first step in this testing involves the examination of the model links theorized to exist. The second step uses statistical analysis to test for those links that are theorized to be nonexistent.

Step 1: Links theorized to exist. In Figure 3.5, there are four causal paths that have been theorized to exist, or, in other words, to be statistically different from zero. There are two regression equations that must be calculated to test the four links. The first equation is that with X_3 as the dependent variable and X_1 and X_2 as independent variables. The second equation contains X_4 as the dependent variable and X_3 and X_1 as independent variables. The standardized regression coefficients that are included in the computer output from the regression analyses are equivalent to the individual path coefficients for the effect of the independent variables on the dependent variable. The significance test that relates to each regression weight indicates whether the path coefficient is significantly different from zero. A coefficient with a significance greater than the prespecified level may be considered to be zero and the model link nonexistent.

Tests of significance are primarily used to examine the existence of a path. However, a further criterion is necessary, especially with large samples. It is possible with large samples for path coefficients of trivial magnitude to be statistically significant. Most authors (James, Mulaik, & Brett, 1982; Pedhazur, 1982) indicate that coefficients less than or equal to .05 should be considered substantively nonsignificant.

As noted above, standardized regression coefficients are used as path coefficients in a causal model. In one particular case, it is more appropriate to use the unstandardized coefficients. This situation occurs when the researcher wishes to compare models with the same variables across populations. In this case, the coefficient should not be manipulated by a sample-specific statistic such as the standard deviation of the coefficient. When the purpose of the research involves comparing variables within a model, the standardized (path) coefficients are more appropriate.

In summary, step 1 in the testing process can be easily accomplished through standard regression procedures, provided the assumptions of path analysis have been met. The process involves solving the regression equations derived from the functional equations and making decisions regarding the links specified based upon the significance of the standardized regression coefficients.

Step 2: Links theorized to be nonexistent. In Figure 3.5, there is only one link, that between X_2 and X_4, that is theorized to be equal to zero. The second step in testing a causal model is to examine whether this theoretical assumption is supported by the data. A regression equation is computed with X_4 as the dependent variable and all other preceding variables as predictors. If the data supports the model, the initial paths, hypothesized to be significant, would enter the equation while the path specified to be zero would, in fact, be zero.

Figure 3.5 has only one path specified as being zero; therefore, only one regression is required to complete the second stage of testing. In more complex causal models, the number of equations necessary in the second step of testing may be equivalent to the number of endogenous variables if there are several paths hypothesized as zero. The absence of more than one link may be tested with each equation.

Assessing fit of data with theory. After statistical analysis is completed, an examination of the model within the context of the theory should be performed. Many researchers find it helpful to visually examine the path model to assess its fit with theory. Each link or lack of a path should be evaluated within the context of the theoretical framework used to generate the model. The value of a particular model or even of a particular path cannot be evaluated solely within the context of the statistical analysis. This type of examination is particularly crucial when the data failed to support links as hypothesized. It is at this point when the researcher must decide whether theory was faulty or whether the fault was with some other problem such as study design errors or measurement errors.

If the researcher decides that the theory needs reformulation, the process of "theory trimming" may be performed at this time. *Theory trimming* refers to the deletion of statistically or substantively nonsignificant paths and is usually used after both steps in the analysis have been completed. Theory trimming involves balancing the criteria for significance against the importance of the path to theory. Decisions to trim the theory are involved with exploratory rather than confirmatory analysis. James, Mulaik, and Brett (1982) note that it is at this point that the researcher is making decisions based upon data and is no longer confirming a model. The researcher is now proposing a new model to be tested with another sample. Of course, the theoretical model and the trimmed model must be evaluated. When evaluating the results of model testing, the researcher must be cognizant of the balance between model parsimony and power. The desirable goal is the most powerful yet least complex solution among all possible solutions.

Summary. Usually, two steps are needed to test a causal model. The first examines the links hypothesized to be significant while the second tests the paths specified to be nonexistent. After these two tests are completed, the results are evaluated. Theory trimming may be used, as necessary, to reformulate theory at this point.

Issues in Model Testing

The next chapter section describes some additional issues in model testing. The first issue to be discussed in this section is model identification because it is crucial to assessing the validity of a tested model or its fit with the data. The section on model identification is followed by tests of and threats to model validity.

Model Identification

Identification, in one sense, has to do with the number of correlations between measured variables. The minimal requirement for identification of model parameters (e.g., path coefficients) is that the number of known correlations between variables must be equal to or greater than the number of parameters to be estimated. It is possible for a causal model to be just identified, overidentified, or underidentified. A *just-identified model* is one in which the number of knowns equals the number of unknowns. An *overidentified model* is one in which the number of knowns is greater than the number of unknowns, while an *underidentified model* has more unknowns than knowns. The overidentified model can be solved for a set of unique parameter estimates. While it is possible to find solutions to the just-identified model, the solutions are not unique (Kenny, 1979). It is not possible, however, to find solutions to the underidentified model.

In a just-identified model, the number of path coefficients to be estimated equals the number of known bivariate correlations between the model variables. The four-variable model in Figure 3.6 is just identified in that there are five paths to be estimated and five correlations that are known between the variables. The astute reader will note that there are actually six correlations known if the non-causal link between variables X_1 and X_2 is considered. However, in determining the identification of causal models, these correlations between exogenous variables are taken as "givens" (Pedhazur, 1982). A manifest variable recursive model is just identified when all the variables are interconnected either by curved noncausal lines or by straight path lines and when all the assumptions about the residuals are viable. This type of model is also called "fully identified."

A way of creating an overidentified model from a just-identified model is to place certain constraints on the model. The most common constraint is that of postulating that some causal paths are equal to zero. Figure 3.7 illustrates the model with the constraint placed such that there is no direct link between X_2 and X_4. Given this constraint, this particular model is overidentified and, therefore, can be solved for unique estimates of the path coefficients.

Figure 3.8 illustrates a model that has the same configuration as the previous two figures; but, in this case, the reciprocal paths yield a model that has a greater number of unknowns than knowns. Unique solutions for the path coefficients cannot be found using the current analysis technique.

The importance of model identification has to do not only with establishing unique estimates of parameters but with testing model validity. The next section briefly reviews two techniques of assessing the fit of the model to the data.

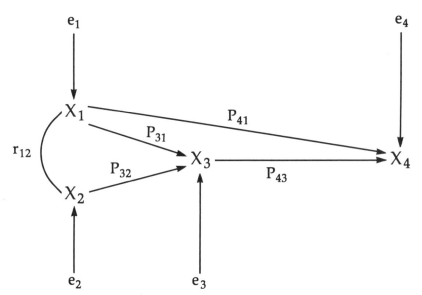

Figure 3.7. An Overidentified Causal Model

Methods to Assess Model Validity

Two strategies for assessing the fit of the model to the data will be addressed in this section. Neither of the procedures to be discussed will tell the researcher whether the model accurately represents theory. The tests, however, provide information about the efficacy of one model as compared with another model. In most cases, the two models under comparison are the fully justified and the theoretically proposed overidentified model. For purposes of this discussion, these will be referred to as the "full" and "reduced" models, respectively.

Reproduction of correlations. The first technique to assess causal model validity is decomposition of correlations. Being able to analyze the components of the correlations among the model variables places the researcher in a much better position to interpret individual relations as well as to describe patterns of variable effects. In fully identified models, the researcher can decompose the path coefficients into unambiguous components.

The correlation between two variables can be broken down into the following components:

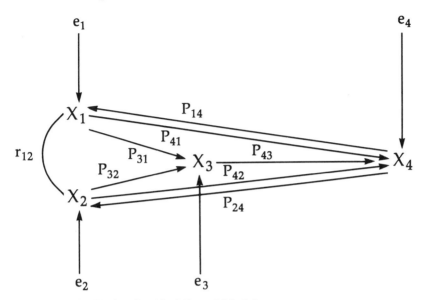

Figure 3.8. An Underidentified Causal Model

(1) *Total effect*: The sum of the direct effect and the indirect effects of a given variable on an outcome variable.

(2) *Direct effect*: The effect of one variable on another without the mitigating effect of intervening variables.

(3) *Indirect effect*: The effect of one variable on another as perceived through an intervening variable.

(4) *Spurious effect*: An artifact between two variables due to the fact that they share a common cause.

(5) *Unanalyzed effect*: The effect of one variable on another that is due to the correlation between two exogenous variables.

Reproduction of coefficients through the use of direct and indirect paths can be used as a test of the validity of a reduced model in comparison with a full model. As mentioned, in the full model, or just-identified model, correlation coefficients may be reproduced no matter how questionable the model may be on theoretical grounds. It is only in overidentified models that the reproduction of the correlations is appropriate for assessment of validity, and this validity is only in relation to a comparison between the fully identified and overidentified models.

There are several excellent reviews of the technique used to reproduce correlations through the tracing of paths (Munro, Visintainer,

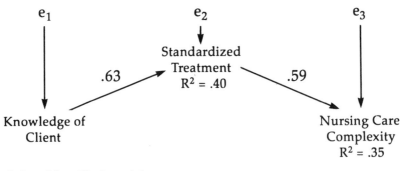

a) Overidentified model.

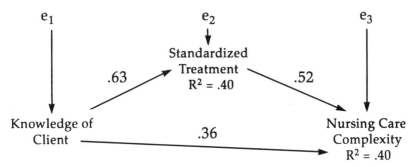

b) Just-identified model.

Figure 3.9. Overidentified and Just-Identified Causal Model

& Page, 1986; Pedhazur, 1982). In brief, correlations are reproduced by adding together the direct, indirect, spurious, and unanalyzable effects of one variable on another. The impact of the direct effect is simply the value of the path coefficient for that link. The other effects are calculated by multiplying the path coefficients for the links making up the indirect path(s), the spurious path(s), or the analyzable path(s).

For the purpose of this section, the technique will be reviewed through an example using Figure 3.9. In Figure 3.9, the results of testing an overidentified model explaining "nursing care complexity" are presented. It was theorized that there was no path between the variables of "knowledge of client" and "nursing care complexity." In part B of the figure, the results due to testing the just-identified model are presented. Table 3.1 gives the results of reproducing the bivariate correlations for both models. If the overidentified model is an accurate representation of the data, the reproduced

TABLE 3.1

Reproduction of Correlation for Causal Models in Figure 3.9

	Knowledge of Client	Standardized Treatment	Nursing Care Complexity
A. Just-Identified Model			
Knowledge of Client	1.00	.63	.69
Standardized Treatment	.63	1.00	.75
Nursing Care Complexity	.69	.75	1.0
B. Over-Identified Model			
Knowledge of Client	1.00	.63	.69
Standardized Treatment	.63	1.00	.75
Nursing Care Complexity	.37	.59	1.00

NOTE: Actual correlations are in the upper triangle of matrix. Reproduced correlations are in the lower triangle.

correlations should approach the magnitude of the actual correlations, or at least those that are calculated from the just-identified model.

In Table 3.1, the upper half of each matrix gives the actual correlations for the bivariate associations between variables. The lower half gives those that have been reproduced for the two models. In part A of the table, the fully identified model is examined. The correlation between "knowledge of client" and "standardized treatment" is simply the value of the path coefficient between the two variables. The correlation between "knowledge of client" and "nursing care complexity" is the sum of the direct path (.36) and the indirect path through "standardized treatment" (.63 × .52).

Note that all three of the correlations have been totally reproduced. The correlation between "standardized treatment" and "nursing care complexity" was calculated by including the spurious effect of the path from "standardized treatment" to "knowledge of client" to "nursing care complexity." In other words, "knowledge of client" is a common cause of both "standardized treatment" and "nursing care complexity," but the causal relationship only flows toward "nursing care complexity" and not in a reverse direction. Spurious relationships are included when reproducing correlations; however, when calculating the total effect of one variable on another, they are ignored. Therefore, the total effect of "standardized treatment" on "nursing care complexity" is .52 rather than .75.

In part B of Table 3.1, the reproduced correlations for the over-identified model are presented. The reproduced correlation between "standardized treatment" and "nursing care complexity" is lower than the actual correlation as is the reproduced correlation between "knowledge of client" and "nursing care complexity." This attenuation indicates that there is a missing path in the model. In other words, the link between "knowledge of client" and "nursing care complexity" should be included in the model. Its absence has resulted in both reproduced correlations being significantly lower than the actual correlation. The logical conclusion is that the theoretically proposed model shown in Figure 3.9, part A, does not fit the data.

Test of overidentified models. The reproduction of correlation coefficients is an effective means of examining the validity of a causal model; however, that technique does not provide a test of the total model in relation to the total just-identified model. A statistical examination of the total model has been proposed that is based on the chi-square distribution (Specht, 1975; Specht & Warren, 1975). This test involves the comparison of a total computed R^2 for the just-identified model. It will be illustrated using the models on nursing care complexity as in the last section.

In Figure 3.9, the R^2 for each of the two model equations are shown. In order to test the full model, a composite R^2 must be computed for both the overidentified and the just-identified models. This is done using the following equation:

$$R^2_c = 1(1 - R^2_1)\ldots(1 - R^2_n)$$

where R^2_c refers to the composite value, R^2_n refers to the R^2 from the nth equation in the model. This composite is formed for both models. The composite for the just-identified model (R^2_{jc}) in Figure 3.9 is

$$R^2_{jc} = 1 - (1 - .40)(1 - .40) = .64$$

The composite for the overidentified model (R^2_{oc}) may be computed similarly

$$R^2_{oc} = 1 - (1 - .40)(1 - .35) = .61$$

The measure of goodness of fit of an overidentified model may be calculated using the following:

$$Q = \frac{(1 - R^2_{jc})}{(1 - R^2_{oc})}$$

When the fit of an overidentified model is perfect, the value of Q would be close to 1.0. The farther away from 1.0, the poorer the fit between the model and the data. For the models in Figure 3.9, the calculated Q value would be .92, indicating a moderate fit of the overidentified model with the data. The statistical significance of Q may be examined by using the chi-square distribution with the following conversion:

$$W = -(N - d)\log_e Q$$

where N equals total sample size, d equals the number of path coefficients theorized to be zero in the overidentified model, and $\log_e Q$ equals the natural log of the goodness-of-fit statistic. W is distributed as χ^2_d. For the Q value calculated from the nursing complexity model, the W could be computed as follows:

$$W = -(629 - 1)(-.08) = 50.24$$

With a W at 50.24 and degrees of freedom equal to 1, the null hypothesis of no difference between the just-identified and the overidentified models would be rejected at $p > .001$. In other words, the overidentified model does not fit the data. The researcher needs either to accept the just-identified model or to develop alternate constraints for the overidentified model.

The W statistic, like many others, is sensitive to sample size. For example, consider the above equation results if the sample size had been equal to 100. In this case, the value of W would have been 7.92. This shows the considerable difference that can result with disparate sample sizes and indicates the caution with which the statistic needs to be interpreted.

This same procedure may be used to test or to compare two varying overidentified models by calculating Q as the ratio of R^2_s between the two models. It is obvious that many different models may fit the same data. The test procedure described above simply provides information on which model is the better fit with data among those selected for comparison.

Threats to Parameter Validity

Parameters that are calculated for a causal model may be inaccurate due to a variety of causes. Two common causes for this problem are multicollinearity and violation of statistical and causal model assumptions. Both of these threats are discussed in the following sections.

Multicollinearity. Multiple regression analysis examines the effect of the independent variable on the outcome variables while taking into account the correlations between a given predictor variable and all other predictor variables, as well as the effect of the other predictor variables on the outcome variable. When all or any subset of the independent variables are correlated, multicollinearity is said to exist. In nonexperimental designs with related independent measures, it is not reasonable to believe that multicollinearity can be totally eliminated. The prudent researcher would do well to seek out the sources of multicollinearity and estimate the magnitude of the resultant problems. Although multicollinearity is problematic, it is not fatal. Kenny (1979) points out that multicollinearity should be considered a necessary trade for being able to make causal inferences with nonexperimental data.

Multicollinearity can result from a number of circumstances. When two independent variables are related, multicollinearity is inevitable, whether the variables are measures of two separate constructs or whether they are both measures of the same concept. In fact, two measures of the same construct are not always better than one measure. If there are high correlations between the multiple measures, the power of one or more hypotheses tests on the beta weights can be markedly reduced. Campbell and Fiske (1959) state that, if the magnitude of the relation between two independent variables is as high as the average of their reliabilities, the measures have no ability to discriminate between different constructs or different domains of the same construct. Care must thus be taken to be sure that highly related variables are not simply multiple measures of the same construct.

Several problems are encountered when multicollinearity exists in an equation. The first problem involves inflated standard errors for path coefficients, which results in unstable estimates of these coefficients. A second problem is that significant variables may not enter the model because shared variance is high. Third, tests of the theoretical importance of each variable are difficult when there are highly related variables in the model. In summary, artifacts in the solution may be introduced by the inclusion of the collinear variables.

Several methods of identifying multicollinearity are proposed and discussed in the following sections of this chapter. One of the most common but ineffective ways of identifying multicollinearity is to examine the simple bivariate correlation matrix. Although Gordon (1968) is frequently cited as a source for defining multicollinearity, he does not actually state a lower bound of correlation coefficient at which multicollinearity is no longer an issue. Most researchers state a point at which a correlation is considered sufficiently high as to present severe problems with parameter estimation. If no significant relationships are found, however, it does not mean that collinearity does not exist. Correlation coefficients only indicate the presence of linear dependencies among two variables. Any linear combination of variables that defines any other variable is also problematic but usually is not located by examining a correlation matrix.

Another way proposed to identify multicollinearity is to examine for reversal of hypothesized signs of path coefficients. However, because sign changes also result from other conditions, such reversals are not sufficient evidence of a multicollinearity problem. Likewise, sign changes may occur when no multicollinearity exists.

An examination of the determinant of the R matrix will also assist in identifying linear dependencies. The closer the determinant is to zero, the greater the problem with linear dependencies. However, the actual source of the linear dependency is not obvious when this method is employed.

A more powerful way to locate the source of multicollinearity is to examine the R^2 of each independent variable regressed on all other independent variables. Pedhazur (1982) provides a simple formula for examining this R^2.

$$R^2_I = 1 - \left[\frac{(1 - R^2)F_I}{(N - k - 1)\beta^2_I} \right]$$

where R^2_I is the R^2 of X_I with all other independent variables; R^2 is the squared multiple correlation of the dependent variable with the independent variables; F_I is the F ratio for testing the significance of the regression coefficient for X_I; b_I is the regression coefficient for

X_1; N is the sample size; and k is the number of independent variables. A high calculated R^2_1 is considered evidence of multicollinearity. A possible strategy to locate the specific sources of dependency, given that R^2_1 is high, is to perform an actual regression analysis. The best predictors of each independent variable can thus be located.

Belsley, Kuh, and Welsh (1980) provide another method to locate key dependencies. Diagnosis of the location of linear dependencies can be made through the use of the Minitab program. In this case, the amount of variance in an independent variable is provided as well as the source of that variance. In the latest edition of SPSS-X, collinearity diagnostics can be performed that provide the same type of information.

Last, locating the source of the dependency does not solve the problem of multicollinearity. A logical option would appear to be the elimination of one of the involved variables from the matrix. However, the variables were selected initially because the model was developed predicated on theory.

Different analysis techniques may also be used to solve the multicollinearity problem. One such technique is ridge regression (Roozeboom, 1979). In recent years, latent variable model analysis has become a popular way to approach the solution of problems of multicollinearity especially when due to multiple indicators.

Violations of assumptions: Residual analysis. As noted earlier, when using multiple regression as the method of analysis in a causal model, assumptions of both the statistical technique and the causal modeling procedure must be met by the data. The assumptions of multiple regression have been well described in a variety of texts. In addition, articles have been published on ways to utilize residuals to examine for possible violations (Verran & Ferketich, 1984, 1987).

In addition to the assumptions of multiple regression, the causal modeling approach has a series of simplifying assumptions. Using the method of residual analysis as described by Ferketich and Verran (1984), it is possible to test some of these assumptions.

Residual analysis is useful in exploring for violations of underlying statistical and causal model assumptions; however, it is an even more powerful tool when exploring the data for further theory development. This approach to model respecification or augmentation utilizes residuals from the theoretical equations in an economical process for determining the value of other variables to the model. Possible errors associated with repeated use of regression analysis for exploration are minimized while data are used to the fullest extent. Examples of this type of model augmentation may be found in Murdaugh and Verran (1987) and Mercer, Ferketich, May, De-Joseph, and Sollid (1988). Because this process is data driven, the resultant augmented model should be tested with another data set. In other words, model augmentation is a form of exploratory rather than confirmatory analysis.

Latent Variable Models

As previously stated, latent variable models have become increasingly important in theory testing and development. Latent variable models have been proposed as the solution to a variety of perplexing problems in behavioral science research. Among these are situations when measurement error exists in a model; when there are multiple measures for a variable; when residuals among equations are correlated, such as in longitudinal designs; and when a nonrecursive model is required by theory. Latent variable analysis, also termed *covariance structure modeling*, is composed of two major components. These components are the measurement model and the structural equation model.

Measurement Model

The measurement model examines the relationships between unmeasured latent variables and measured manifest variables. A simplistic way of viewing the measurement model is to think of it as a form of confirmatory factor analysis (James, Mulaik, & Brett, 1982; Loehlin, 1987). The latent variable in a model is considered an unmeasured common factor while the manifest variables are the measured indicators of the factor. In the measurement portion of a latent variable model, the latent variable is considered the cause of the manifest variables that are indicators of the unmeasured construct. Multiple indicators are used in this aspect of latent variable analysis if the latent variable can be indexed in a variety of ways and/or if the various indices are measured with error. In latent variable models, when only one manifest variable is included for a latent variable, it is considered a perfect indicator of the construct and none of its variance can be attributed to either random or nonrandom error. Bentler (1980) notes that choosing the right number of manifest variables for each latent variable is an art. In theory, the more indices, the better; in practice, the larger number of manifest variables, the more difficult it is to fit the model to the data.

In the measurement model, when manifest variables are considered nonperfect indicators of the latent variable, the fit of the model is tested to determine whether the measured variables are related to latent variables in the manner specified. As noted, this examination resembles a confirmatory factor analysis.

Structural Equation Model

Once the fit of the measurement model is assured, the fit of the causal model can be determined by estimating the paths between and among the latent variables. Because the latent variables are considered to be perfectly reliable (James, Mulaik, & Brett, 1982), the estimated parameters are regarded as unbiased, hence the results of the structural equation model are more meaningful than those that would result from the analysis of a pure manifest variable model.

The structural equation model in latent variable analysis may contain both latent and manifest variables. A manifest variable would be included when it is the only index of a construct. It is important to point out, however, that models that contain multiple operational measures of an abstract concept are not latent variable models unless the measurement portion of the analysis is performed and a composite latent variable is created. Many researchers include multiple indicators of constructs but they treat them as separate manifest variables in testing a causal model. As mentioned earlier, this practice could result in multicollinearity among the independent variables in regression equations.

Analysis Methods

There are a number of analysis approaches to the examination of latent variable models. Among the best known are the LISREL program proposed by Jöreskog (Jöreskog & Sörbom, 1981) and EQS by Bentler (Bentler, 1985). While some general conventions have been developed for pictorially representing a latent variable model, they vary depending on the specific analysis program used. The pictorial representative should be consistent with the analytic procedure selected.

Latent variable analysis provides an excellent approach for the solution of some of the difficulties encountered in manifest variable causal modeling. However, the advantages of the technique are accompanied by some inconvenience. For instance, because the two models in a latent variable analysis result in an underidentified system, a series of constraints are required to obtain results. Constraints involve the selection of specific paths or variable variances that are restricted to specified values. A knowledge of both the theory and the mathematics involved in the program are necessary to make the restrictions and interpret the results accurately. A further difficulty is that the combination of both a measurement model and a structural equation model requires large samples to achieve stable estimates. The required sample sizes can often reach levels such that the efficiency of the study is reduced due to the cost of collecting the data.

There are a number of reasons to choose latent variable analysis for examining a causal model. However, the researcher is advised to invest the time necessary to adequately understand the theory underlying the analysis program. Some authors have suggested the use of a confirmatory factor analysis followed by multiple regression with composite variables calculated from factor scores as latent variables. This procedure allows the examination of latent variable models without the sophisticated knowledge required for programs such as LISREL or EQS. It must be emphasized, however, that sophisticated analysis techniques also provide sophisticated meaningful results.

The use of these programs in nursing research will only increase in the future as they are intuitively applicable to many aspects of nursing science. The researcher who is planning to frequently utilize the technique of causal modeling would be well advised to become familiar, through self-study, with the theory of latent variable analysis as well as the details of the commonly used analysis programs.

This chapter was designed to provide an overview of causal modeling. The reader is urged to explore topics of interest in further detail because this coverage could not be exhaustive. There are many interesting and informative texts on each of the topics covered. Causal modeling is a useful approach for nursing research when experimental designs cannot be used because of the clinical situation under study. It cannot, however, be performed without careful planning and attention to the underlying theory and to the assumptions and hazards of the analytic procedure. The effort can, however, be rewarded with a greater understanding of the subtleties and complexities of the phenomena under study.

Chapter Summary

Causal modeling is used to examine causal sequences with nonexperimental data.

The causal model design meets the conditions for causal inferences through the process of theoretical development rather than by control and manipulation of experimental protocols.

A *causal model* is a set or sets of interrelated hypotheses that attempt to explain the occurrence of phenomena.

Theory to be tested in a causal model must be well supported with previous research for causal analysis using nonexperimental data to be appropriate.

Conventional representation of causal models serves the purpose of easing communication among professionals and disciplines.

A *manifest variable* is a measured or observed variable that is most commonly used in causal models.

A *latent variable* is an unmeasured, unobserved abstract construct commonly indexed by several manifest variables.

A *recursive model* differs from a *nonrecursive model* in that the causal flow is only in one direction.

A *structural equation* is a mathematical formulation of a cause-and-effect relationship, assuming that the causal agents are unique determinants of the effect.

When writing functional equations, there will be exactly p functional equations for p endogenous variables.

In testing a causal model, the two basic steps are, first, to examine whether proposed links are supported and, second, to examine whether proposed absent links are actually zero.

In order for an adequate test of the model to be performed, measurement error in the independent variables must be minimized.

Theory trimming may be performed as part of the exploratory aspect of model respecification.

Model identification is important in testing model validity and in considering whether estimations are unique.

Two methods to test overidentified models are reproduction of correlations and the use of composite R^2 to compare results with the just-identified model.

Multicollinearity and violation of statistical and causal model assumptions are threats to estimate validity.

Latent variable models are useful when there is measurement error, multiple indices of a variable, correlated residuals among equations, or the presence of a nonrecursive model.

References

Asher, H. B. (1983). *Casual modeling*. Beverly Hills, CA: Sage.

Belsley, D. A., Kuh, E., & Welsh, R. E. (1980). *Regression diagnostics: Identifying influential data and sources of collinearity*. New York: John Wiley.

Bentler, P. M. (1980). Multivariate analysis with latent variables: Causal modeling. *Annual Review of Psychology, 31*, 419-456.

Bentler, P. M. (1985). *Theory and implementation of EQS, a structural equations program*. Los Angeles: BMDP Statistical Software.

Billings, R. S., & Wroten, S. P. (1978). Use of path analysis in industrial/organizational psychology: Criticisms and suggestions. *Journal of Applied Psychology, 63*, 677-688.

Bohrnstedt, G. W., & Carter, T. M. (1971). Robustness in regression analysis. In H. L. Costner (Ed.), *Sociological methodology 1971*. San Francisco: Jossey-Bass.

Campbell, D. T., & Fiske, D. W. (1959). Convergent and discriminant validation by the multitrait-multimethod matrix. *Psychological Bulletin, 56*, 81-105.

Cohen, J. (1988). *Statistical power analysis for the behavioral sciences*. Hillsdale, NJ: Lawrence Erlbaum.

Cohen, J., & Cohen, P. (1983). *Applied multiple regression/correlation analysis for the behavioral sciences* (2nd ed.). Hillsdale, NJ: Lawrence Erlbaum.

Cook, T. D., & Campbell, D. T. (1979). *Quasi-experimentation: Design and analysis issues for field settings*. Chicago: Rand McNally.

Ferketich, S. L., Verran, J. A. (1984). Residual analysis for causal model assumptions. *Western Journal of Nursing Research, 8*, 41-60.

Gordon, R. (1968). Issues in multiple regression. *American Journal of Sociology, 73*, 592-616.

Griffin, L. J. (1977). Causal modeling of psychological success in work organizations. *Academy of Management Journal, 20*, 6-33.

James, L. R., Mulaik, S. A., & Brett, J. M. (1982). *Causal analysis: Assumptions, models, and data*. Beverly Hills, CA: Sage.

Jöreskog, K. G., & Sörbom, D. (1981). *LISREL V: Analysis of linear structural relationships by the method of maximum likelihood: User's guide*. Uppsala, Sweden: University of Uppsala.

Kenny, D. A. (1979). *Correlation and causality*. New York: John Wiley.

Loehlin, J. C. (1987). *Latent variable models*. Hillsdale, NJ: Lawrence Erlbaum.

Mercer, R. T., Ferketich, S., May, K., DeJoseph, J., & Sollid, D. (1988). Further exploration of maternal and paternal fetal attachment. *Research in Nursing & Health, 11*, 83-95.

Munro, B. H., Visintainer, M. A., & Page, E. B. (1986). *Statistical methods for health care research*. Philadelphia: J. B. Lippincott.

Murdaugh, C. (1981). Problems in doing research: Measurement error and attenuation. *Western Journal of Nursing Research, 3*, 252-256.

Murdaugh, C. L., & Verran, J. A. (1987). Theoretical modeling to predict physiological indicants of cardiac preventive behaviors. *Nursing Research, 36*, 284-291.

Nunnally, J. C. (1978). *Psychometric theory* (2nd ed.). New York: McGraw-Hill.

Pedhazur, E. J. (1982). *Multiple regression in behavioral research*. New York: Holt, Rinehart & Winston.

Roozeboom, W. W. (1979). Ridge regression: Bonanza or beguilement? *Psychological Bulletin, 86*, 242-249.

Specht, D. A. (1975). On the evaluation of causal models. *Social Science Research, 4*, 113-133.

Specht, D. A., & Warren, R. D. (1975). Comparing causal models. In D. K. Heise (Ed.), *Sociological methodology 1976* (pp. 46-82). San Francisco: Jossey-Bass.

Stember, M. L. (1986). Model building as a strategy for theory development (pp. 103-110). In P. L. Chinn (Ed.), *Research methodology: Issues and implementation*. Rockville, MD: Aspen.

Thorndike, R. (1978). *Correlational procedures for research*. New York: Gardner.

Turner, M. E., & Stevens, C. D. (1971). The regression analysis of causal paths. In H. M. Blalock, Jr. (Ed.), *Causal models in the social sciences* (1st ed., pp. 75-100). Chicago: Aldine.

Verran, J. A., & Ferketich, S. (1984). Residual analysis for statistical assumptions of regression equations. *Western Journal of Nursing Research, 6*, 27-40.

Verran, J. A., & Ferketich, S. L. (1987). Testing linear model assumptions: Residual analysis. *Nursing Research, 36*, 127-130.

4

The Design and Analysis of
Time-Series Studies

IVO L. ABRAHAM AND MARCIA M. NEUNDORFER

*The necessity for studying change over time . . . is mandated by what
we want to know about our interventions.*

Nursing is concerned with change. In nursing practice, we try to
bring about change in the health status of patients and their families.
In nursing education, we strive to promote changes in what students
know and how students know. Nurse-managers attempt to innovate
the delivery of care. Yet, in nursing, we are not always aware that we
are "changers" or "change agents," committed to improving today's
clinical, educational, and administrative practices in the function of
tomorrow. Rather, we tend to think about today, without recognizing
that what we do today affects how things will be tomorrow. Or we
focus too much on what we should be doing tomorrow, ignoring that,
to achieve tomorrow's goals, we have to do something today.

Not all changes in nursing are literally from today to tomorrow,
yet they are from one time point to another. In many cases, we can
speak of a sequence of time points, say from time 1 to time 2 to time
3, all the way to some end point time n. In critical care environments,
the intervals between time points may be as small as a few seconds.
In community health nursing, the time intervals could be several
days or weeks; for instance, the intervals could be defined as the time

NOTE: Preparation of this chapter was supported by grant 1R01NR01566 from the
National Center for Nursing Research, National Institute of Health.

between home visits. In nursing management, budget cycles could serve as time intervals. And, in education, we may choose graduation cycles as time points. What is important, then, is that nursing is *temporal*, and that studying nursing is *studying change over time*.

The relative lack of attention to nursing as a discipline of change is reflected in our research methods and dominant approaches to analyzing the data from our research. Many studies are cross-sectional, capturing a state as it exists at one point in time, isolated from what preceded and followed that state. Other studies, where change over time is studied, identify only two time points: before something was done (e.g., a patient teaching intervention) and after it was done. In only a small minority of studies do we see more detailed observations over time, reflecting an interest in investigating the *course* of change over time.

This chapter focuses on designing and analyzing intervention studies that measure change over time. The emphasis is on studying not only whether or not change occurred (*presence* versus *absence of change*) but also the course of this change (*process of change*). Indeed, our concern in nursing is not only whether some intervention had an effect; we also want to know how this change came about and what this tells us about how the intervention does what it does. This twofold focus on studying change over time will allow us to study the *efficacy* of our interventions (did it have an effect?) as well as the *manifestation* of the change process (what type of effect does the intervention have?).

This twofold conceptual focus on studying change translates itself into research methodology, as follows. The challenge is to design and implement studies with minimal threats to validity that allow us to investigate changes *within* groups and changes *across* groups. Specifically, we want to ascertain whether subjects receiving a particular intervention do better than those not receiving the intervention, receiving an alternative intervention, or receiving the same intervention in modified form. We also want to examine what the intervention *did* to our experimental subjects and how this evolved over time. Similarly, we want to investigate what not receiving the intervention, or receiving alternative or modified interventions, did to our comparison subjects.

This chapter describes a perspective on the measurement of change that encompasses investigation of both the process and the outcome of change through time-series designs. We argue that this will maximize the informativeness of data collected over time and will answer questions about change more appropriately. Although we focus predominantly on clinical research, the principles and techniques presented in this chapter can be readily applied to nursing services research and research in nursing education. First, we discuss the importance of studying change over time in nursing. In a subsequent section, we introduce the definition of *time series* and discuss the objectives of this research paradigm. In that section, we also describe four dimensions along which effects over time can be described as well as two dimensions along which change processes can be compared. This is followed by a technical section in which we review conventional approaches to studying change and offer an alternative statistical model for analyzing change within (time-series analysis) and across (time-profile analysis) groups. The final two sections present procedural descriptions of time-series analysis and time-profile analysis.

The Study of Change in Nursing

As we have already pointed out, the research and analysis strategies for studying change in nursing have not always maximized the informativeness of investigations. Time-series design and analysis (hereafter, we will refer to the integration of time-series design and analysis as *time-series studies*) itself is a relative newcomer to the nursing research literature. Metzger and Schultz (1982) described the potential contributions of time-series studies to nursing research. Clinton (1986) discussed several conceptual and technical issues in designing time-series studies in clinical research. In another paper, she and her associates (Clinton et al., 1986) drew upon their experiences in conducting time-series research and recounted the human factors that influence the implementation of such research. Jirovec (1986) presented the mathematical explication of ARIMA models.

This does not mean that nurse-researchers do not recognize the importance of studying change over time. For instance, a recurrent theme at the *Invitational Conference on Statistics and Quantitative Methods in Nursing* (Abraham, Nadzam, & Fitzpatrick, 1989a) was the need for more longitudinal research. Several scientists emphasized the influence that this epistemology could have on research in medical-surgical nursing (Leidy, 1989; Roberts, 1989), nursing care of children (Krowchuk, 1989; Lobo & Ross-Alaolmolki, 1989), psychiatric nursing (Jones & Jones, 1989), and gerontological nursing (Buckwalter, 1989; Whall, Booth, & Jirovec, 1989). Others called for the integration of time-series methodology into doctoral curricula

(Abraham, Nadzam, & Fitzpatrick, 1989b; Brogan, 1989). Contributions to Volumes 1 through 6 of the *Annual Review of Nursing Research* typically echo this call for more longitudinal research.

The issue is not just that we need *more* studies of change over time; instead, we also need *more informative* methods for studying change. Indeed, a conventional perspective on the measurement of change prevails in nursing research. Pretest-posttest and repeated measures designs dominate, and, consequently, such statistical techniques as the *t*-test for correlated observations (also known as the "paired *t*-test"), analysis of covariance (ANCOVA), repeated measures analysis of variance (RM-ANOVA), and their complements also dominate. It is not that these designs and statistical models are inappropriate; their use is often appropriate in particular studies. Yet, in other studies, they may unduly restrict the information that can be distilled from the research. Further, these conventional approaches are frequently misapplied as designs and/or as statistical methods—which, of course, is scientifically intolerable.

The necessity for studying change over time in as detailed as possible a way is mandated by what we want to know about our interventions. Indeed, when researchers and clinicians attempt to change the health of subjects/patients, their interest goes beyond the mere fact of whether health has changed or has not. They might like to know the answers to such questions as these: Does the change persist after the treatment has been terminated or is there decay over time? When do the clinical changes occur, during or after the intervention? Do changes occur immediately after treatment implementation or is there a time lag? Are the changes gradual or abrupt? Do they follow a linear course? Can a cycle of increases and decreases in status be detected? If there are such fluctuations, are they related to changes in treatment, or are they due to extraneous influences? Are there seasonal factors confounding the process of change? Do control subjects show clinically relevant changes during the study? Is there a clinically and statistically significant change once confounding effects are neutralized? These are questions about the process of change as it occurs within a given group of subjects over time.

The following questions pertain to differences between treatment and control groups in the process of change: How do treatment and control subjects differ in their responses over time? Do they differ only in outcome, with treatments showing change and controls no change, or are the between-group differences a matter of intensity, with treatment subjects showing the same effects as control subjects but at a higher level of intensity?

Studying Events over Time

Time series

Definitions. A time series is involved when we "have multiple observations over time" (Cook & Campbell, 1979). *Time-series designs* refer to a group of designs in which multiple observations are made longitudinally. These observations can be *retrospective,* as in studies in which data recorded in the past are analyzed. The observations can also be *prospective*; in this case, a study is designed with multiple observations scheduled for future time points. There is flexibility as to on whom data can be collected. It can be on the *same* subjects over time or on different but similar *cohorts* of subjects sampled at each time point. A time series can be *interrupted* by a treatment, in which case it is referred to as an *interrupted time series* (Cook & Campbell, 1979; Glass, Wilson, & Gottman, 1975). Alternatively, the time series can be without manipulations and can thus be a *continuous time series.* Treatments, if applied, can be short in duration or spread over a segment of the time series.

Cook and Campbell (1979), building upon Campbell and Stanley (1963) and Glass, Wilson, and Gottman (1975), offered a most thorough argument in favor of time-series research in field settings, and they reviewed specific designs. Two design variants are of particular interest to clinical research in nursing. The first one, the *interrupted time-series design with a nonequivalent no-treatment control group time series,* features a treatment and no-treatment group observed longitudinally. The treatment group receives an intervention at a certain point in time. In Cook and Campbell's (1979) X-O notation, where X denotes a treatment and O an observation, the design can be diagramed as follows:

$$O\ O\ O\ O\ O\ X\ O\ O\ O\ O\ O\ O\ O$$

$$O\ O\ O\ O\ O\quad O\ O\ O\ O\ O\ O$$

This design may be extended to three or more groups in which all but one receive a different treatment.

The second variant, not considered by Cook and Campbell (1979) yet particularly applicable to nursing, involves a treatment administered to some subjects over time with observations made at several times before, during, and after the treatment. A control group, which receives no treatment, is observed at similar time points. This *inter-rupted time-series design with removed treatment and with a no-treatment control group* is diagramed as follows:

$$O \; O \; O \; O \; X \; O \; O \; O \; O \; O \; \overline{X} \; O \; O \; O$$

$$O \; O \; O \; O \quad O \; O \; O \; O \; O \quad O \; O \; O$$

Note how, in the top row, the treatment is introduced after a few baseline observations, carried out during a period of time during which several observations are made, and then removed to be fol-lowed by more observations. In our opinion, this design, and its extension to three or more groups, is one of the most clinically and specifically informative designs for clinical research.

Time-series analysis refers to the statistical models for the analysis of time series. These models analyze aspects of the *process of change within a given group*. For example, in the second design diagramed above, two analyses would be performed: one on the time series of the treatment group and one on the time series of the control group.

Threats to the Validity of Time-Series Designs

Cook and Campbell (1979) distinguished between four types of validity of research designs and described possible threats to each. The challenge to any researcher is to eliminate, or at least minimize, these potential threats to the scientific and technical integrity of a study. We refer to the Cook and Campbell (1979) text for a review of possible threats to the different types of validity. Our discussion here is limited to those threats specific to time-series designs that we consider pertinent and that have been identified by Cook and Camp-bell (1979).

(1) Statistical conclusion validity. The first type of validity is statis-tical conclusion validity. It "refers to inferences about whether it is reasonable to presume covariation given a specified [alpha] level and the obtained variances" (Cook & Campbell, 1979, p. 41). This type of validity is concerned with the adequacy and appropriateness of the statistical analysis performed on the data, in particular, whether they permit inferences about covariation (e.g., does receiving versus not receiving a group therapeutic intervention affect depression and cognition among long-term care residents?). While all possible threats to statistical conclusion validity may apply to time-series

designs, the most pertinent threats are low statistical power and violation of statistical assumptions.

With regard to *low statistical power*, it must be recognized that time-series analysis is based on covariation over time, specifically in the form of autocorrelation and autocovariance (to be discussed later in this chapter). This requires sufficient subjects in first place, but also an alpha level that is not too tolerant. Some may argue that an alpha of .05 is too tolerant, yet, in young sciences like nursing, where so much remains to be explored, such an alpha level might be defensible.

Each statistical test has *assumptions that cannot be violated* to apply the test appropriately. Time-series analysis is no exception to this. The assumptions may not be as stringent as those for other, more conventional tests for analyzing change data, yet they exist, must be met, and cannot be violated.

Perhaps not a threat to statistical conclusion validity per se, *adequate statistical reporting* merits mentioning here as well. Like so many other advanced statistical techniques, time-series analysis implies a series of decisions (if not judgment calls) that must be made by the researcher. Often, there are no quantitative criteria to guide this decision making and the researcher has to rely upon his or her own experience and insight or that of a statistician. However, the decisions must be made and they must be defended. Thus, when reporting a time-series analysis, it is essential to review the entire analysis process, clarify the decisions that needed to be made, detail the decisions that were made, and describe the rationale for each of the decisions.

(2) *Internal validity.* When two variables (e.g., longitudinal treatment and longitudinal outcome variables) are found to covary, we must assess "whether there is any causal relationship between the two and, if there is, to decide whether the detection of causality" (Cook & Campbell, 1979, p. 50) is from the treatment to the outcome. The task in assuring internal validity is to assure that there is no alternative explanation for the covariation. Time-series designs are sensitive to particular threats to internal validity, which may indeed provide such alternative explanations.

Maturation exists when subjects grow and mature over the course of the time series, whether intellectually, experimentally, or otherwise. *Testing* occurs when subjects are administered the same measurement devices over time and become familiar with them. *Instrumentation* occurs when changes in measurement strategies cause changes in responses. This threat can occur when researchers try to avoid testing effects by switching over to alternative measurement strategies. It can also occur when there is a change in conceptualization and operationalization of constructs over time, a threat not uncommon in retrospective time-series designs. Researchers must carefully weigh the likelihood of each of these threats when planning and executing a time-series study.

History is a pervasive problem in longitudinal research. This threat exists when, during the course of the time series, an event takes place that is unrelated to the treatment. While the likelihood of history effects can be mitigated by careful planning and execution of the research, the unpredictable is always possible. Cook and Campbell (1979) advise using no-treatment control groups, assuming that these controls would also experience the same event. If this is impossible or if controls are not affected by historical events, the only recourse left to the researcher is to attempt to statistically eliminate the effects of history using some of the methods described later in this chapter.

Selection is a potent threat to the internal validity of time-series studies. This threat exists when there are substantive differences between experimental and control subjects. This threat should especially be considered when subjects are not randomly assigned to the conditions. It may also be a problem when cohorts of subjects are used longitudinally, and cohorts at some time points end up being different from those at other time points. Finally, selection is a severe threat in the case of subject attrition or mortality over time. Attrition and mortality change the constitutions of subject groups, including those established by randomization. In fact, from the moment even one subject drops out of a time-series study, randomized as well as nonrandomized samples are changed and cease to be what they were at the inception of the study. The solution recommended by Cook and Campbell (1979), which we have found to be helpful in our time-series study with old and frail long-term care residents, is to perform a double statistical analysis of the time series: one with all subjects, including those who dropped out, and one with only those subjects who completed the time series.

(3) Construct validity. This type of validity is threatened when "what one investigator interprets as a causal relationship between theoretical constructs labeled *A* and *B*, another investigator might interpret as a causal relationship between constructs *A* and *Y* or between *X* and *B* or even between *X* and *Y*" (Cook & Campbell, 1979). Of all the threats to construct validity cited by Cook and Campbell (1979), not one stands out as being particularly more

problematic in time-series studies. Indeed, all the threats should be considered equally.

(4) External validity. External validity is concerned with the extent to which a research design permits "(1) generalizing *to* particular target persons, settings, and times, and (2) generalizing *across* types of persons, settings, and times" (Cook & Campbell, 1979, p. 71; our italics). As in the case of construct validity, not one of the threats to external validity identified by the authors stands out as being particularly more problematic than others in time-series studies. They should all be considered while planning and executing time-series studies.

Objectives of Time-Series Design and Analysis

Four characteristics of time-series design and analysis can contribute to a better understanding of change processes (see also Chatfield, 1984):

(1) Description of change processes. Change can be described in two complementary forms, both of which should be used. *Visual description,* in the form of plotting and exploratory data analysis (Chambers, Cleveland, Kleiner, & Tukey, 1983; Tukey, 1977), provides an initial assessment of the effects and variations that characterize the change process under study. It helps researchers in familiarizing themselves with their data. It also offers an avenue for detecting and managing outliers (Kleiner, Martin, & Thomson, 1979). *Statistical description,* the second form, concerns the statistical significance of variations over time in the data. Here, we assess whether what we see in the visual description is statistically significant or nonsignificant. Indeed, what appears significant on a plot, in fact, may be statistically nonsignificant, due to an extraneous influence, or may be an artifact of the scaling of the plot.

(2) Explanation of time-dependent associations among variables. Time-series analysis permits us to analyze associations among variables manifested over time. In other words, it is possible to explain variation over time in one variable as a function of the variable at an earlier time. In clinical research, the use of multiple outcome variables is common. If the study over time of each variable by itself were complemented by the study of interrelationships between the multiple variables over time, findings could be much more informative. Such comprehensive analyses "may lead to a deeper understanding of the mechanism which generated a given time series" (Chatfield, 1984, p. 8).

(3) Anticipation of future changes. Research is not only concerned with assessing change processes as they are manifested in a chosen time period. Instead, we may want to estimate how this change process might continue beyond the time period studied; in other words, we may want to anticipate future changes. *Forecasting* and *prediction* are terms used interchangeably to denote systematic approaches to the estimation of how changes over time may extend beyond the time period investigated.

(4) Monitoring of change processes. In their seminal work on time-series analysis, Box and Jenkins (1968, 1976) demonstrated how time-series approaches can be used for monitoring or controlling change processes. By applying certain statistical methods, it can be evaluated whether a time series deviates from an anticipated time series, or, in our terminology, whether a change process strays from what we expected the change process to look like.

Interpreting Effects over Time

Cook and Campbell (1979) described three dimensions along which effects over time can be observed. We add a fourth dimension, which consists of integrated effects.

Type of Effect

This first dimension along which effects can be interpreted has to do with the basic characteristics and manifestations of the effect. An *intercept or level effect* exists when there is a change in the mean values. Graphically, this type of effect is expressed by a change in the intercept (or level) of the plot: The graph shows a sudden "jump" up or down (Figure 4.1). This indicates that there is a sudden change in the intensity of subjects' responses. Figure 4.1, section 1A, depicts this type of effect.

A *slope,* or *drift, effect* refers to changes in the slope of the plot. There is no "jump" up or down, as in an intercept effect. Instead, slope effects indicate alterations in the rate with which change takes place (Figure 4.1, section 1B).

A *variance effect* refers to situations in which the variance in the data changes over time. Figure 4.1, section 1C, shows a time series in which variances increased during the administration of an intervention. This reflects a widening of the range and variance of subject responses due to the treatment. Conceptually, this means that sub-

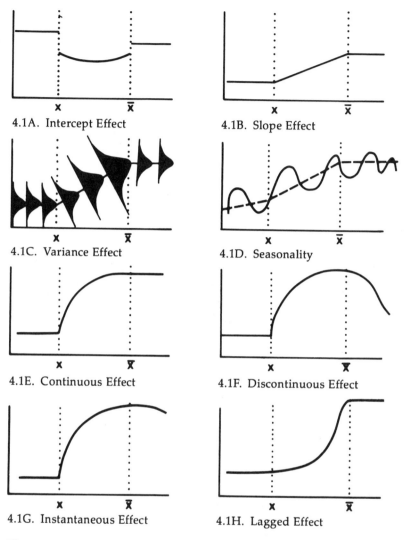

4.1A. Intercept Effect

4.1B. Slope Effect

4.1C. Variance Effect

4.1D. Seasonality

4.1E. Continuous Effect

4.1F. Discontinuous Effect

4.1G. Instantaneous Effect

4.1H. Lagged Effect

Figures 4.1A–4.1H

jects generally benefited from the treatment but not all of them did so equally. In fact, often, variance effects indicate that the treatment yielded heterogeneity among subjects before anything else.

Seasonality is a fourth type of effect. It is characterized by the regular and cyclical recurrence of a change pattern (Figure 4.1, section 1D). The term *seasonality* originated in economic research, where, often, effects related to seasons have been noted. It has since broadened in meaning and now generally refers to cyclical effects, regardless of whether they coincide with particular seasons.

Permanence of Effect

This second dimension of effects involves the assessment of the degree of decay of effects after completion of the treatment. Effects persisting beyond the intervention are termed *continuous* (Figure 4.1, section 1E). Conversely, *discontinuous effects* are those that decay once the treatment has been removed from the time series (Figure 4.1, section 1F).

Type of Impact

This third dimension assesses how effects occur relative to the introduction of treatment. The impact of an intervention may be immediate, in which case it is defined as *instantaneous* (Figure 4.1, section 1G). Often, however, a time lag is noted between the introduction of a treatment and the occurrence of change. This is termed a delayed or *lagged impact* (Figure 4.1, section 1H).

Integrated Effect

The three dimensions along which effects can be studied are interrelated, and different types of effects can occur concurrently. Therefore, we add the fourth dimension of "integrated effects." A slope effect may be lagged and continuous, or instantaneous and discontinuous, or lagged and discontinuous. Similarly, effects of the intercept and variance type can be integrated. Seasonal effects can be continuous and, therefore, recur even in the absence of treatment, or they may be discontinuous, in which case the researcher is faced with the task of determining the relationship between seasonal and treatment-related variation. When linked to the latter, seasonals may also conform to instantaneous or lagged response patterns.

Comparing Change Processes over Time

There are two dimensions to comparing the change processes of subgroups of subjects over time: (a) the comparability of the change process and (b) the differential intensity of these processes.

Comparability of Change Processes

This dimension is concerned with the question: "Are the change processes the same or are they different?" Ideally, when we study the effects of a treatment using a two-group design, we would expect the plots of experimental and control subjects to be different in shape. If, however, the plots are similar in shape, we would infer *comparability* of subject responses (see Figure 4.2, section 2A). This indicates that the change processes of subjects were similar. Figure 4.2, section 2B, shows an instance of *noncomparability* of change processes.

Figure 4.2, section 2C, illustrates the situation in which two different treatments are compared with a third group that receives no treatment. The assessment of comparability here is obviously more complex than in the two-group case. Analysis begins with the overall comparison of the shapes of the three time profiles, assessing the extent to which differences in shapes of the profiles exist. This is followed by pairwise comparisons of profile shapes: Treatment I with control subjects, Treatment II with control subjects, and Treatment I with Treatment II subjects. Extensions can be made for studies with four or more groups.

Differential Intensity of Change Processes

The change processes of groups may differ in levels of intensity. In studies with experimental and control subjects, the differential intensity may simply be that the experimental subjects changed and the controls did not. However, in studies in which different treatments or treatment levels are compared, differential intensity becomes a primary interest. Figure 4.2, section 2D, shows a situation in which a placebo treatment did not have an effect, the experimental treatment was effective, and no-treatment subjects did not change.

Designing Time-Series Studies

In this section, we review some of the conventional approaches to the measurement of change. We also introduce an alternative statistical model for the analysis of time-series designs.

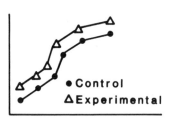

4.2A. Similarity of two
time profile shapes

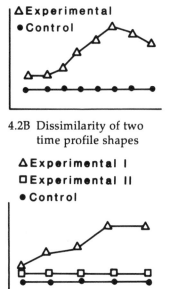

4.2B Dissimilarity of two
time profile shapes

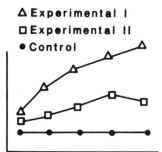

4.2C. Three group design
with two treatments
and one control

4.2D. Three group design with
one treatment, one placebo,
and one control

Figures 4.2A–4.2D

Conventional Approaches to Studying Change

The reviewed conventional designs and their complementary statistical analyses allow researchers to confirm or disconfirm that there has been a change. In other words, these designs permit judgments about the *outcomes* of change. In many cases, this is perhaps all an investigator wants to know. If not, then more sophisticated research designs and statistical analyses are needed. In what follows, we review several of these approaches. We describe the essentials of each briefly, assuming that the reader is familiar with the more general details. We also critique each approach along the following dimensions: (a) aspects of change a technique is designed to measure (i.e., the technique's appropriate application) and those it cannot measure (i.e., inappropriate application); (b) research aims and designs that lead to violations of statistical assumptions; and (c) sensitivity of the approach to threats to internal validity.

Pre-Post Designs with *t*-Test for Correlated Observations

Descriptions. Studies employing the pretest-posttest design typically rely upon the *t*-test for correlated observations (also known as
the paired *t*-test) to assess whether subjects changed significantly on
a dependent variable following a treatment. The unit of measurement used in the statistical analysis is the difference between pretest
and posttest scores.

Critique. The sensitivity of the paired *t*-test to the detection of
change is limited. First, as the unit of measurement is the difference
in scores between pretest and posttest, the paired *t*-test implicitly
assumes that subjects have similar pretest scores. For example, in
studying the effect of an intervention on depression in long-term care
residents, if some subjects' depression scores decreased from 19
(extremely high) to 15 (high) and other subjects' depression scores
decreased from 11 (moderate) to 7 (low), the difference score in both
cases equals 4. That these equal change scores actually represent
clinically different changes goes undetected.

Second, the paired *t*-test is the least sensitive of any of the conventional techniques to the *process* of change. Its applicability is limited
to the dichotomous assessment of outcome, that is, whether or not
change, in fact, occurred. The paired *t*-test presumes that change is
a (quasi-)linear event occurring proportionately and in equal install-
ments from pretest to posttest. Thus it cannot detect graduality in
change or other aspects of the process of change as it occurs from
time 1 to *time 2*.

Third, the paired *t*-test, by being limited to assessing change at two
time points, cannot investigate what occurred between the two time
points. For instance, a given paired *t* value may indicate that subjects
did not differ between pretest and posttest. However, it is very
possible that changes occurred; the change simply may not have
persisted until the time when the posttest observations were made.
Further, control subjects may have demonstrated a Hawthorne effect, which had, however, diminished by time 2. Another possibility
is that subjects may indeed have responded to the treatment but that,
without reinforcement at the appropriate time, the effect had already
diminished at the posttest observation. Finally, other extraneous
influences on the responses may have occurred between *time 1* and
time 2. All these scientifically and clinically significant observations
on the *pattern* of change are lost with the pretest-posttest design
using the paired *t*-test for analysis.

Pre-Post Designs with Analysis of Covariance

Description. Because of the many limitations of the paired *t*-test for analyzing data from pre-post studies, analysis of covariance (AN-COVA) is frequently used as an alternative. The ANCOVA approach applies to designs with two or more groups observed before and after treatment implementation. In ANCOVA, pretest scores are used as a covariate in the estimation of posttest scores. The adjusted posttest scores are used for between-group comparison.

As reviewed by Huitema (1980), eight assumptions govern AN-COVA, and violation of any of them compromises or invalidates the ANCOVA. The assumptions are these:

(1) random selection from a population and random assignment to treatment and control conditions;

(2) homogeneity of within-group regressions;

(3) statistical independence of covariate and treatment variables;

(4) fixed and error-free covariate values;

(5) linearity of within-group regressions;

(6) normality of adjusted dependent variable scores on covariate scores;

(7) homogeneity of variances of the adjusted posttest scores; and

(8) fixed treatment levels.

Critique. Meeting all ANCOVA assumptions is often impossible, particularly in the case of pre-post designs. Random selection (assumption 1), which is most often unfeasible, may be disregarded if generalization to the population is not intended (Huitema, 1980). Random assignment, however, remains a prerequisite.

From a statistical point of view, homogeneity of within-group regressions (assumption 2) and homogeneity of the variances of the adjusted scores (assumption 7) are the most important assumptions. However, they may be unattainable because a pre-post design was used. Consider the case of a two-group pre-post study in which some subjects receive a treatment and others do not. Unless confounding occurred, control subjects should show minimal changes; if change in the control subjects occurs nonetheless, the change should be due to random variation. The adjusted posttest scores for control subjects can then be expected to be densely distributed around their adjusted mean posttest score, resulting in a relatively low variance coefficient. In contrast, because of manipulation, treatment subjects can be expected to vary more on their adjusted posttest scores. Consequently, adjusted posttest scores will be distributed more widely around the mean. This wider distribution of scores will be expressed in a relatively higher variance coefficient. The assumption of homogeneity of variance would thus be violated. Furthermore, because of the greater variability in scores for the treatment group, the slope of the regression line representing the scores of treatment subjects is likely to differ from the control group regression line, leading to violation of the assumption of homogeneity of within-group regressions (assumption 2).

In sum, by its very nature, the pre-post design often yields data that are not fit for consideration under the ANCOVA model. Although several alternative statistical strategies have been developed to adjust the ANCOVA model for heterogeneity of regression slopes (Huitema, 1980; Johnson & Neyman, 1936; Pothoff, 1964; Robson & Atkinson, 1960; Steel & Federer, 1955), they are largely unable to do so due to the bias inherent in the pre-post design.

Assumptions 3, 4, and 8 of the ANCOVA model are more easily met when applying ANCOVA to pre-post data. Violation of assumption 6 is possible, yet it can be verified statistically and can often be corrected through transformations.

Finally, the assumption of a linear relationship between covariate and posttest scores (assumption 5), while easy to meet, poses a conceptual problem. By selecting a pre-post design with ANCOVA, investigators conclude, often prematurely, that the process of change is linear without considering the possibility of nonlinearity. Unless there is uncontestable evidence of a linear change process, alternative approaches that are more explorative and speculative about the pattern of change should be implemented in addition to ANCOVA.

Even if all the assumptions of ANCOVA were met, the analysis still would only have revealed whether or not the treatment had an effect. ANCOVA is quite insensitive to the actual process of change and the detection of extraneous influences occurring between the two time points.

Pre-Post Designs with Analysis of Variance on the Gain Scores

Description. In analysis of variance on the gain scores (ANOVA-GS), the general analysis of variance (ANOVA) model is applied in order to examine differences between groups on the mean change. Change is defined as a gain score. An ANOVA is done on the mean gain scores for each group. In the case of three or more groups, multiple post hoc comparisons may be done. The general assumptions for the ANOVA model apply. Kenny (1975) proposed a Standardized Analysis of Variance on Gain Scores to be used when groups are likely to change at different rates.

Critique. Like the paired *t*-test, the ANOVA-GS implies the absence of variability within the pretest scores, limiting its relevance to situations in which subjects (and groups) have similar pretest scores. Like the paired *t*-test and ANCOVA, this technique merely detects a difference between groups in gains from pretest to posttest and, therefore, reveals little about the process of change. The influence of extraneous variables cannot be assessed. Furthermore, it has long been established that the ANOVA-GS is statistically less accurate than the ANCOVA (Cox, 1957; Feldt, 1958) and, consequently, leads more readily to Type I error.

Repeated Measures Analysis of Variance

Description. RM-ANOVA has been advocated for use in studies with two (i.e., pre-post; Brogan & Kutner, 1980) or more (Winer, 1971) observations over time. Typically, in an RM-ANOVA design, subjects serve as their own controls over time: The observation of the subject at time 1 is the control for the observation of the same subject at time 2, and so forth. Winer (1971; see also Kirk, 1982) warned that the design and its statistical analysis should be limited to studies in which the same subjects are observed under all the k treatments so that $p = k$ observations on each subject are obtained. In other words, this orthodox view posits that *each observation point (p) coincides with a different treatment (k)*. The number of observations (p) then equals the number of treatments (k). RM-ANOVAs are often complemented by a trend analysis of polynomial orthogonals in which the goodness of fit of linear and nonlinear (cubic and quadratic) curves in representing data over time is determined (see, e.g., Edwards, 1985; Kirk, 1982; Neter & Wasserman, 1974; Winer, 1971).

In addition to the assumptions for the general ANOVA model, RM-ANOVA is governed by the requisite of compound symmetry (Edwards, 1985; Hyunh & Feldt, 1970):

(1) the assumption that the experimental errors for each treatment/observation are independent and randomly distributed with equal variances and

(2) the assumption that correlations among observations for the various treatments have equal population correlation coefficients.

Critique. There is a pervasive tendency to ignore the orthodox RM-ANOVA requisite that each observation be paired with a specific treatment. RM-ANOVA is frequently applied to designs with multiple observations but only one or a few manipulations (McCall & Appelbaum, 1973). For example, the investigator makes several pretest observations, conducts a treatment, then makes several posttest observations. Using an (orthodox) RM-ANOVA to (unorthodoxly) analyze such time-series data violates both aspects of compound symmetry. Because not all observations are paired with experimental manipulations, independence of error components in each of the observations cannot be presumed (the first assumption of compound symmetry). Further, correlations among observations at different time points may not be uniform, violating the assumption of equality of population correlation coefficients (the second assumption of compound symmetry).

If only one or a few observations are paired with manipulations, changes in dependent measures will tend to occur more around the time(s) of manipulation and less at other points in time. The inconsistency will result in heterogeneity of variances, which, in turn, will cause correlations among observations to differ across time points.

As a complement to RM-ANOVA, trend analysis allows investigators to describe changes in the dependent variable over time and clarifies the variable's direction and intensity. This technique has more to offer in terms of informativeness and documentation of the process of change than the conventional approaches described so far. A permissible deviation from the orthodox RM-ANOVA occurs when observations do not coincide with treatments but are made *between* treatments. In this type of design, the study begins with an observation, after which manipulations and observations are alternately made. The study ends with a final observation, making the number of treatments k equal to $p-1$ observations. Brogan and Kutner (1980) have defended this approach as a technique for pre-post data.

Statistical Model

In the remainder of this chapter, we present a statistical model that enables researchers to document in detail change over time within and between groups. This model combines time-series analysis with time-profile analysis for studying, respectively, within-group change processes and between-group comparisons of these change processes.

The two statistical techniques are described procedurally, as opposed to mathematically, the latter being impossible within the scope
of one chapter (however, we do make reference to some leading
sources). The emphasis is on understanding each technique for the
purpose of drawing scientific inferences about clinical processes.
Therefore, a conceptual discussion is given here, focused on the
inferential activities involved. We have included flowcharts to illustrate the different steps that must be taken. Rectangles indicate
actions to be taken. Diamonds indicate decisions to be made and
should be read as questions. Rectangles with dotted lines indicate
inferences drawn from the analyses.

The next two sections should be seen as general introductions to
time-series and time-profile analyses. Within the scope of this chapter, it is impossible to go into the mathematical models of the different techniques and approaches. The goal instead is to give the reader
an orientation to the paradigms. We have included several references
to excellent textbooks on time-series and time-profile analyses; and
it might not be unwise to solicit the participation of a statistician.

Time-Series Analysis:
Analyzing Within-Group Differences

Figure 4.3 presents the flowchart for analyzing the time series of a
given group. This chart pertains to time-series analysis using probability models (for excellent reviews and mathematical explications,
though varying in sophistication and complexity, see Anderson,
1971; Box & Jenkins, 1976; Chatfield, 1984; Cox & Lewis, 1966; Gottman, 1981; Kendall, 1976). However, the principles described here
can be readily adapted to the so-called spectral analysis of time series
(see Anderson, 1971; Bloomfield, 1976; Koopmans, 1974).

Plotting and Transformations of Data

The first step is the visual description of the time series. This is
achieved by plotting scores on the dependent variable over time.
Visual inspection of this plot, using procedures for exploratory data
analysis (Chambers, Cleveland, Kleiner, & Tukey, 1983; Tukey, 1977),
gives an initial impression of the nature of the data, such as the
presence/absence of change, seasonality, and type of effects.

Chatfield (1984) stressed plotting as a means for evaluating the
need for data transformation. Transformation is indicated if, longi-

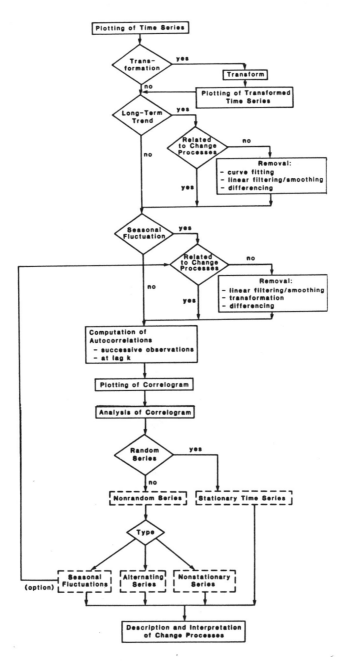

Figure 4.3

tudinally, the variance increases or decreases proportionally to increases and decreases in the mean. Transformation is also indicated if the data diverge from normality yet are assumed to be distributed normally. Transformed data are replotted over time.

Secular Trend

The plot, original or transformed, is then examined for secular trend, that is, long-term change in mean values, possibly due to extraneous factors. For instance, if one wishes to trace childbearing practices over the last half century, it is important to recognize that white, upper-middle-class primiparas today tend to be older than even a decade ago. Consequently, childbearing practices within this group may differ just because these women are often more "life-experienced and/or educated." Note also that a secular trend may be a seasonal cycle in disguise, not apparent to the investigator because the cycle's wavelength exceeds the time series (Granger, 1966).

A secular trend should be assessed for its scientific relevance, that is, its relationship to the change process being studied. If the trend is indeed an important aspect of the phenomenon of concern, it should be analyzed as an integral part of the change process and the time series. In contrast, if it is truly extraneous and confounds the time series, it should be removed.

In intervention research, the distinction between a relevant trend and a confounding one can be difficult to make. In fact, a trend effect is expected due to the manipulation. The complete removal of any trend present in the time series will violate the statistical conclusion validity of the study. A trend related to the intervention should not be removed, only the (secular) trend related to extraneous sources of variance.

There are three major approaches to the removal of a secular trend from a time series. In *curve-fitting*, a function is fitted to the data, and the residuals (i.e., the difference between observed and predicted values) are estimated. The residuals reflect the fluctuations related to the trend. Time-series analytic procedures are performed on the newly established time curve. For trend removal, any type of curve may be fitted, with polynomial (linear, quadratic, cubic), logarithmic, and logistic curves being most common.

In *linear filtering*, a time series with trend is converted into a "smooth" time series devoid of trend-related fluctuation. This is done by means of a linear operation in which each original score is transformed into a weighted score. Weights are chosen on the basis of the extent to which a given score is confounded by the trend. Thus highly affected scores will be given relatively low weights, and less affected scores will receive higher weights. As linear filtering "moves" the values of the means for each time point, it is often called a *moving average operation* (see Kenny & Durbin, 1982, and Kendall, 1976, for reviews and mathematical explications of the different linear filters).

The final trend management technique is *differencing*, an approach particularly favored by Box and Jenkins (1976). In differencing, a given time series is transformed into a new one by subtracting the observations at one time point from those at a subsequent time point. The new time series still represents the original change processes, although no longer in their "raw" format. Differencing is particularly helpful in intervention research for it removes a secular trend without affecting trend effects related to the independent variable of interest. McCain and McCleary (1979) provide an excellent review of differencing techniques that is particularly suited to nonmathematicians.

Seasonality and Other Cyclical Variations

In addition to secular trends, it is imperative to examine seasonal fluctuations and other cyclical variations early on in the time-series analysis. As in the examination of a secular trend, this begins with the evaluation of the relationship of the cycles to the change processes being studied. If seasonality is indeed a characteristic, it should be analyzed as such. However, if it is an undesirable influence that could not be otherwise controlled, its removal is indicated. Linear filtering, or *smoothing*, whether or not in conjunction with logarithmic transformation, is often sufficient for dealing with seasonality. More complex seasonals can be eliminated through differencing. While their effects are different, the management of secular trends is quite similar to that of seasonal trends.

Autocorrelations

The next step consists of computing the sample autocorrelation coefficients. These coefficients describe the correlations between observations at different time points. *Successive autocorrelation* is the association between two temporally adjacent time points (e.g., between times 4 and 5). Coefficients may also be computed for nonadjacent time points, in which case they are referred to as *autocorrela-*

tions at lag k (k = 2, . . . p, where *p* is the number of observations over time). Values may range from –1.00 to +1.00. A positive value reflects change in the same direction and a negative value reflects change in the opposite direction. Autocorrelations reflect the covariation between time points (the *autocovariance*).

Correlogram

Although a time series can be evaluated through its autocorrelation coefficients, visualization is very helpful. In a *correlogram*, autocorrelation coefficients are plotted against their lag. A region around value zero is identified to indicate the critical value to be attained for statistical significance. Figure 4.4 shows a hypothetical correlogram for an intervention study. Note the trend effect over time; the trend, however, progressively decreases in intensity, even to the point of nonsignificance.

Analyzing a correlogram consists of evaluating the extent to which it represents a random series. A series is said to be *random* or *stationary* if, after the management of undesired trend and seasonality, "there is no systematic change in mean (no trend), [and] if there is no systematic change in variance" (Chatfield, 1984, p. 14). A series of this type indicates the absence of change over time. In a correlogram, it shows a succession of autocorrelation coefficients located mainly within the region of statistical nonsignificance. Those located outside this region should be at arbitrary lags for the series to be considered random. Kendall (1976), among others, described various tests of randomness to complement visual inspection, and their use is recommended in the case of seemingly arbitrary coefficients of statistical significance.

If the correlogram and the subsequent tests suggest that the series is nonrandom, the presence of change over time can be inferred. Statistically, three types of nonrandom series are possible: nonstationary, alternating, or seasonal. First, a *nonstationary* time series is one with true trend. The consistent changes in means that characterize this type are ascribed to factors related to the phenomena of concern. Nonstationary series, a variant of which can be seen in Figure 4.4, are very common in intervention research.

The second type, an *alternating* series, is a nonrandom series in which the direction of changes in means over time alternates from being positive to negative, back to positive, and so on, without showing the regularity of seasonality. Also, the alternating pattern is believed to be a true effect and related to the study variables. Some-

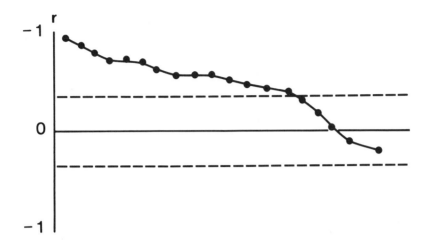

Figure 4.4

what common in intervention studies, alternating time series are often difficult to describe and interpret conceptually.

Finally, a nonrandom series can be *seasonal*. Assuming that any undesirable seasonality was removed at earlier stages, the finding that a nonrandom process is seasonal indicates that the observed effect is truly cyclical in its occurrence. However, this cannot be concluded blindly, and the possibility that seasonality is confounding the data even at this late stage in the analysis should be considered. As shown in the flowchart, there is the option of reevaluating the seasonal fluctuations.

Time-series analysis concludes with the description and interpretation of the observed processes, whether indicative of change or not. This is done through the sequential analysis of the autocorrelation coefficients, preferably in conjunction with the plot of the (transformed) time series and the correlogram. This will allow the investigator to assess the different characteristics of within-group change identified earlier. Statistical modeling techniques are used to describe the time series quantitatively (see, e.g., Box & Jenkins, 1976; Chatfield, 1984; Cox & Lewis, 1966; Kendall, 1976; McCain & McCleary, 1979).

Earlier, we criticized conventional approaches to the description of change for their insensitivity to the detection of extraneous sources of variance. In particular, it was argued that these methods offer little assistance in the consideration of Hawthorne effects and other threats to the internal validity of a study. It should be apparent that time-series design and analysis provide the investigator with sufficient detail to assess the presence of change among subjects who are not expected to change in the first place. Further, even if confounding influences are present, time-series analysis contains provisions to *identify* and to *treat* them. The effects of secular and seasonal trends, whatever their origin, can be neutralized with relative ease. Because, most often, nursing research is conducted under suboptimal conditions, extraneous sources of variance cannot always be controlled. Time-series analysis offers post hoc strategies for dealing with undesired effects that were either uncontrollable or could not be anticipated a priori.

Time-Profile Analysis:
Comparing Change Processes Across Groups

Figure 4.5 depicts the flowchart for performing between-group comparisons using time-profile analysis. A conceptual presentation is given here; for mathematical explication, see Harris (1985).

Observations over time on a given subject can be represented as a time profile. Similarly, observations over time for a group of subjects can be represented as a time profile of mean values. Time-profile analysis consists of three *hierarchical* procedures in which the time profiles of means of different subsamples are compared for similarities and differences in shape and level. It permits a detailed comparison of change processes along dimensions identified earlier as important to clinical research and practice.

In keeping with our preference for graphic methods for data analysis, time-profile analysis begins with the plotting of the time profiles of the different groups being compared. This consists of plotting the *adjusted* time series of each group; that is, the time series from which secular trends and seasonal fluctuations unrelated to the phenomena under study have been removed.

In profile analysis, three null hypotheses are tested in hierarchical dependency to each other. Progression to the next hypothesis is possible only if the previous one was retained. Tested are the hypotheses of parallelism, coincidence, and flatness.

The null hypothesis of *parallelism* assesses whether the time profiles have similar shapes. *Similarity* is defined as being within boundaries of statistical nonsignificance. This test concerns the overall similarity of change processes across groups. Geometrically, similar-

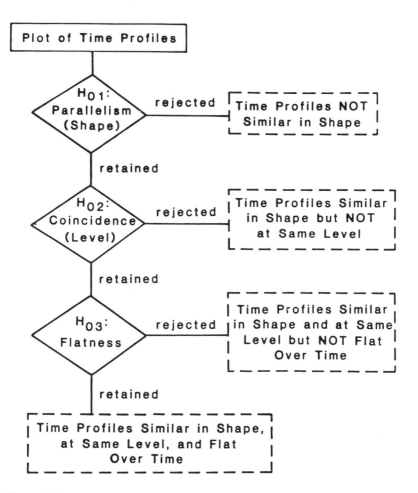

Figure 4.5

ity exists if profiles and their segments maintain parallel positions (see Figure 4.2, section 2A). If the null hypothesis is rejected (the shapes are not parallel), it is inferred that the time profiles, and, therefore, the change processes, differ (see Figure 4.2, sections 2B and 2C).

If, however, the null hypothesis of parallelism is retained, it is known that the profiles are similar in shape. The next question, then, is whether the similarly shaped change processes occur at the same level of intensity. In other words, are the profiles coincident in space, occupying approximately the same geometrical location? For instance, are the profiles in Figure 4.2, section 2A, so to speak truly "one on top of the other" or is the small space between them sufficient to be statistically significant? In conceptual terms, is the phenomenon of change occurring at the same level of intensity for both groups or do the control subjects manifest the same change process at a lower level of intensity?

These questions are answered by testing the hypothesis of *coincidence*. If rejected, the conclusion is that time profiles are similar in shape but not at the same level. Retention indicates that, in addition to being similar in shape across time, change processes also are similar in intensity. Retention permits testing of the third null hypothesis, flatness of effect.

The *flatness* hypothesis assesses whether the pooled profile (pooled because groups did not differ anyway) is flat. Its retention indicates that no change occurred over time. If rejected, one concludes that the groups had profiles with similar shapes, that these profiles reflect processes at the same level of intensity, and that there was no change over time.

References

Abraham, I. L., Nadzam, D. M., & Fitzpatrick, J. J. (Eds.). (1989a). *Statistics and quantitative methods in nursing: Issues and strategies for research and education*. Philadelphia: W. B. Saunders.

Abraham, I. L., Nadzam, D. M., & Fitzpatrick, J. J. (1989b). Statistics in nursing curricula. In I. L. Abraham, D. M. Nadzam, & J. J. Fitzpatrick (Eds.), *Statistics and quantitative methods in nursing: Issues and strategies for research and education*. Philadelphia: W. B. Saunders.

Anderson, T. W. (1971). *The statistical analysis of time series*. New York: John Wiley.

Bloomfield, P. (1976). *Fourier analysis of time series: An introduction*. New York: John Wiley.

Box, G. E. P., & Jenkins, G. M. (1968). Some recent advances in forecasting and control. Part I. *Applied Statistics, 17*, 91-109.

Box, G. E. P., & Jenkins, G. M. (1976). *Time series analysis, forecasting, and control* (2nd ed.). San Francisco: Holden-Day.

Brogan, D. R. (1989). A statistician's view on statistics, quantitative methods, and nursing. In I. L. Abraham, D. M. Nadzam, & J. J. Fitzpatrick (Eds.), *Statistics and quantitative methods in nursing: Issues and strategies for research and education*. Philadelphia: W. B. Saunders.

Brogan, D. R., & Kutner, M. H. (1980). Comparative analyses of pretest-posttest designs. *American Statistician, 34*, 229-232.

Buckwalter, K. C. (1989). Increasing rigor and meaningfulness in gerontological nursing research. In I. L. Abraham, D. M. Nadzam, & J. J. Fitzpatrick (Eds.), *Statistics and quantitative methods in nursing: Issues and strategies for research and education*. Philadelphia: W. B. Saunders.

Campbell, D. T., & Stanley, J. C. (1963). Experimental and quasi-experimental designs for research on teaching. In N. L. Gage (Ed.), *Handbook of research on teaching*. Chicago: Rand McNally.

Chambers, J. M., Cleveland, W. S., Kleiner, B., & Tukey, P. A. (1983). *Graphical methods for data analysis*. Belmont, CA: Wadsworth.

Chatfield, C. (1984). *The analysis of time series: An introduction* (3rd ed.). London: Chapman & Hall.

Clinton, J. (1986). Conceptual and technical issues in using time-series methodology in clinical nursing research. In P. L. Chinn (Ed.), *Nursing research methodology: Issues and implementation*. Rockville, MD: Aspen.

Clinton, J., Beck, R., Radjenovic, D., Taylor, L., Westlake, S., & Wilson, S. E. (1986). Time-series designs in clinical nursing research: Human issues. *Nursing Research, 35*, 188-191.

Cook, T. D., & Campbell, D. T. (Eds.). (1979). *Quasi-experimentation: Design and analysis issues for field settings*. Chicago: Rand McNally.

Cox, D. R. (1957). The use of a concomitant variable in selecting an experimental design. *Biometrika, 44*, 150-158.

Cox, D. R., & Lewis, P. A. W. (1966). *The statistical analysis of series of events*. London: Chapman & Hall.

Edwards, A. L. (1985). *Multiple regression and the analysis of variance and covariance*. New York: Freeman.

Feldt, L. S. (1958). A comparison of the precision of three experimental designs employing a concomitant variable. *Psychometrika, 23*, 335-353.

Glass, G. V., Wilson, V. L., & Gottman, J. M. (1975). *Design and analysis of time-series experiments*. Boulder: Colorado Associated University Press.

Gottman, J. M. (1981). *Time series analysis*. Cambridge: Cambridge University Press.

Granger, C. W. J. (1966). The typical shape of an econometric variable. *Economometrica, 34*, 150-161.

Harris, R. J. (1985). *A primer of multivariate statistics* (2nd ed.). New York: Academic Press.

Huitema, B. E. (1980). *The analysis of covariance and alternatives*. New York: John Wiley.

Huynh, H., & Feldt, L. S. (1970). Conditions under which mean square rations in repeated measures designs have exact F-distributions. *Journal of the American Statistical Association, 65*, 1582-1589.

Jirovec, M. M. (1986). Time-series analysis in nursing research: ARIMA modeling. *Nursing Research, 35*, 315-319.

Jones, S. L., & Jones, P. K. (1989). A statistical evaluation of the psychiatric nursing research literature. In I. L. Abraham, D. M. Nadzam, & J. J. Fitzpatrick (Eds.), *Statistics and quantitative methods in nursing: Issues and strategies for research and education*. Philadelphia: W. B. Saunders.

Johnson, P. O., & Neyman, J. (1936). Tests of certain linear hypotheses and their application to some educational problems. *Statistical Research Memoirs, 1*, 57-93.

Kendall, M. G. (1976). *Time series*. London: Griffin.

Kenny, D. A. (1975). A quasi-experimental approach to assessing treatment effects in the nonequivalent control group design. *Psychological Bulletin, 82*, 345-362.

Kenny, P. B., & Durbin, J. (1982). Local trend estimation and seasonal adjustment of economic and social time series. *Journal of the Royal Statistical Society, A, 145*, 1-41.

Kirk, R. E. (1982). *Experimental design*. Belmont, CA: Wadsworth.

Kleiner, B., Martin, R. D., & Thomson, D. J. (1979). Robust estimation of power spectra. *Journal of the Royal Statistical Society, B, 41*, 313-351.

Koopmans, L. H. (1974). *The spectral analysis of time series.* New York: Academic Press.

Krowchuk, H. V. (1989). Implications for design, sampling, measurement, and statistical analysis in parent-child nursing research. In I. L. Abraham, D. M. Nadzam, & J. J. Fitzpatrick (Eds.), *Statistics and quantitative methods in nursing: Issues and strategies for research and education.* Philadelphia: W. B. Saunders.

Leidy, N. K. (1989). Toward methodological proficiency in medical-surgical nursing research. In I. L. Abraham, D. M. Nadzam, & J. J. Fitzpatrick (Eds.), *Statistics and quantitative methods in nursing: Issues and strategies for research education.* Philadelphia: W. B. Saunders.

Lobo, M. L., & Ross-Alaolmolki, K. (1989). Statistics and quantitative research methods in nursing care of children. In I. L. Abraham, D. M. Nadzam, & J. J. Fitzpatrick (Eds.), *Statistics and quantitative methods in nursing: Issues and strategies for research education.* Philadelphia: W. B. Saunders.

McCain, L. J., & McCleary, R. (1979). The statistical analysis of the simple interrupted time-series quasi-experiment. In T. D. Cook & D. T. Campbell (Eds.), *Quasi-experimentation: Design and analysis issues for field settings.* Chicago: Rand McNally.

McCall, R. B., & Appelbaum, M. I. (1973). Bias in the analysis of repeated-measures designs: Some alternative approaches. *Child Development, 44*, 401-415.

Metzger, B. L., & Schultz, S. (1982). Time series analysis: An alternative for nursing. *Nursing Research, 31*, 375-378.

Neter, J., & Wasserman, W. (1974). *Applied linear statistical models.* Homewood, IL: Irwin.

Pothoff, R. F. (1964). On the Johnson-Neyman technique and some extensions thereof. *Psychometrika, 29*, 241-256.

Roberts, B. L. (1989). Statistics and quantitative methods in medical-surgical nursing. In I. L. Abraham, D. M. Nadzam, & J. J. Fitzpatrick (Eds.), *Statistics and quantitative methods in nursing: Issues and strategies for research and education.* Philadelphia: W. B. Saunders.

Robson, D. S., & Atkinson, G. F. (1960). Individual degrees of freedom for testing homogeneity of regression coefficients in a one-way analysis of covariance. *Biometrics, 16*, 593-605.

Steel, R. G. D., & Federer, W. T. (1955). Yield-stand analyses. *Journal of the Indian Society of Agricultural Statistics, 7*, 27-45.

Tukey, J. W. (1977). *Exploratory data analysis.* Reading, MA: Addison-Wesley.

Whall, A. L., Booth, D., & Jirovec, M. M. (1989). Statistics and quantitative methods in gerontological nursing research. In I. L. Abraham, D. M. Nadzam, & J. J. Fitzpatrick (Eds.), *Statistics and quantitative methods in nursing: Issues and strategies for research and education.* Philadelphia: W. B. Saunders.

Winter, B. J. (1971). *Statistical principles in experimental design.* New York: McGraw-Hill.

PART II

Nonstatistical Approaches for Theory Building

5

The Case Study Approach

SALLY A. HUTCHINSON

> To generalize is to be an idiot. To particularize is the lone distinction
> of merit. General knowledges are those that idiots possess.
> —William Blake (1808)

Blake's declaration is rather extreme but it does highlight his belief in the value of the particular. A case study as an intensive investigation of an individual, a program, an institution, a community, or a decision is an investigation of the particular. Nurses take care of individuals with particular problems, needs, wishes, and goals. For nursing research to be useful, it must speak to practicing nurses. Case studies aid in our aim to understand particulars, increasing the knowledge base of our practice. They reveal greater social complexities through a systematic, holistic approach. Particulars are then used to build theory for nursing practice; such theory ultimately will involve generalizations that, contrary to Blake's rhetoric, should be explanatory, predictive, and useful.

Although the case study strategy is criticized for being "soft" science due to numerous uncontrolled variables, frequent ambiguity of design, and inherent bias, when executed with systematic rigor, it has much to offer the nursing profession. By illuminating human experience and real-life problems, the case study method provides a service neglected by many other "scientific" approaches.

Case studies in the fields of psychiatry, psychology, sociology, anthropology, political science, and organizational behavior are revered as classics today, responsible for altering those disciplines' views of the world. As a developing science, nursing can learn from those more mature fields. Freud (1938) generated his theory of psychoanalysis from case studies of his clients. Anna O., a woman diagnosed with hysteria, became miraculously symptom-free when she talked about her feelings (catharsis). In clinical psychology, case studies have been the main source of fundamental insights. The theory of operant conditioning was developed and refined as Skinner (1959) and his colleagues studied interventions with animals and people. Anthropological and sociological studies of communities in various parts of the United States and abroad (Gans, 1962; Lynd & Lynd, 1929) taught much about the interplay of people, culture, and society. We also learned about types of people—*The Cocktail Waitress* (Spradley & Mann, 1975), *The Jackroller* (Shaw, 1967), *The Professional Thief* (Sutherland, 1937)—and their unique ways of viewing and living in the world. In anthropology, case studies moved away from the "etic" norms of structural-functionalism to the "emic" realities of actual behaviors and personal interpretation. Studies in political science have revealed useful information about domestic and foreign policy (Allison, 1971; Neustadt, 1960) while studies in organizational behavior have shed light on institutions (Weppner, 1983).

In nursing in the 1960s, case examples ("Mrs. Jones Takes A Bath") populated the nursing literature and were used as teaching exemplars as is common in law and public policy. Clinical case studies of patients from different clinical units are frequently presented at case conferences with the goals of illustrating nursing diagnoses or care plans. The case study as scientific research is less available in the nursing literature, partly because of the difficulty in doing one well and partly because the strategy is generally not taught in nursing research courses due to our predominant focus on quantitative methods. In most nursing texts, the case study approach either is not mentioned or is discussed within a few paragraphs; however, Schultz and Kerr in *Nursing Research Methodology* (Chinn, 1986) offer a chapter; Woods and Cantanzaro (1988) discuss the case study method as one example of hypothesis-generating research; and Wilson (1989) provides a few pages on the case study method. Another reason for the lack of identified published nursing case studies is semantic. Some studies fit the criteria of case studies yet are not labeled as such (see Hutchinson, 1983; Wilson, 1986).

The purpose of this chapter is to discuss the case study strategy, to relate the strategy to the phases of the research process, and to provide exemplars of case studies from nursing and other research. With a closer look at this unique strategy, we can expand our research repertoire and contribute relevant holistic, humanistic studies to the professional literature, providing more data to undergird our practice and future research.

Theoretical Issues and Assumptions

According to Yin (1984, p. 23), who wrote most definitively on the subject of case studies, the case study is "an empirical inquiry that investigates a contemporary phenomenon within its real-life context; when the boundaries between phenomenon and context are not clearly evident; and in which multiple sources of evidence are used." Interestingly, many studies that use phenomenological, grounded theory and ethnographic methods also meet these criteria and, therefore, could qualify as case studies. However, all qualitative studies are not case studies, neither are all case studies qualitative. Yin (1984) recognizes two conditions of qualitative research that do not always apply to case studies: (a) researchers' close observations of a natural setting and (b) an atheoretical stance at the initiation of the research. Qualitative research in sociology and anthropology, however, is not always atheoretical but may rely on theories of culture, kinship, and social class. Examples of qualitative and quantitative case studies are presented later in the chapter.

Case studies are especially useful in examining "how" or "why" questions when the researcher cannot manipulate events and when the focus is on a contemporary phenomenon within a real-life context (Yin, 1984, p. 13). Diverse types of data (e.g., interview, document analysis, and surveys) aid in achieving the depth and breadth of evidence required to answer how and why questions. And it is the required depth and breadth of evidence that supports the case study as an approach or strategy rather than a definitive method with clear structured directions. The idea of a strategy/approach suggests a flexibility that is essential to case studies and to answering how and why questions.

In any study, the researcher's general philosophical orientation influences the process of inquiry (DeGroot, 1988). The selected research question and/or purpose guides the research, and a thorough literature review will yield sufficient data for an argument that

Box 5.1. Examples of Types of Case Studies

Descriptive	The purpose is to describe the implementation of primary nursing on a medical unit in a 500-bed teaching hospital.
	The purpose is to describe the use of a structured relaxation program with patients who experience cholecystectomy.
Exploratory	The purpose is to explore relevant variables in staff's decisions to place psychiatric patients in seclusion.
	The purpose is to explore caregivers' experiences in caring for family members with Alzheimer's disease.
Explanatory	The purpose is to explain patients' anger.
	The purpose is to explain how and why a 10-year-old child died from child abuse.

supports a particular type of study. Because case studies may be the strategy of choice in research that has the purpose of exploring, describing, or explaining phenomena, they have the ability to answer a variety of questions. Note some examples of types of case studies in Box 5.1.

Depending on the researcher's decision, other research designs or strategies may also be used instead of the case study or as part of the case study. When events can be manipulated, a quasi-experimental or experimental design is preferred because of the ability to control variables and thus measure the effects of a specific intervention. These designs, also able to answer a how or why question, test existing theory. When events are noncontemporary, the historical approach is appropriate. Survey designs assess a specified population in order to describe behaviors or attitudes.

Case Studies and Case Histories

Sociologists Strauss and Glaser (1970) differentiate between case histories and case studies, which other authors do not, yet it is significant for our understanding and doing of research (see Table 5.1 and Box 5.2). The more clear we can be about what it is that we are doing, the better research we can design and conduct. The goal of a case history is to "get the fullest possible story for its own sake" (Strauss & Glaser, 1970, p. 182). Theory may or may not be applied to the story (see Box 5.3). This story can be an experience in a person's

TABLE 5.1

A Comparison of Case Studies and Case Histories

	Case Histories	*Case Studies*
Topic	A life experience or an event, decision, program, institution, organization.	A life experience or an event, decision, program, institution, organization.
Purpose	To present the fullest possible story.	To describe, verify or generate theory.
Relevance of Theory	Minor focus (from none to minimal).	Major focus.
Style	Descriptive/narrative.	Analytical/abstract.

life (an illness, a loss, a career change) or an actual biography of someone's life. Sutherland's (1937) book on the professional thief, Festinger, Reichen, and Schechter's (1956) study of a cult that predicted a cataclysmic flood, and Shaw's (1967) book on a delinquent boy are examples. Life histories, so well known in anthropology, are one kind of case history (see Box 5.4). Watson and Watson-Franke

---

Box 5.2. An Example of a Case History That Is Called a Case Study

In a study by Wolcott (1967), (one of a series on education and culture) the author contributes an ethnography of a North American Indian village on a small island and its school. As is true of most ethnographies, much descriptive information is presented about a designated problem. Interpretive generalizations are made. The Spindlers, well known anthropologists and editors of the education and culture series, view the studies as useful resources for comparative analysis and "for stimulating thinking and discussion about education that is not confined by one's own cultural experience" (Wolcott, 1967, p. v).

Interestingly the Spindlers call their group of monographs, case studies. A careful examination of several studies suggests that, according to the Strauss and Glaser's (1970) criteria, they are more like case histories because attention is given to full description and the aim is not to verify, test or generate theory. With the recognition of different criteria for the case study and the case history, previous works may be reevaluated and reclassified. The purpose in this of course is only that we be clear and have a full understanding of the terms we are using.

Box 5.3. An Example of a Case History Without Theory

In *Eleven Blue Men, and Other Narratives of Medical Detection,* Rouché (1946) presents a classic collection of brief medical case histories. The discovery of trichinosis, leprosy, air pollution and other public health problems in various patients is dramatized in different examples of physician as sleuth. The theory is absent but the logical problem-solving process is clear. Probably, if the book were written today, epidemiological theories would be relevant in comparative analysis of the cases.

(1985) advocate life history research because it reveals human responses and viewpoints within the context of culture. Life histories can provide information about cultural patterns, cultural change, and cultural deviance. They can be autobiographical and biographical. "The best life history documents have a sensitivity and a pace, a dramatic urgency, that any novelist would be glad to achieve" (Becker in Shaw, 1967, p. 5). Other kinds of case histories also examine one social unit, but the unit may be a group, a community, a nation, a status, an organization, a relationship, a type of behavior, or a process (Strauss & Glaser, 1970).

Case studies, in contrast, do not focus on a complete story but have as their aim the analyses of single or multiple cases so as to describe, verify, or generate theory. In *The 36-Hour Day,* Mace and Rabins (1981) use medical knowledge and social-psychological knowledge about patients with Alzheimer's Dementia (AD) as the descriptive theory that structured their educative case study for families who care for AD patients. Vignettes documenting caregivers' experiences support and illustrate the theory. As Mace and Rabins' work indicates, the case study is more abstract, more conceptual, than the case history. Case studies either are theory driven (they describe or test a

---

Box 5.4. An Example of Life Histories

In *Life Histories of African Women* (Romero, 1988), seven life histories of African women from different geographical areas in Africa were presented. The authors are from seven different disciplines revealing a variety of methods and questions. For example, one of the life histories is auto-biographical, told in the first person with the theoretical commentary confined to an introduction. Other histories told in the third person have integrated theoretical comments throughout the story. Historical documents and oral tradition are used in several of the histories.

---

theory) or clearly aim to generate theory, whereas case histories provide detailed data that may or may not be linked to theory.

Strauss and Glaser's (1970) case history, *Anguish: A Case History of a Dying Trajectory*, is a poignant description of a 54-year-old woman with cancer who experienced a lingering death in the hospital. After a theoretical introduction in Chapter 1, the authors take three chapters for rich description: "The Death," "The Pain," "The Last Days"— each of which reveals interactions with and around the patient through the dialogue of Strauss, a student-nurse, and a nurse-researcher, the latter two of whom kept copious notes over the four-month period. At the end of each section is a brief theoretical comment on the chapter in which Glaser and Strauss's previously generated theories of pain, dying trajectories, and awareness of dying are applied. Mrs. Abel comes alive for the reader; her anguish is palpable. The theoretical applications illuminate the social complexity of pain and death and propose social-psychological explanations for the anguish. The discussion is contextual, revealing the interaction and the interplay among staff/patient/hospital environment. Martinson (1976) presents a case history about home care for dying children. Mothers and fathers, nurses, a physician, a chaplain, and a social worker tell their stories and offer varied perspectives on care of the dying child. Theoretical and research literature is interwoven with descriptive material. The final section of the book is titled "Theoretical Considerations for Health Professionals"; the aim is theory generation.

Case histories are needed in nursing because they force us to be linked cognitively and affectively to real patients and real situations. Thus both the hypothesis-generating and nursing practice implications are considerable. One cannot read *Anguish* without being touched by both the patient's and the nurses' experiences. Nurses are "privileged" in their communications with patients, which permit use of the case history. Strauss and Glaser (1970) write clearly on the practical contributions of the case history, which suggest a general reform of terminal care. As befits their perspective, they are interested in making the care more compassionate and thus more focused on the social-psychological aspects of dying (Strauss & Glaser, 1970, p. 178). Like the Spindlers' (1978) case histories in anthropology, case histories in nursing can serve the purpose of comparative analysis, highlighting differences and similarities across cultures. As nurses travel, study, and consult in different cultures, knowledge of the environment, and recognition that West-

---

Box 5.5. An Example of a Case History in Nursing

Blake's (1964) study *Open Heart Surgery in Children* is a classic in nursing. She studied children with operable cardiac defects to learn ways to improve patient care. She cared for six children and observed them at their homes and during clinic visits and studied two other children who were cared for by other nurses. In her published work, she presents a case history of a four-year-old girl "to portray the way in which a child and her parents react to and deal with hospitalization, nursing care, and treatment for multiple septal defects, and to demonstrate a method of studying patient care" (Blake, 1964, p. 2.).

Data analysis revealed descriptive interpretation including stages the child passed through postoperatively. Theoretical commentary appeared in the beginning of the report in the form of a brief literature review. Blake used participant observation in that the nurses studied the children as they cared for them. Responding to guiding questions, they carried notebooks to record notes about their own feelings and observations and the child's behaviors and interactions. Erikson's recently published article "Youth and the Life Cycle" raised questions that guided the data analysis. This case history is descriptive with no integration of theory; in the final chapter, hypotheses are presented along with suggestions for further research, and on how to use the present study for teaching.

---

ern nursing cannot alter an environment without understanding it and adapting to it, is vital to success.

Ideas for case histories may derive from nurses' work with patients with a unique experience (the young man who contracted AIDS through motor vehicle trauma in Africa—Breo, 1989), or with a typical experience (depression, grief, intractable pain). (See Box 5.5 for a case history in nursing.) Nurses could learn much from studying the "bubble boy," who was immunologically suppressed since birth and who lived in a plastic bubble, a germ-free environment within a hospital, for his entire life. Surely, this dramatic example would have illuminated much about social and psychological isolation, nurse/patient/family relationships, and institutionalization. Understanding patient experiences guides the way for further research and theory extension. Recognizing the case history method as a viable research strategy should heighten researchers' sensitivity to important "stories" that they come across in research and/or practice.

Before beginning a case study or case history, a researcher assesses the reason for studying a particular phenomenon and the best way to go about doing it. A case history is useful for exposing problems because many different issues come to the fore. No one issue is treated in systematic fashion, but if the investigator is good, she or he presents the information in an enlightening way. The case study sacrifices comprehension about an episode/individual to focus intensely on theory and its usefulness in explaining events. Both the case history and the case study add to one another and contribute to knowledge building in different ways.

Case Histories and Their Relation to Theory

A major issue concerns the type of theories that can be applied to case histories. Because theories are at different levels of abstraction (substantive/middle-range or formal/grand), the more formal or grand theories may be difficult to apply to a case history that provides minute details about human behavior (see Box 5.6). Theories that are best able to illuminate and explain case history data should be used, and this requires that researchers seek diverse types of theories in nursing and the social sciences. A combination of theories may be useful, or one major theory may be more effective, in explaining the case history. Either way, the theory(s) become clarified, extended, and made relevant because of the relationship with practice. With theory, meaning is made of experiences, behaviors, and events. What appears idiosyncratic in the case history is moved into a broader frame of reference, thus becoming more useful and applicable to other situations.

If the theory doesn't fit the case history exactly, the researcher can return to the case history and look for data that may help expand the theory. If gaps in the theory become known, this recognition can suggest ideas for further research. Sometimes theories can be "found" in the data and expanded with other cases. In *Anguish*, Strauss and Glaser discovered a subtheory of "lingering hospitalized dying." This theory helped to explain aspects of Mrs. Able's case history and can explain some other patients' histories. Once there is understanding of a phenomenon, suggestions for interventions arise naturally. Theory and practice are affected.

Recently, in my research on "nurses who violate the nurse practice act," I discovered a nurse who had 20 circumstances in which he physically and mentally abused patients and coworkers in violent

Box 5.6. An Example of a Case History That Uses Grand Theory

Sutherland's (1937) case history, *The Professional Thief*, was actually written in part by an experienced thief who responded in writing to questions from Sutherland. In addition, Sutherland spent seven hours per week for twelve weeks discussing what the thief wrote. Theft is explained as a profession, as a social institution and as a group way of life; theft is a culture with tradition, codes of behavior, status, and organization. Sutherland proposed that only by understanding the culture can strategies for the control of theft be developed. He proposed several hypotheses at the end of the case history: that professional thieves constitute a group that has the characteristics of other groups and that these group characteristics are not pathological; that tutelage by professional thieves and recognition as a professional thief are essential and universal elements in the definition, genesis, and continued behavior of the professional thief (Sutherland, 1937, p. viii). Sutherland views his study as incomplete description and explanation but as a beginning work in problem definition and in setting the stage for future research. The book is divided into two parts. Part I is written as a descriptive account by the thief and annotated by Sutherland. Part II is a 22 page theoretical interpretation that uses concepts from grand sociological theory to explain the case history, such as the profession of theft as a complex of techniques, as status, as consensus, as differential association, and as organization. This book was written using grand theory for interpretation because of the status of sociological theory at that time.

ways. He tied a nurse to a chair, threw water on a restrained patient, brought martial arts weapons and a gun to work, and picked up a retarded patient by the head. Surely, a case history of his nursing career would offer much toward the understanding of how a person like this remained in nursing for as long as he did without experiencing legal or administrative actions. In this example, the case material for a case history was "found" in the interviews for another study (Hutchinson, 1990).

Journalistic case histories can contribute to our data base. The book *The Long Dying of Baby Andrew* (Stinson, 1979) is not a case history in the pure sense because the theoretical analyses are lacking, but it is a moving journalistic account by Andrew's parents of his death in a neonatal intensive care unit. Because of this book, nurses and physicians and any other readers are forced to change their perceptions of neonatal care and of parental experiences in neonatal units. Nurses could apply theory (for example, ethical theories, communications theory, decision-making theory) to the case history, which would highlight the variety of problems that occurred throughout Andrew's brief life. The decision-making processes, in particular, require theoretical analysis.

Using *Anguish* as a model, nurses who generate grounded theories could do a case history that can be explained by their theory. Mishel and Murdaugh's (1987) theory described family adjustment to heart transplantation and the processes used to cope with continual unpredictability. A case history of such a family would be a great contribution to nursing science, particularly if it were analyzed by the substantive theory, revealing the strengths and limitations of the theory via illustrating a patient's (family's) problems. Because unpredictability is present for many patients, learning more about this concept is sure to benefit nursing theory and practice.

Like the case study, the case history may rely on diverse methods, depending on the research question and/or purpose. Although a case history usually refers to one case, multiple cases may be used with a theory that integrates them all. Case histories are usually long, due to their goal—"the fullest possible story." If multiple case histories were used, they would probably be shorter. Also, the analysis of several case histories would focus on comparisons among them, for example, a patient with a lingering dying trajectory and a patient with a brief dying trajectory, a dying trajectory in the hospital and a dying trajectory that occurs at home or in a nursing home. The theory explains the selected points in the case history, which is unlike the case study in which the analyst uses the data to search for concepts that describe, verify, or generate theory.

Case Studies and Their Relation to Theory

Lijphart (1971, p. 692) distinguishes six "ideal types" of case studies. Classifying case studies in this way helps us look closely at the connection between the research and the theory. The types include the following:

(1) Atheoretical—the focus is on the case itself (this would be a case history according to Strauss & Glaser, 1970). The term is actually inaccurate because theoretical ideas inevitably guide the study, even if they are unarticulated.

(2) Interpretive—theoretical propositions or conceptual models (Fawcett, 1984; Parse, 1987) are used to guide the data analysis. "Although not empirically testable, conceptual models or paradigms serve as heuristic devices or springboards for developing theories" (Moody & Hutchin-

---

Box 5.7. An Example of a Deviant Case Analysis

In Neustadt's (1960) book *Presidential Power*, he attempts to derive lessons for how to rule effectively by looking at enlightening episodes from three different presidencies. He links the material from the presidencies to a common theme, the difficulty in effecting policies even when you have enormous power. Making decisions that are rightfully yours are very difficult. Auxiliary skill is necessary to effect your will; legal and constitutional obstacles are not the primary obstacles. Thesis 1 is to persuade the reader through different incidents to feel this forcefully. Thesis 2 offers some insight on what power is really. The author provides training in the acquisition and use of power. The book is more like a case history because of the underdeveloped or unarticulated alternative explanations.

---

son, 1989). A case study can be considered a case history if the propositions are few and loosely connected and if the emphasis is on detailed description.

(3) Hypothesis generating—here the goal is theory building. Hypotheses are formulated and tested in difficult cases in an effort to develop theoretical explanations, like Yin's (1984) "explanation building" that will be discussed later in this chapter.

(4) Theory confirming and

(5) Theory informing—an established theoretical framework guides the study and this framework is either supported or not supported by the data, like Yin's (1984) "pattern matching," which will be discussed later. The theoretical propositions are tested by the data. Such research is also called causal hypothesis-testing research (Diers, 1979).

(6) Deviant—the deviant case study is an examination of a case that the researcher recognizes deviates from the typical, established generalizations. The aim is to find why and how deviant cases are deviant and, by doing this, to identify new relevant variables. Meier and Pugh (1986) see deviant case analysis as a way to understand treatment failures. Kayser-Jones and Kapp (1989, p. 353) provide an excellent example with their study that illustrates "how a mentally impaired but socially intact nursing home resident, who had no one to act as an advocate for her, was denied appropriate treatment for an acute illness which ultimately resulted in her death." Neustadt's (1960) study *Presidential Power* (see Box 5.7) also illustrates deviant case analysis. He believes that negative examples are the most illuminating (see also Weppner, 1983).

Lijphart (1971) views types 3 (hypothesis generating) and 6 (deviant) as contributing the most to theory development. Type 3 generates new hypotheses and Type 6 "refines and sharpens" existing hypotheses. Types 4 (theory confirming), 5 (theory informing), and 6 (deviant) all use comparative analyses, and, in Type 6, the comparative analysis involves the deviant case (experimental group) being compared with the "normal cases" (control group).

Case Study Designs

Because a typology of case study designs has not been generated, the researcher has to make certain decisions regarding design that are fundamental to the execution and completion of quality research. The phenomenon studied can often be "fuzzy" or ambiguous due to the focus of the case study strategy (contemporary, real-life phenomenon, unclear boundaries between phenomenon and context, many sources of evidence) and, therefore, certain guiding questions help decrease the confusion and clarify the focus:

- What is the research question(s)? The question(s) must be clear and be unaltered throughout the study. This is vital because the temptation is often to follow ideas and information that often are not directly linked to the original questions and data collection strategies. A clear focus is essential to clear research. A study with a research question about the nature of nurse-patient interaction in labor and delivery should not have findings that emphasize nurse-physician interaction.
- What is the research purpose? To test, verify, or generate theory? To provide a complete rendition of a problem? How does the theory fit with the purpose?
- What is being studied? A person, an intervention, a program, a decision-making process? Or are several "units of analysis" being examined? Is the study in the neonatal intensive care unit (NICU) about a baby who was dying or about the staff decision-making processes?
- Where does the case begin and where does it end? If we study how a team of physicians/nurses/parents decide to terminate life support on an infant, where does the case study begin? At the birth of the baby or two months later when he was readmitted to the NICU?
- Are data collection strategies aimed to achieve reliability and validity? Or, to use the more appropriate terms for qualitative research, *truth*

value, applicability, consistency, neutrality (Lincoln & Guba, 1985). For example, if we plan to study elders' perspectives of an intergenerational geriatric remotivation program, we need to think about how we can establish that our findings about the elders' perspectives will have truth value. Will our findings be applicable in other contexts. If the same or similar elders were studied in the same or similar context, will there be consistency of findings? Will our findings be based on informants' responses and not our own biases?

Will the data analyses yield information relevant to the research question? If the research question is a how or why question, using only descriptive statistics for data analysis is inadequate. Appropriate quantitative and/or qualitative methods of analysis need to be selected to answer all research questions.

Once these questions are pondered, a design should be selected. Case study designs can be single or multiple, holistic or embedded (Yin, 1984). (See Figure 5.1.) Single cases of one person or event are appropriate if (a) the case represents a critical test of existing theory, (b) the case is unique or rare, or (c) the case is "revelatory," something never studied before (Yin, 1984, p. 47). The single case design may be holistic or embedded. Embedded designs are those in which several units of analysis are studied via different data collection and analysis strategies, while holistic designs provide a more global or abstract approach to an institution, individual, or event. The nature of the research question determines whether an embedded or holistic design is more useful. As with any design, each has strengths and limitations. The holistic design may be too abstract, not yielding much relevant data, while the embedded designs may suffer from a focus on minutiae that are not well linked to the context, thus altering the original focus.

Some researchers use multiple case (also called comparative) designs if the research purpose requires it. However, Yin (1984) cautions that the logic for multiple case studies is not the sampling logic used in other research designs (e.g., surveys, experiments) that look for incidence of phenomena. Rather, replication logic is used, which means that each case is considered as a single experiment, and the data analysis is not the "within-experiment" analysis but is that used for cross-experiments. Instead of looking for "incidence" of phenomena, which is not relevant in case studies, the replication logic is directly linked to a theoretical framework that predicts certain occurrences in specific situations. For example, a multiple case replication

	Single-Case Designs	Multiple-Case Designs
Holistic (single unit of analysis)	TYPE 1	TYPE 3
Embedded (multiple units of analysis)	TYPE 2	TYPE 4

Figure 5.1 Basic Types of Designs for Case Studies

SOURCE: Yin, R. (1984). *Case study research: Design and methods* (p. 46). Beverly Hills, CA: Sage.

design would be used to present the implementation of primary nursing in hospitals with different organizational structures (decentralized, centralized). Theory(s) could predict the outcomes. After an analysis of each case study, based on the predictive theory, the researcher then can do a cross-analysis, looking for patterns. Then theory can be modified and implications for practice developed. The multiple case study may use a holistic or embedded design, depending on the research questions and theoretical framework.

Waltz and Bausell (1981, pp. 135-136) propose the following general steps in designing a case study:

(1) State the objectives, the purpose, of the case study in observable, behavioral terms.

(2) Identify the unit of study: individual, group, or community.

(3) List the characteristics, relationships, processes that will direct the investigation, at least initially.

(4) Review the literature.

(5) Determine how subjects will be selected and identify potential data sources.

(6) Specify the available data collection methods and plan as much as possible how data will be collected.

(7) Develop a tentative scheme for organizing the findings into a coherent, well-integrated description of the unit.

(8) Plan for reporting results.

(9) Anticipate hypotheses for further study that may result from the case study.

A problem with case study research, as is true of much qualitative research, concerns the possible shift in focus that comes with the required flexibility of case situations. The flexibility is useful, but if it shifts too far away from the original plan, a new study needs to be designed or the final product suffers from a lack of integration, logic, and theoretical relevance. Keeping the focus of case studies clear can be difficult because the case study method often looks at complex social phenomena. Therefore, researchers have to constantly reexamine their designs, research questions, theoretical frameworks, and data collection strategies to prevent losing the focus. Documenting changes and their rationale during the course of the study is essential, helping to provide a road map for researchers and, in the future, for readers who want to understand and/or replicate the study.

Data Collection

Yin (1984) advocates pilot studies to illuminate problems, suggest modifications, and investigate protocols for clarity of data collection. He repeatedly emphasizes the difficulty in doing good case studies due to the ongoing interaction between the data and relevant theory(s). Data may yield insights about gaps in theory, and theory may guide data collection. As leads are followed and shifts are made, the researcher must continually reassess the design and theoretical framework (if there is one) to be certain the new plans are linked to them. If not, a new design and framework may be needed. For more information, see Chapter 7 in Volume 1.

Because of the complexity of case studies, data collection strategies that often deal with multiple types of data need to be carefully planned and written out. Depending on the research purpose, these strategies may include such diverse activities as in-depth interviews, surveys/questionnaires, participant observation, direct observation, document analysis, and retrieval of archival records. Such varied methods may yield qualitative and quantitative data. Triangulation of data is one of the strengths of the case study in that one source (e.g., documents) can confirm or refute evidence found with another source (interviews or participant observation). Thus findings that are suggested by a preponderance of evidence from multiple data sources are more likely to be accurate than those that rely on one source. Because the different data sources tap different kinds of information—behavioral, cognitive, attitudinal—the case study's depth and breadth are potentially great.

Each data collection strategy needs to be planned to decrease loopholes; a rationale for each strategy and its relationship to the theoretical framework and research question is of fundamental importance. This way, the sources of data and methods for acquiring data are linked to specific research questions. Consequently, it should be possible to answer all questions, and all data collected should have relevance to the study. Flexibility, however, is also important and involves the freedom to alter research questions and data collection strategies. The secret to success resides in thinking through and documenting each strategy. Data that appear "extraneous" at one point may assume great significance as the findings gel.

In embedded and multiple case designs, the level and nature of questions are varied. For example, in an intergenerational geriatric remotivation study, some of the questions focused on individuals (the elders' and children's responses to the program), some focused on the intervention (which activities worked better and why), and some focused on the context (the nature of the nursing home milieu). Because multiple cases were involved, questions were asked across cases. At the end of the study, questions about recommendations and program alteration were appropriate. Keeping these varied questions and varied units of analysis clear and focused is a difficult task requiring constant reassessment.

Data Recording

Good data recording methods for each strategy used are vital for retrievability of data. Each type of data will require a different type of data recording. For example, field notes from participant observation may be kept in large notebooks ready for use with the Ethnograph or some other computerized program for qualitative data analysis. Survey, archival, or questionnaire data that yield quantitative data needs to be in tables/files; interview data may be kept along with participant observation data if they are clearly distinguished as interviews. Guiding questions or concepts from the theoretical framework may serve as headings for data to aid in organization. A face sheet that lists all the types of data is useful for easy reference (see Box 5.8).

Accurate and careful data recording is tedious but ultimately is absolutely necessary for retrievability of data. When the case study is finished, it enhances truth value because each source of evidence

---

Box 5.8. An Example of a Face Sheet

---

1. Participant observation data

2. Documentary material   Census data
                                    City and county records
                                    Court files
                                    School records
                                    State biennial reports
                                    Yearbooks
                                    Two daily papers
                                    Democratic & Republican dailies
                                    Democratic Weekly
                                    Organizations' minutes (Board of
                                        Education, missionary societies,
                                        Ministerial Association, The Federated
                                        Club of Clubs, the Woman's Club, the
                                        Library Board, The Humane Society)
                                    School examination questions
                                    Two detailed personal diaries
                                    Histories of state, county & city
                                    City directories
                                    Maps
                                    Chamber of Commerce publications
                                    High school annuals

3. Compilation of statistics   Wages
                                    Steadiness of employment
                                    Industrial accidents
                                    Nearness of residence to plant
                                    Promotion
                                    Club memberships
                                    Church membership, contributions and
                                        attendance
                                    Library and periodical circulation
                                    Attendance at motion picture theaters
                                    Ownership and use of automobiles

4. Interview data

5. Questions   Club memberships and activities
                                    High school life
                                    Public issue

SOURCE: Lynd, R. and Lynd, H. (1929).

can be linked to pieces of the case study narrative, increasing auditability and construct validity.

Research Teams

Often, a team of researchers is necessary to carry out the case study protocols. In an effort to maximize communication and efficiency, team meetings are set up on a regular basis. In an ongoing evaluation study of an intergenerational geriatric remotivation program, the team met weekly in the beginning when the responsibilities of the researchers were planned, twice a month during data collection, and weekly toward the end when data analysis was especially complex. The meetings were problem-solving and strategy-planning sessions and were tape-recorded and transcribed. Methodological insights and changes were documented to increase auditability. The multiple research purposes and each of the researcher's roles were redefined and clarified. The meeting tone was one of negotiation and collaboration.

Data Analysis

Data analysis of case studies is inevitably complex due to the diversity of data, making the achievement of a coherent, unified product more difficult. As with all research, an analytic strategy is chosen, preferably at the beginning of the research. Yin (1984) proposes the strategy of using theoretical propositions that guide the case study as the framework of the write-up. In *The Silent Dialogue* (1968), a classic social-psychological study on the professional socialization of baccalaureate nursing students, Oleson and Whittaker began with existential theory and wrote the chapters in accordance with this theory. The three levels of existence (environmental, relational, and inner) are demonstrated in chapters on the institution of nursing and the nursing school, termed "environmental"; the role and student culture, termed "relational"; and the self, termed "inner."

Another analytic strategy is that of straight description (Schatzman & Strauss, 1982). In Viditch and Bensman's (1958) classic community study *Small Town in Mass Society*, the chapter headings in-

---

Box 5.9. An Example of a Case Study That Uses Pattern Matching

In *Essence of Decision, Explaining the Cuban Missile Crisis*, Allison (1971) compares and contrasts three frameworks ("conceptual lens") and their attempts to explain the Cuban missile crisis. He notes that using the three different lenses allows us to see "what each magnifies, highlights, and reveals as well as what each blurs or neglects." Each of these conceptual chapters is followed by a case study that is explained by the preceding conceptual chapter. In a "conclusion," he discusses the differences in interpretation and he ponders if the models and case studies depict different answers or different questions. He wonders, "and where do we go from here?" Implications and issues for future research follow.

---

dicate the straight descriptive approach: "Social, Economic and Historical Settings of the Community," "Springdale's Image of Itself," "The Major Dimensions of Social and Economic Class." Using Strauss and Glaser's (1970) criteria for case histories and case studies, the straight descriptive approach presents more like a case history. Because case studies aim to be more analytic and in the service of generating, verifying, or testing theory, the analytic strategies need to be more than descriptive. For example, a researcher may aim to generate a grounded theory and, therefore, would use an analytic strategy that permits this. If theory is to be verified, the theoretical propositions would be appropriate to structure the data analysis.

Dominant Modes of Analysis

There are as many methods of data analysis as there are types of data. A plan for each type of data analysis needs to be made at the beginning of the study. Yin (1984) advocates three dominant modes of analysis:

Pattern matching. Pattern matching, similar to descriptive analysis and a way to verify theory, refers to taking a theoretical pattern or arrangement of variables and comparing it with the pattern found in the data. Depending on the study question and theoretical framework, the investigator can predict patterns of independent and dependent variables. Allison's (1971) study (see Box 5.9) is an excellent example of pattern matching. In an earlier work, Festinger, Reichen, and Schechter (1956) set out hypotheses and then discussed them within a lengthy detailed description of a small cult. This cult pre-

Box 5.10. An Example of a Case Study That Uses Explanation Building

Timetables, by Julius Roth (1963), is a theory-generating case study that conceptualized how patients with tuberculosis view their lengthy time in a hospital or TB ward. Data collection occurred in five hospitals where Roth was either a patient being treated for TB or a social science observer. He noted the extreme importance of time, how patients and physicians have different timetables, and how this difference results in conflict and bargaining. Roth then describes other career timetables including those of polio convalescents, psychiatric patients, and business executives. A final chapter addresses the study of career timetables and includes numerous theoretical propositions that were generated from his multiple sources of data. He postulates that career timetables define and affect human behavior.

dicted a cataclysmic flood and was convinced that true believers would be rescued by flying saucers. Although this work is more like a case history, because of minimal theory, it is an example of pattern matching because of the authors' use of hypotheses. Because qualitative data are used in most case studies, the precision of the experimental design is lacking; Yin (1984) calls for more precise techniques.

Explanation building. Used in explanatory case studies, explanation building aims to generate theory (see Box 5.10). The investigator examines the data without preconceived notions, without a particular theoretical stance, and, by a process of analysis, arrives at theoretical propositions and perhaps even a theoretical framework. To do this well, specific methods for data analysis are necessary. For example, coming from a sociological perspective (Glaser, 1978; Glaser & Strauss, 1967; Strauss, 1987), grounded theory aims at generating social-psychological processes that form the basis for substantive, or formal, theories. Coming from an anthropological perspective, the ethnographic method (Spradley & Mann, 1979) can, with the interpretation of a good investigator, yield conceptual explanations for phenomena. Both of these methods generally rely on qualitative data (interviews, participant observation, documents) but are also able to use quantitative data. Both build explanations through a process of comparing each piece of the data with every other piece (called the constant comparative method in grounded theory), looking for patterns, themes, and their relationships. In explanation building, the patterns emerge from the data with the theoretical sensitivity of the

Box 5.11. An Example of a Time-Series Analysis in Nursing
In 1975, a clinical nursing study entitled "Failure to Thrive in a Child with Down's Syndrome" by Barbara Durand was published in *Nursing Research*. Fourteen pages were allotted, compared to the usual three pages. The article's structure included an extensive literature review followed by the case history with sections on observation and evaluation (history, medical work-up, nursing assessments). The hypothesis and care plan came next, followed by data collection and data analysis. This clinical study was a case history of a 5-year-old boy with Down's Syndrome and failure to thrive. An individualized nursing care plan based on developmental theory was used for a period of 17 days and resulted in improvement in seven of nine criteria: height, weight, amount of sleep, active mobility, awareness of the environment, prelanguage vocalizations, and self-stimulating behavior. The finding dramatically demonstrated that nursing interventions on physical and behavioral patient outcomes can be measured and suggest that nursing care can be the primary therapy in children with failure to thrive as a result of deprivation (Durand, 1975, p. 284). The author describes her attempt to use principles of experimental research in a clinical, "uncontrolled" setting.

researcher, whereas, in pattern matching, the pattern is imposed on the data and the question of whether or not the empirical data fit the imposed pattern is addressed.

Time-series analysis. Metzgar and Schultz (1982) suggest that time-series analyses are appropriate yet unused methods of research in nursing. They are especially appropriate because so many nursing judgments and interventions rely or are based on "rate, pattern, and change" (Metzgar & Schultz, 1982). (See Box 5.11.) Time-series analysis can follow numerous patterns that are described in great detail in books on experimental psychology (see Herson & Barlow, 1976; Kazdin, 1980). These experimental and quasi-experimental studies rely on quantitative data. Interestingly, qualitative studies in which a grounded theory is generated frequently reveal phases or stages of interaction and behaviors (see Hutchinson, 1987,1990; Wilson, 1982). When coding domains are used as a step in the ethnographic method, the researcher may choose a key domain that involves a sequence. For example, X is a step in parents' learning to care for a critically ill child. An entire ethnographic study could be based on strategies of caregiving.

Yin (1984), referring to experimental time-series analysis, notes that there are simple time series with one dependent or independent

---

Box 5.12. An Example of a Single Case Time-Series Analysis

In this single case time-series analysis, a severely depressed 56-year-old woman was hospitalized for arrhythmia control. Previously, she had experienced a stroke, a myocardial infarction, and had four recent hospital admissions. In an effort to prepare the patient for open heart surgery, Blyth & Erdahl (1986), clinical social workers, used the three phases of stress inoculation-education and cognitive preparation, skill acquisition, and application training. To evaluate change, a self-report depression inventory and a daily behavioral checklist were used. The test scores revealed marked improvement in levels of depression at each testing point and a marked decrease in the level of disturbed behavior. The authors describe "a clinically significant improvement in the patient's mood and behavior" (Blythe & Erdahl, 1986, p. 272), that were supported by evaluations from the patient, her family, and physicians.

---

variable and more complex time series with more variables and thus a more complex pattern over time. Researchers initiate the study with hypotheses that predict a trend over time or with hypotheses that predict different trends. They are seeking to find the relationship of variables over time. In the more complex studies, different variables may be predicted to have different patterns over time. The aim of time-series analysis is to look for causal inferences. In this way, behavioral changes can be predicted. A quality study requires clearly defined variables and clearly defined time sequences.

Time-series analysis should not be compared with the single case experimental design, also called a case study by some. Time-series analyses used with case studies have no experimental controls (if they did, they would be experimental studies) but rather rely on much anecdotal information. Kazdin (1981) views case studies and experiments on a continuum that reflects the degree to which specifically adequate influences can be shown. Meier and Pugh (1986, p. 198) discuss time-series analysis in single-subject research, which "uses repeated administration, withdrawal and/or modification of the intervention with one subject over time, during which multiple observations of a dependent variable are made" (also Holm, 1983). (See Box 5.12.)

Hayes (1981) notes three general strategies for single case designs: within, between, and combined. The "within" strategy refers to examining one patient over time in response to some intervention. There is one series of data points. For example, a burn patient

receives hypnosis prior to each debriding. "Between" strategies involve two or more series of data points over time. For example,
patients' verbalizations may be measured during the time the nurse
sits in a chair and talks with the patient versus when the nurse stands
up and talks with the patient. Depending on the research question,
the treatments may be done simultaneously or alternately. Combined
strategies use comparisons made between and within a series of
measurements. For example, a patient with severe nutritional problems is offered two types of diet (between) and his family is present
during some meals and not during others (within).

Numerous authors (Barnard, 1983; Hayes, 1981; Holm, 1983; Meier
& Pugh, 1986) advocate the use of the time-series case study for
clinical problem solving. Hayes (1981) advocates that practitioners
examine their practice and make it scientific by (a) taking systematic
repeated measurements, (b) specifying their own treatments, and (c)
recognizing the design strategies they are already using, and, at
times, use existing design elements to improve clinical decision
making (Hayes, 1981, p. 194). Unlike the controlled rigor of experimental designs, the time-series analysis in case studies may have to
be used with practical measures that have little control. To be overly
rigorous in clinical situations is often unrealistic and impossible and
prevents good research from being completed. Flexibility is necessary, including changing the focus or the presumed relevant variables. Hayes called this using "design elements" instead of pure
designs. Creativity is far more important than rigidity. Metzgar and
Schultz (1982, p. 375) state:

> Prediction to the individual from the individual has many implications
> for nursing practice. It allows the uniqueness of the individual concept
> to exist as a basis for nursing care and provides a framework for
> assessing change, not as a deviation from an aggregate mean, but as an
> alteration in a unique but consistent pattern.

A major point in using time-series analysis is that "dense data sets"
are required as the interrelationship of the data is what is important
(see Chapter 4). That is, observations over time cannot be viewed or
analyzed as independent observations but must be seen as a piece of
a pattern. Consequently, this method is, as are all other case study
methods, expensive in time and money. The benefit should be revealed in its predictability of clinical practice and usefulness in
clinical decision making.

Incomplete Modes of Analysis

Yin (1984, pp. 114-118) describes additional modes of analysis that he calls "incomplete" because they must be used along with the dominant modes of pattern matching, explanation building, or time-series analysis. These "lesser" modes include the following:

Analyzing embedded units. A researcher can use any appropriate strategy to analyze a smaller part of the larger study, such as a survey, historical analysis, or a case history. Of importance is that these techniques and the resulting data analysis do not become the focus of the study. Analysis of the embedded units occurs within each case (unlike survey data that is pooled or historical data that derives from numerous informants or documents). The embedded units solve a piece of the research and ultimately must be related to the larger study via the dominant analytic modes.

Making repeated observations. Similar to time-series analysis, this strategy is different because it may occur at different sites or with different cases. It is a "lesser" mode because it contributes one piece of the total information; it alone does not answer the research questions.

Doing a case survey. If numerous case studies are available—not typical as yet in nursing—the researcher develops a survey instrument and uses it with the various case studies; thus it is essentially a cross-case and secondary case analysis. As with the other two lesser modes, the case survey strategy is only a part of the larger study.

Validity/Reliability

The appropriate concerns for case studies—construct, internal and external validity, and reliability—depend on the nature of the design and the methods of analysis. Consequently, the topic of validity and reliability will be subdivided into sections based on the variable types of designs and methods of analysis used in case studies.

Construct validity and internal validity for pattern matching and explanation building. Construct validity in case studies that use pattern matching and explanation building refers to how closely the concepts or framework (in the literature or "discovered" in the data) fit the people, event, or program that was studied. Construct validity in qualitative research is discussed in more detail by numerous authors (Lincoln & Guba, 1985; Sandelowski, 1986), but for our purposes it is important to know that the issue needs to be addressed and that one useful method of checking construct validity is to return to the informants and ask them if the report accurately portrays their world. For example, Sutherland took his manuscript on professional thieves and had the thief who wrote it with him, four other thieves, and two former detectives read it and suggest corrections.

To address internal validity, a researcher looks for rival hypotheses. Patton (1980) suggests that this means searching for other explanatory schemes or other ways to arrange the data that would yield different findings. The idea is not to disprove the alternate hypotheses but to look for data that support them.

Construct validity/reliability for lesser modes of analysis. Each instrument used to analyze embedded units, to make repeated observations, or to do a secondary analysis across cases will need to be assessed for reliability and validity. The standard rules apply.

Reliability in pattern matching and explanation building. Because these data analysis strategies are generally used with qualitative data, the reliability measures of quantitative data are not appropriate. Miles (1979) quotes Guba (1979):

> Certain kinds of reliability must be intentionally violated in order to gain a depth of understanding about the situation (i.e., the observer's behavior must change from subject to subject, unique questions must be asked of different subjects . . . there is an inherent conflict between validity and reliability—the former is what fieldwork is specially qualified to gain, and increased emphasis on reliability will only undermine that unique function.

As mentioned earlier, Lincoln and Guba (1985) propose that terms such as *truth value, applicability, consistency,* and *neutrality* are more appropriate for qualitative research than the terms *reliability* and *validity* that are used to evaluate quantitative research.

Internal validity for time-series analysis. A term used in experimental designs, *internal validity* refers to whether or not manipulation of an independent variable causes changes in the dependent variable(s). Kazdin (1981) points out that, with experimentation, a researcher can rule out threats to internal validity, that is, alternative rival hypotheses. He proposed several ways to increase the internal validity of case studies (Kazdin, 1981, pp. 185-188) that use time-series analysis and thus have to be concerned about alternative hypotheses:

- Type of data: Use objective data and not just anecdotal data. Make the data collection systematic and quantitative as this increases control.

- Assessment occasions: Do not just collect data before or after treatment. Aim for continuous assessment over time before and/or after treatment so as to be sure that it is not the assessment itself that initiates change. If assessments occur prior to treatment, the researcher can make predictions about the future.

- Past and future protections: If behavior is stable over time and if treatments bring changes, the intervention may have caused the change. If the researcher can predict what the problem should be like in the future (e.g., cancer) and if the patient gets better, the treatment was probably responsible. If the problem will probably improve with time (e.g., depression/grief), it is more difficult to evaluate the intervention. Because of the stability of chronic problems, they are easier to evaluate than acute problems.

- Time and effect: If changes occur immediately and dramatically (magnitude) after the intervention, the intervention probably was causal.

- Number and heterogeneity of subjects: The greater the number of subjects and the more heterogeneous the group who respond after intervention, the more likely it is that the intervention caused the change.

See Box 5.13 for an example of inferences drawn from a single case. This case could be evaluated on the previously presented criteria. Kazdin's (1981) criteria for assessing the internal validity of case studies that use time-series analysis are most useful in confronting the problem of rival hypotheses. Researchers need to think about what possible rival hypotheses could account for the results and how they could be studied in the future.

External validity/generalizability. One of the many criticisms of case studies is their lack of generalizability because they are based on one event or one or a few people in a particular place and time. Due to the idiosyncratic nature of the study, generalizability to other populations is considered to be poor. However, as Yin (1984) points out, there is another kind of generalizability—analytic generalizability—that case studies have. The theories and/or conceptual frameworks that are generated in case study research can be used when examining other situations. For example, in one study (Hutchinson, 1983), the substantive theory of "covering" emerged: a self-protective process that prehospital care workers (including nurses) use to survive the uncertainty and visibility inherent in their jobs. "Covering" is described in detail, including its dimensions, properties, and phases.

Box 5.13. An Example of Inferences Drawn from a Single Case

Fetal brain damage is a documented result of phenylketonuric mothers' biochemical abnormalities. Research on pregency in phenylketonuric women and on the fetus after the mother is treated is rare. Farquhar's (1974) study of the baby of a phenylketonuric mother suggests that a fetus may not suffer the brain damage, failure to grow, and malformations if the mother eats a special diet beginning in the twentieth week of gestation. The timing of the diet is significant because introducing the diet in early pregnancy causes extreme nausea and vomiting. Farquhar cautions accepting the findings as final and, due to the severity of the problem, requests replications. Replications help ascertain if the hypotheses about diet and timing of diet explain the events that occurred in this case. Data analysis and interpretation from single cases serve as precursors to theory.

Covering as a process that we all use at one time or another can be applied to other situations, such as working in the emergency room, being a student, or being handicapped. Understanding if and how covering is used in different places and at different times gives us insight into human behavior. Whether covering is relevant or not—that is, is generalizable to multiple situations—is determined by further research. In this way, a body of knowledge is built; our understanding of the theory is expanded by examining it with different cases; and our understanding of different cases is expanded by looking at them in relation to the theory of covering. Nursing science needs to increase its repertoire of relevant theories—what they are and how and where they fit. Analytic generalization is especially useful in generating, expanding, and verifying theories. Processes may be generalizable even if specifics are not.

Stake (1978) suggests that generalizing to a population is not always essential. He advocates "naturalistic generalization," whereby the case study is generalized to a single case. Nurse-clinicians can then determine if a case is generalizable or not. In order to do this, the case study must provide a detailed and complete description. Generalizations from a single case may shed light on a patient's response or nonresponse to an intervention.

Although single-subject case studies, by definition, violate the requirements for generalizability, such as random sampling and a statistical sample of population variability, replications are most useful in moving toward generalizability (Meier & Pugh, 1986). Holm (1983) suggests two levels of replication: (a) selecting subjects with characteristics similar to the original subjects and (b) systematically verifying variables that were previously held constant. Research protocols must be the same with all subjects, and the clinical setting needs to be as constant as possible (Holm, 1983, p. 254).

Ethics

In all case study research, the usual ethical considerations revealed by standardized informed consent apply. Subjects need to be informed of the research purpose and of their right to refuse participation, to withdraw, and to have anonymity and confidentiality, and they must be made aware of possible risks and benefits. However, case study ethics are more complex than those of most research because of the multiple sources of data. Each source of data has ethical considerations, often including different informed and administrative consent. For example, time-series analysis with one patient may necessitate informed consent from the patient, a family member, the physician, and nursing administration. The patient needs to be aware of what the intervention(s) is and if and how it will be varied. Because a time-series analysis case study is less controlled than an experimental design, the ethical issues of withholding treatment at different times may not arise. If they do, they need to be addressed.

Hayes (1981) believes that the involved clinician who is systematically collecting data and varying treatment is more effective and contributes more to patient care than a clinician who is not doing research. Learning from one patient can be transferred to others. On the other hand, a caregiver who is also doing research needs to have sufficient self-awareness to deal with the potential conflict of interest. Decisions such as what treatment to try, when to do it, when to alter it or withdraw it, and how to evaluate it do raise ethical questions.

Due to their complexity, the ethics of interviews and participant observation are examined by numerous authors (Field & Morse, 1985; May, 1979; Wilson, 1989). Munhall (1988) suggests that informed consent in interviews and participant observation is not static, as implied by a form that is signed and then filed away, but is an ongoing process (process consenting). The mutual give-and-take nature of such qualitative research, the complexity of the social environment, and the multiple levels of communication that occur require that the researcher continually assess "ethics." It is the integrity of the researcher and his or her openness to talk with and negotiate with informants about ethical considerations that is the sine qua non of ethical research. Ultimately, and in unusual situations, this may mean not documenting certain events or dialogue and even not publishing a piece of the data analysis (see Becker, 1969). Munhall (1988, p. 6) advocates that, in both quantitative and qualitative research, we start by "reflecting, knowing and bracketing out what our clinical means and ends are." Such clarity about our own motives provides a beginning for the ongoing negotiation and collaboration that need to be a part of all case study research.

For an interesting dialogue about the ethics of a case study, see the final chapter of Viditch and Bensman's (1958) book, *Small Town in Mass Society*. The study aroused so much furor that journal articles and newspaper editorials reported on the case and published a discussion among experts and numerous involved people. As with all ethical problems, there are no easy answers and the ethical problems (e.g., confidentiality, anonymity) that plagued Viditch and Bensman still exist today. Yin (1984) suggests that case studies that report on a single case (individual, unit, institution) are most open to criticism from the participant(s) while case studies that use multiple cases with aggregate, unidentifiable data are more likely to avoid criticism and accusations of unethical behavior from the participants.

Writing up the Case Study

Case studies can be seductive; ideally they are interesting, dramatic, and intellectually stimulating as they portray social phenomena from a new and different perspective. Although there are numerous ways to present case studies, depending on the research question(s) and methods of data analysis, caution is required due to the inherent complexity of case studies. If the necessary precautions were taken throughout—careful documentation of methodological strategies, including changes of focus; organization of different types of data; frequent evaluation of perspective/focus—the write-up should proceed fairly smoothly in spite of the massive and diverse data case studies generate. See Table 5.2 for Lincoln and Guba's (1985) suggestions about the content of a case study report.

Identifying the audience is a critical question. What is the significance of the case study and to whom is it significant? This helps the researcher identify the audience and write to that audience. Yin (1984) reminds us that the report of the case study is excerpted from

TABLE 5.2

Content of the Case Study Report

Aspects	Intention	Implementation	Modification
Substantive Considerations			
Problem			
Context or setting			
Transactions—processes relevant to the problem			
Saliencies—important elements studied in depth			
Outcomes (Lessons)—working hypotheses			
Methodological Considerations (Placed in Appendix)			
Investigator(s)—credentials, biases			
Methods/Design			
Trustworthiness—description of measures to ensure and assess validity, reliability.			

SOURCE: Adapted from Lincoln, Y. and Guba, E. (1985, p. 362).

the vast data base; it is not *the* data base. Patton (1980, p. 304) suggests three steps: (a) assembling the raw case data; (b) constructing a case record in which the data are condensed, organized, and edited; and (c) writing the case study narrative.

As the diverse pieces of data are analyzed, reports can be written, meaning that the final write-up of all the triangulated data often does not begin without fairly complete reports. The methods section may be written throughout the research process; the bibliography should be constantly updated; and data analysis of the qualitative data occurs simultaneously with data collection. Consequently, part of the final report is available, at least in draft form.

Guba and Lincoln (1981, p. 374) discuss the different possibilities for writing the case study report:

- Case studies may be written with different purposes in mind, for example, to chronicle (temporally and sequentially), to render (description), to teach (instructional material), to test (specific theories/hypotheses). A case may have several purposes.

- Case studies may be written at different analytic levels, including a merely factual level, an interpretive level, and an evaluative level.
- Both the researchers' analysis and write-up of the case report will vary according to the purpose and level of the case study. For example, a simple factual chronicle will be analyzed differently and will read much differently than an evaluative study in which the researcher does complex data analysis and makes judgments based on the data.

Studying the structure of published case studies in all disciplines is a way to become knowledgeable about possible structures. In fact, in planning case studies, an awareness of the structures can be inspirational. For example, the structure of Allison's (1971) *Essence of Decision Making* (see Box 5.10) would be ideal for examining a variety of nursing theories and their explanation of a particular clinical problem. Depending on the research question/purpose, a researcher can choose a structure prior to the initiation of the study or can wait until the data are analyzed. In case studies that are explanatory and aim for theory generation, the structure would not be determined until the study's completion. For specific details about varieties of case report structures, see Yin (1984).

The case study report is a major and difficult effort. The aim is to unify the fragments so as to present a clear portrait of a person, event, program, decision, or institution. This is a difficult goal but one that is important for the development of nursing science.

Evaluation of Case Studies

Case studies can be evaluated in part according to the typical criteria for evaluating research.

- Do the research questions/hypotheses have scientific merit? Relevance for nursing science?
- Is the study inductive (to generate theory), deductive (to test theory), or a combination?
- Is the design appropriate for the questions/hypotheses?
- Is the sample appropriate?
- Is the sample size adequate?
- Are the rights of human subjects protected?

- Are data collection strategies explicit, relevant, and appropriate to the research focus?
- Are changes in the research strategies and the rationale for the changes documented?
- Are theoretical and personal biases and assumptions discussed?
- Are the data collection strategies reliable and valid (if quantitative)? Auditable and credible (if qualitative)?
- Are the methods for data analyses clear?
- Are the data analysis methods appropriate to the questions/hypotheses and type of data?
- Are the theoretical, statistical, and clinical significance of the findings discussed?

Along with these more general criteria, case studies, because they often aim to generate theory, require further evaluation criteria that specifically address the quality of the generated theory and the relationship of the theory and the research. When the relationship of theory and research is clear, the differentiations of case histories and case studies can be made. Strauss and Glaser (1970, p. 189) suggest the following questions:

- What is the amount of theory used? Ideally, a solid theory with several key constructs or concepts is generated or is tested in case studies.
- Does the theory work, that is, explain the major behavioral and interactional variations of the substantive area? A quality theory can predict what happens under certain conditions.
- What is the level of generality of the theory? Is the theory a grand or formal theory that is quite abstract or is the theory more substantive, explaining an empirical area of inquiry? Substantive theories are more directly linked to empirical data and, are therefore, easier to test and easier to generate. They tend to be more useful and have clear implications for practice. Abstract theories are more difficult to understand and are less clearly linked to the data.
- What is the source of the theory? Is it derived from logic? Is it a derivation of existing theories in a different area? Is it grounded in data? The more the theory is grounded in data, the more useful and coherent it is.
- What is the degree of systematization of the theory? Is the theory loose, for example, containing bits and pieces from different theories, or is it

well integrated? The aim is for well-integrated theories rather than loose, unsystematized groupings of theoretical propositions.

- Is the theory dense? Or is it "thin"? Dense theories are complex and richly descriptive; thin theories provide inadequate explanations of behavior. Are the analytic constructs supported by the data? Ideally, enough data are used to illuminate and support the constructs. Having too much data is boring, unnecessary, and distracting; having too little is not useful in illustrating the analytic points.

- Is the theory relevant to the social scene under investigation? People in the scene are most important in determining the relevance of a proposed theory. If they say the theory is "right on," then the theory is relevant.

- Is the theory modifiable, that is, able to capture the fluctuating nature of social life? For example, if certain variables are changed, the theory should be able to be altered to fit the group or setting.

- Finally, does the case study do what it set out to do—provide a holistic in-depth study of a complex social phenomenon?

Summary

The case study approach provides a holistic, humanistic, intense, and systematic examination of complex social phenomena. Complex social phenomena are the essence of nursing practice. Consequently, the fit of the method for nursing is clear. Case studies are useful in examining nursing interventions with one or a few patients, in decision making about patient care, in implementation of programs, in extreme or typical cases, and in failures or successes as well as for myriad other problems in nursing practice. This chapter provides a review of the relevant methodological literature, refers the reader to references for further, more detailed study, and offers examples from numerous descriptions that should serve to whet our appetites for the diversity of questions and designs that case studies encourage. In addition, the examples are models, or propositions, that will enable us to increase our research repertoire; to test, modify, extend, and generate theory; and to positively affect nursing practice.

References

Allison, G. (1971). *Essence of decision making: Explaining the Cuban missile crisis.* Boston: Little, Brown.

Barnard, K. (1983). The case study method: A research tool. *MCN, 8*(1), 36.

Becker, H. (1969). Problems in the publication of field studies. In G. McCall & J. Simmons (Eds.), *Issues in participant observation* (pp. 260-288). Menlo Park, CA: Addison-Wesley.

Blake, F. (1964). *Open heart surgery in children* (Public Health Service publication no. 2075). Washington, DC: Public Health Service.

Blyth, B., & Erdhl, J. (1986). Using stress inoculation to prepare a patient for open-heart surgery. *Health and Social Work, 11*(4), 265-274.

Breo, D. (1989). Confronting the rarest AIDS infection, a young man makes a cry from the heart. *Journal of the American Medical Association, 262*(10), 1383-1387.

Chinn, P. (Ed.). (1986). *Nursing research methodology: Issues and implementation.* Rockville, MD: Aspen.

DeGroot, M. (1988). Scientific inquiry in nursing: A model for a new age. *Advances in Nursing Science, 10*(3), 1-21.

Diers, D. (1979). *Research in nursing practice.* Philadelphia: J. B. Lippincott.

Durand, B. (1975). A clinical nursing study: Failure to thrive in a child with Down's syndrome. *Nursing Research, 24*(4), 272-286.

Erikson, E. (1960). Youth and the life cycle. *Children, 7,* 43-49.

Farquhar, J. (1974). Baby of a phenylketonuric mother. *Archives of Diseases in Childhood, 49,* 205-208.

Fawcett, J. (1984). *Analysis and evaluation of conceptual models of nursing.* Philadelphia: F. A. Davis.

Festinger, L., Reichen, H., & Schechter, S. (1956). *When prophecy fails.* Minneapolis: University of Minnesota Press.

Field, P., & Morse, J. (1985). *Nursing research, the application of qualitative approaches.* Rockville, MD: Aspen.

Freud, S. (1938). *The basic writings of Sigmund Freud.* New York: Modern Library.

Gans, H. (1962). *The urban villagers.* New York: Free Press.

Glaser, B. (1978). *Theoretical sensitivity.* Mill Valley, CA: Sociology Press.

Glaser, B., & Strauss A. (1967). *The discovery of grounded theory.* Chicago: Aldine.

Guba, E. (1979). *Investigative journalism as a metaphor for educational evaluation.* Unpublished paper written for Northwest Regional Educational Laboratory, Portland, OR.

Guba, E., & Lincoln, Y. (1981). *Effective evaluation.* San Francisco: Jossey-Bass.

Hayes, S. C. (1981). Single case experimental designs and empirical clinical practice. *Journal of Consulting and Clinical Psychology, 49*(2), 193-211.

Herson, M., & Barlow, D. (1976). *Single-case experimental designs: Strategies for studying behavior.* New York: Pergamon.

Holm, K. (1983). Single subject research. *Nursing Research, 32*(4), 253-255.

Hutchinson, S. (1983). *Survival practices of rescue workers: Hidden dimensions of watchful readiness.* Lanham, MD: University Press of America.

Hutchinson, S. (1986). Chemically dependent nurses: The trajectory toward self-annihilation. *Nursing Research, 35,* 196-201.

Hutchinson, S. (1987). Toward self-integration: The recovery process of chemically dependent nurses. *Nursing Research, 36,* 339-343.

Hutchinson, S. (1990). Responsible subversion: A study of rule bending among nurses. *Scholarly Inquiry for Nursing Practice: An International Journal, 4*(1), 3-17.

Kayser-Jones, J., & Kapp, M. (1989). Advocacy for the mentally impaired elderly: A case study analysis. *American Journal of Law & Medicine, 14*(4), 353-376.

Kazdin, A. (1980). *Research design in clinical psychology.* New York: Harper & Row.

Kazdin, A. (1981). Drawing valid influences from case studies. *Journal of Consulting and Clinical Psychology, 49*(2), 183-192.

Lijphart, A. (1971). Comparative politics and the comparative method. *American Political Science Review, 65*, 682-693.

Lincoln, Y., & Guba, E. (1985). *Naturalistic inquiry.* Beverly Hills, CA: Sage.

Lynd, R., & Lynd, H. (1929). *Middletown.* New York: Harcourt, Brace & World.

Mace, N., & Rabins, P. (1981). *The 36-hour day: A family guide to caring for persons with Alzheimer's disease, related dementing illnesses, and memory loss in later life.* Baltimore, MD: Johns Hopkins University Press.

Martinson, I. (1976). *Home care for the dying child: Professional and family perspectives.* New York: Appleton-Century-Crofts.

May, K. (1979). The nurse as a researcher: Impediment to informed consent? *Nursing Outlook, 26*, 36-39.

Meier, P., & Pugh, E. J. (1986). The case study: A viable approach to clinical research. *Research in Nursing and Health, 9*, 195-202.

Metzgar, B., & Schultz, P. (1982). Time series analysis: An alternative for nursing. *Nursing Research, 31*(6), 375-378.

Miles, M. (1979). Qualitative data as an attractive nuisance: The problem of analysis. *Administrative Science Quarterly, 24*, 590-601.

Mishel, M., & Murdaugh, C. (1987). Family adjustment to heart transplantation: Redesigning the dream. *Nursing Research, 36*(6), 332-338.

Moody, L., & Hutchinson, S. (1989). Relating your study to a theoretical context. In H. Wilson (Ed.), *Research in nursing* (pp. 275-332). Menlo Park, CA: Addison-Wesley.

Munhall, P. (1988). Ethical considerations in qualitative research. *Western Journal of Nursing Research, 10*(2), 150-162.

Neustadt, R. (1960). *Presidential power.* New York: John Wiley.

Oleson, V., & Whittaker, E. (1968). *The silent dialogue.* San Francisco: Jossey-Bass.

Parse, R. R. (1987). *Nursing science major paradigms: Theories and critiques.* Philadelphia: W. B. Saunders.

Patton, M. (1980). *Qualitative evaluation methods.* Beverly Hills, CA: Sage.

Romero, P. (Ed.). (1988). *Life histories of African women.* London: Ashfield.

Roth, J. (1963). *Timetables.* New York: Bobbs-Merrill.

Roueche', B. (1947). *Eleven blue men.* Boston: Little, Brown.

Sandelowski, M. (1986). The problem of rigor in qualitative research. *Advances in Nursing Science, 8*(3), 27-37.

Schatzman, L., & Strauss, A. (1982). *Field research.* Englewood Cliffs, NJ: Prentice-Hall.

Schultz, P., & Kerr, B. (1986). Comparative case study as a strategy for nursing research. In P. Chinn (Ed.), *Nursing research methodology: Issues and implementation* (pp. 195-220). Rockville, MD: Aspen.

Shaw, C. (1967). *The jackroller.* Chicago: University of Chicago Press.

Skinner, B. (1959). *Cumulative record.* New York: Appleton-Century-Crofts.

Spindler, G., & Spindler, L. (1978). *Urban anthropology in the United States: Four cases.* New York: Holt, Rinehart & Winston.

Spradley, J. (1980). *Participant observation.* New York: Holt, Rinehart & Winston.

Spradley, J., & Mann, B. (1975). *The cocktail waitress, woman's work in a man's world.* New York: John Wiley.

Stake, R. (1978). The case study method in social inquiry. *Educational Researcher, 7*(1), 5-8.

Stinson, R., & Stinson, P. (1979). *The long dying of baby Andrew.* Boston: Little, Brown.

Strauss, A. (1987). *Qualitative analysis for social scientists.* New York: Cambridge University Press.

Strauss, A., & Glaser, B. (1970). *Anguish: A case history of a dying trajectory.* Mill Valley, CA: Scientology.

Sutherland, E. (1937). *The professional thief.* Chicago: University of Chicago.

Viditch, A., & Bensman, J. (1958). *Small town in mass society.* Princeton, NJ: Princeton University Press.

Waltz, C., & Bausell, R. (1981). *Nursing research: Design, statistics, & computer analysis.* Philadelphia: F. A. Davis.

Watson, L., & Watson-Franke, M. (1985). *Interpreting life histories: An anthropological inquiry.* New Brunswick, NJ: Rutgers University Press.

Weppner, R. (1983). *The untherapeutic community.* Lincoln: University of Nebraska Press.

Wilson, H. (1982). *Deinstitutionalized residential care for the mentally disordered.* New York: Grune & Stratton.

Wilson, H. (1986). Presencing—social control of schizophrenics in an antipsychiatric community: Doing grounded theory. In P. Munhall & C. Oiler (Eds.), *Nursing research: A qualitative perspective* (pp. 131-144). Norwalk, CT: Appleton-Century-Crofts.

Wilson, H. (1989). *Research in nursing* (2nd ed.). Menlo Park, CA: Addison-Wesley.

Wolcott, H. (1967). *A Kwakiutl village and school.* New York: Holt, Rinehart & Winston.

Woods, N., & Cantanzaro, M. (1988). *Nursing research: Theory and practice.* St. Louis: C. V. Mosby.

Yin, R. (1981). The case study crises: Some answers. *Administrative Science Quarterly, 198a*(26), 58-66.

Yin, R. (1984). *Case study research: Design and methods.* Beverly Hills, CA: Sage.

6

Foundational Inquiry

JUDITH BAIGIS-SMITH

The aim and value of foundational inquiry consists of making issues clearer.

In this chapter, an explanation of foundational inquiry is presented and a research agenda for foundational issues in nursing is suggested. The chapter is organized around the following key ideas and concepts: (a) what foundational inquiry is, (b) an analytic approach to foundational inquiry, (c) a synthetic approach to foundational inquiry, and (d) foundational issues in nursing such as these: What is health? What is the relationship between health and culture? Is nursing a science? And the question of the nature of diagnosis.

Foundational inquiry can be approached analytically or synthetically. The common feature for either approach is an emphasis on clarity and argumentation. The aim and value of foundational research consists in making issues clearer.

Analytic Approach

As the name implies, this approach involves analyzing the phenomenon, the issue, or the situation into components that are simpler or at least clearer. Such analysis could then clarify the problem as a whole. Consider, for example, the issues surrounding drug testing.

We can determine upon analysis that these issues ought to be separated into (a) issues of health and safety and (b) issues of criminality. Answers to questions concerning health and safety may not be answers to questions concerning criminality. Assessing drug-testing proposals or programs would need to be separated into at least two sets of concerns. Once its most important components are analyzed, methods to resolve or at least address the problem rationally and logically should be forthcoming.

Synthetic Approach

While the analytic approach examines the components of the problem, the synthetic approach, in contrast, tries to characterize the overall structure of the problem by identifying broad general features it shares with other problems. For example, human immunodeficiency virus (HIV) infection can be viewed as part of the more general phenomenon of disabling or handicapping conditions. People who test seropositive for HIV are then seen as disabled or potentially disabled or handicapped. Within this context, they are eligible for the same kind of protection provided other disabled or handicapped people. They can then be treated in the schools and the workplace as any other disabled or handicapped people are. They should not be thrown out of either setting just because they are HIV antibody positive. In this approach, arguments will often turn on the usefulness of the proposed analogy. The usefulness of the analogy is judged according to the light it sheds on the problem that generated the inquiry. Furthermore, because analogies are only analogies, one may need to show that certain features of the problem under examination are unimportant. Thus, according to the above example, the mechanisms or nature of HIV infection are not important features for proper social treatment of the disease; what is important is only that it is a debilitating, impairing condition.

Foundational inquiry, and qualitative research generally, are done when quantitative methods are not useful or applicable or appropriate. Important questions need to be addressed in nursing, but such questions will not always be answerable using the methods of quantitative inquiry. I'll outline several issues that I think are foundational issues for nursing and suggest either the analytic or the synthetic approach in exploring them.

Foundational Issues for Nursing

What Is Health?

The major issue for nursing is this: What constitutes health? Health is one of four concepts viewed as central to the development of nursing knowledge (Crowley, 1985; Fawcett, 1978; Newman, 1983), and so it is a directive aim in nursing practice. Yet there are a variety of definitions of *health* that vary according to the perspective of the respondent. Health is, for example, viewed in terms of physiology, *health* being thus defined as the optimal functioning of organ systems (Boorse, 1977). It is also viewed psychologically, *health* being thus defined as positive self-concept and self-esteem. There are also a variety of definitions that emphasize ideas, such as high-level wellness, well-being, and expanding consciousness (Dunn, 1961; Newman, 1986). How can such a problem be clarified (see Box 6.1)?

The clarification of the idea of health using the analytic approach can be undertaken (a) by resolving the multiple views of health into a small number of distinctive concepts, and, if possible (b), by reconciling seeming differences among the ideas. I've used this approach in my previous work (Smith, 1981, 1983, 1988) to identify and assess four ideas of health that I consider to underlie the four important models of health. All of the ways that health professionals might think of health can be resolved into these four types or models of health. They are called the clinical model, the role-performance model, the adaptive model, and the eudaimonistic model of health.

The clinical model is accepted as the directive aim of much of contemporary nursing and medical practice. When relief from pain is attained and the signs and symptoms of disease are no longer present in the body or mind, the task of medicine is complete. The patient is restored to health.

Health as role-performance has social and psychological dimensions. The role-performance model requires people to be socially fit. Accordingly, people who assume a role in society and fulfill the requirements of that role are healthy.

The adaptive model requires that people possess capacity for adjustment to changing circumstances through growth, expansion, and creativity. Thus the adaptive model views people in relation to their social and natural environments, and health signifies the effective functioning of these systems.

The eudaimonistic conception of health extends the idea of health to embrace capacities and activities in cultural enterprises such as

Box 6.1. Abstract: The Idea of Health (Smith, 1986)

Based on intensive studies of the relevant literature (readings highlighting the seminal issues on health in nursing, medicine, public health, and philosophy), I have identified what I consider to be the four important ideas of human health. All of the ways professionals in the health sciences (nursing, medicine, social work, physical therapy, and so on) may think of health can be resolved into these four types or models of health. These four models differ mainly in the degree to which they engage not merely the physiological but also the social and psychological qualities of life. The four models of health are the clinical model, role-performance model, adaptive model, and eudaimonistic model.

An analysis and critical appraisal of these four concepts of health were undertaken through an examination of the representative literature. Thus the clinical model was explored insofar as it is implicit in much of medical practice, through current critical studies of the limitations of this model. The role-performance model was studied through some of the writings of Talcott Parsons and others. The study of the adaptive model focused on the writings of Rene Dubos, and the examination of the eudaimonistic model of health was focused on the writings of Abraham Maslow. This foundational inquiry regarding the "idea of health" provides direction for future scientific work.

music, art, and religion. This idea describes the healthy person as the self-actualizing, fulfilled and fulfilling, loving personality.

These ideas of health are presented as four ways of conceiving the health-illness continuum and as four models of health care. These models were chosen because of their significance as directive ideas in the practice of health professionals and because they play a significant role in the writings of a number of important contemporary researchers. One outcome of the inquiry was the recognition of the progressively inclusive character of these four ideas of health. It appears that the eudaimonistic model of health embraces the concerns of the other three and can be viewed as an ideal of human health. The clarification of the idea of health can provide direction for the development of programs of empirical research (see Box 6.2).

What Is the Relation Between Health and Culture?

Any analysis of the idea of health cannot be separated from considerations of the variations in that idea due to cultural mores. To explore such diversities in the health-illness concept, it would be

---

Box 6.2. Directions for Future Research (Smith, 1986)

- Phase I: Development of a survey questionnaire containing items that tap each of the four models of health as well as items related to demographic variables known to be correlated with each model of health.
- Phase II: Survey of health professionals and their patients to determine their primary conceptions of health and the relation of their conceptions to clinical activities and treatment outcomes.
- Phase III: Nationwide survey of various ethnic and racial groups representative of the United States population, to determine their conceptions of health and their health status as measured by variables reflecting all four models of health.
- Phase IV: Use of methods of health education to reorient individuals in schools and communities to a broadened and more progressive conception of human health.
- Phase V: Resampling of selected groups following health education programs to determine any changes in health status and conceptions of health.

---

useful to consider illness in three dimensions: (a) the recognition of a condition as illness, (b) the treatment approved within a culture or cultural subgroup, and (c) the person accepted as the healer within that culture (Smith, 1986).

(1) Anthropological and sociological studies have disclosed numerous instances of cultural diversity in the practice of "medicine." Conditions of the body that in Western European culture would at once be identified as illness are tolerated as normal, that is, healthy states, among other peoples of the world (Paul, 1955). Such disparities have been reported even among different economic and educational strata of technologically advanced societies (Koos, 1954). Illnesses that are present at a high incidence in a population tend to be regarded as normal and tolerable. In other words, they are regarded as a kind of healthy condition (Strole et al., 1962).

(2) It is well known that, in so-called primitive cultures, the treatment of illness often includes some form of magic as well as certain techniques based on knowledge and experience of the folk culture. A full understanding of such primitive medicine requires some fine distinctions between magic and empirical techniques. But the need to make these distinctions, which Malinowski (1948) explored with reference to his Polynesian studies, is not confined to these remote

"primitive" societies. Similar patterns of culture may be detected among certain strata of advanced societies (Montagu, 1957). A number of institutionalized religions whose doctrines are based on a supernaturalistic worldview continue to function in modern technological civilizations. Many of them impose upon their worshipers certain restrictions and prohibitions on food, dress, and behavior that may deviate or conflict with the practice of scientific medicine. Thus the doctrines of the Jehovah's Witnesses are in opposition to blood transfusions. Christian Science is viewed by its followers as a system of divine healing and in it disease is regarded as an erroneous appearance or an illusion that can be dispelled by spiritual understanding and faith in the scriptures or word of God. Christian Scientists thereby dispense with or reject scientific medical therapy.

(3) It is not uncommon even in highly civilized societies to find sick people seeking relief through the services of a priest, a "reader," or a mystical transcendental guru as an alternative to a scientific medical practitioner. The occasionally reported cures effected by these nonscientific healers tend to encourage confidence in their services.

An analysis of the differences among science, magic, and religion in relation to medicine is appropriate here, along with consideration of the problems entailed in more effective popular medical and health education in cultivating the ideals of community health.

Is Nursing a Science?

This kind of question explores the status of nursing. At a high level of abstraction, nursing is an organized effort to secure a good end for human life. This may be one of the aims of practice. Without such an aim, nursing practice is untargeted and, perhaps, fruitless. In exploring this question, it would be useful to analyze the characteristics of a science and to show how nursing does or does not meet them. If nursing is a science, what kind of a science is it? What are the problems it addresses, that is, what are the "scientific" problems in nursing? What kinds of problems (social, economic) are not addressed by this conception of nursing as a science? If medicine is a relationship of healing prompted by a need (Pellegrino & Thomasma, 1981, p. 173), as well as a science of practice with a set of principles governing healing, what is the science of nursing?

In raising this kind of question, one would need to show how this question is not simply one concerning professional status but one concerning more serious problems having to do with the relationship between nursing and other disciplines like physiology, biology, and psychology.

What Is the Nature of Diagnosis?

The synthetic approach of foundational inquiry can be used to clarify the nature of diagnosis by showing that it is a procedure that conforms to the hypothetical-deductive method of scientific inquiry. Diagnosis follows the patterns of scientific method in explaining some observed fact. The problem is to account for or find the cause of the observed sign and symptom of disease. This procedure calls for the invocation of as many plausible hypotheses as possible. A final decision is made in favor of the hypothesis that best meets the further tests of the inquiry. Each of the hypotheses involves a conception of some disease. But such conceptions need not apply only to the clinical model of health and disease mentioned above but to the other models as well. Hypotheses are drawn from the fund of knowledge that the clinician has of various diseases. In some instances, none of the hypotheses fits the observed facts. In that case, the clinician is faced with a new disease for which a new structure has to be invented.

A person generally seeks care under two conditions: (a) a person has a complaint or some abnormality and the clinician tries to explain its cause—this is clearly a problem-solving situation—or (b) a person goes to a clinician and asks to be told what condition he or she is in. In this instance, the clinician tries to determine if there are any abnormalities. If there are, the clinician is back to the first case—trying to explain causes. Within this context, then, one must be able to show that diagnosis is a form of problem solving that reflects scientific inquiry.

Conclusion

Because the crucial features of both the analytic and the synthetic approaches to foundational inquiry are argument and clarity, good background preparation for this work consists in recognizing the standard logical fallacies and in knowing why they are bad arguments (Fearnside & Holther, 1959). I'll give one example of a logical fallacy.

In the genetic fallacy, one confuses the justification for a position with the motivation for holding that position. In this fallacy, one can, for example, argue against the holder of the argument rather than the argument itself. To criticize Freudian theory by pointing to Freud's neuroses is an example of the genetic fallacy. Freud could have all kinds of neuroses; nevertheless, his views may be true. The genetic fallacy is an irrelevant criticism of a position and the proper response to it is "so what?"

Summary

There are a number of ways that foundational inquiry can contribute to advancing nursing science and theories for nursing practice. Foundational inquires are undertaken with the aim of clarifying ideas central to nursing and can be useful in developing programs of empirical research. As in all research methods, there are accepted standards for conducting foundational inquiries so that they will be accepted within a discipline's community of scholars.

Point-Counterpoint

(1) Identify two foundational issues in nursing and discuss how you might proceed with the analysis. Which approach would you use, analytic or synthetic?

(2) Review the article by Rodgers (1989) and Chapter 5 in Volume 1. How is concept analysis different from and similar to foundational inquiry.

(3) Review the study published by Smith (1986), focusing especially on the recommendations made for future directions for research (see Box 6.2). What other recommendations might be made? Also review the Laffrey (1986) Health Conception Scale, which was based on the four models of health identified by Smith. Critique the tests and development of this instrument. With what populations might this instrument best be used?

References

Boorse, C. (1977). Health as a theoretical concept. *Philosophy of Science, 44,* 542-573.

Crowley, M. E. (1985). Toward greater specificity in defining nursing's metaparadigm. *Advances in Nursing Science, 7*(4), 73-81.

Dunn, H. L. (1961). *High-level wellness.* Arlington, VA: R. W. Beatty.

Fawcett, J. (1978). The "what" of theory development. In the National League for Nursing, *Theory development, what, why, how?* New York: National League for Nursing.

Fearnside, W. W., & Holther, W. B. (1959). *Fallacy—the counterfeit of argument*. Engle-wood Cliffs, NJ: Prentice-Hall.

Koos, E. (1954). *The health of Regionville: What the people thought and did about it*. New York: Columbia University Press.

Laffrey, S. C. (1986). Development of a health conception scale. *Research in Nursing and Health, 9*, 107-113.

Malinowski, B. (1948). *Magic, science and religion and other essays*. Glencoe, IL: Free Press.

Montagu, M. F. A. (1957). *Anthropology and human nature*. Boston: Porter Sargent.

Newman, M. A. (1983). The continuing revolution: A history of nursing science. In N. L. Chaska (Ed.), *The nursing profession: A time to speak* (pp. 385-393). New York: McGraw-Hill.

Newman, M. A. (1986). *Health as expanding consciousness*. St. Louis: C. V. Mosby.

Paul, B. D. (1955). *Health, culture, and community*. New York: Russell Sage.

Pellegrino, E., & Thomasma, D. C. (1981). *A philosophical basis of medical practice*. New York: Oxford University Press.

Rodgers, B. (1989). Concepts, analysis and the development of nursing knowledge: The evolutionary cycle. *Journal of Advanced Nursing, 14*, 330-335.

Smith, J. A. (1981). The idea of health. *Advances in Nursing Science, 3*(3), 43-50.

Smith, J. A. (1983). *The idea of health: Implications for the nursing professional*. New York: Columbia University, Teachers College Press.

Smith, J. A. (1986). The idea of health: An example of foundational inquiry. In P. Munhall & C. Oiler (Eds.), *Nursing research: A qualitative perspective*. New York: Appleton-Century-Crofts.

Smith, J. B. (1988). Public health and the quality of life. *Journal of Family and Community Health, 10*(4), 49-57.

Strole, L., Langner, T. S., Michael, S. T., Oplen, M. K., & Rennie, T. (1962). *Mental health in the metropolis: The midtown Manhattan study*. New York: McGraw-Hill.

7

Hermeneutic Inquiry

JANICE L. THOMPSON

The person with understanding does not know and judge as one who stands apart and unaffected but rather as one united by a specific bond with the other.

—Gadamer (1975)

The purpose of this chapter is to provide a brief introduction to hermeneutic philosophy and to discuss the application of hermeneutics in nursing research. This chapter explores philosophical hermeneutics as a contemporary philosophy that is beginning to shape nurses' understanding of research, education, and practice. Like other philosophies, hermeneutics expresses a Western worldview about knowledge, understanding, experience, and inquiry. But hermeneutics offers different insights about the relationship between inquiry and practice, about the links between understanding and action, and thus addresses questions that are central to nursing. As a philosophy, hermeneutics joins other contemporary schools of thought in providing us with both time-honored and radically new understandings of the research process.

AUTHOR'S NOTE: I wish to thank David Allen, Nancy Diekelmann, and Patricia Benner for their careful reading and assistance with this work.

Nursing and Hermeneutics in the 1980s

The term "philosophical hermeneutics" is not commonly used in nursing contexts, and, even among nurses who have a strong background in philosophy, this field may not be well known. This is understandable because, until the 1970s, discussions of hermeneutics were concentrated in the humanities, appearing primarily in Continental philosophy, theology, and literary criticism. But, beginning in the 1970s, there were increasing references to hermeneutics in research methods literature found in the social sciences. This methodological literature discussed hermeneutics as a philosophy that redefines the scope and nature of the social sciences (Bauman, 1978; Bernstein, 1976; Polkinghorne, 1983; Ricoeur, 1981). In these discussions, social scientists argued that their disciplines could not rely on empiricism for an adequate philosophical foundation. Interpretive sociology and social anthropology were two fields that saw in hermeneutics an alternative philosophy, one that could provide an appropriate self-understanding for their approaches to human experience.

In this methodological literature, hermeneutics was recognized as a philosophy that supports an interpretive approach to people through research methods that focus on meaning and understanding in context (Geertz, 1979; Mischler, 1979). These discussions in the social sciences were part of a growing controversy in the United States that struggled with the limits of empiricism and the need for philosophical alternatives in the human studies. Because nurses practiced and studied during these years, we have been affected by these discussions, and they have come to inform our understanding of our own research agenda.

The growing interest in hermeneutics in nursing may seem puzzling to scholars in the humanities and other fields. But among practitioners in applied disciplines and among scholars in the social sciences, the turn to hermeneutic philosophy has occurred as part of a larger crisis that has seriously challenged the authority of positivism as an adequate philosophical grounding for both science and practice.

> The "crisis" in contemporary social science . . . has become the necessary starting point for all works on contemporary social and political theory. But . . . it is by no means self-evident what that crisis is, or how it should be characterized. Although attacks on positivist social science and proposals for alternative conceptions have become commonplace in the

literature of social and political theory, no resolution of the debate has been forthcoming. . . . The positivist research program in the social sciences that has been seriously discredited in recent decades still serves as the basis for most social scientific research. It has not been replaced by any of the alternative programs that have been proposed, first, because no unanimity exists as to which of these alternatives should be adopted and secondly, because none of these alternatives offers what appears to social scientists to be a viable methodology for social scientific research. As a result, as many have argued, the social sciences are cast adrift without a theoretical anchor. (Hekman, 1986, p. 1)

This erosion of positivism has occurred across a broad range of disciplines, including nursing, in part as a result of other postmodern philosophies, such as feminism, critical theory, and deconstruction. These are contemporary schools of thought that critique empiricist assumptions in science and view the rise of scientism as a distorted cultural phenomenon. One outcome of this cultural critique of empiricist science has been a turn to other philosophical traditions and a renewed interest in what other philosophies have to say to nursing about knowledge and inquiry.

During the 1980s, interest in hermeneutics has grown steadily, and now, hermeneutic philosophy is cited as an important philosophical alternative to empiricist and historicist accounts of science (Hekman, 1986). The implications of this historical development are important, because they suggest that hermeneutics may be emerging not just as a philosophy that applies to the humanities and to some social sciences but as a philosophy that applies equally to the philosophy of the natural sciences and to practice disciplines. In the last decade, for example, the following hermeneutic insights have been identified in the philosophy of science.

In contemporary reexaminations of the social disciplines there has been a recovery of the hermeneutical dimension, with its thematic emphasis on understanding and interpretation. This is also what has been happening in the postempiricist philosophy and history of science. . . . There is, however, a much stronger and much more consequential sense in which the hermeneutic dimension of science has been recovered. In the critique of naive and even of sophisticated forms of logical positivism and empiricism; in the questioning of the claims of the primacy of the hypothetical-deductive model of explanation; in the questioning of the sharp dichotomy that has been made between observation and theory (or observational and theoretical language); in the insistence on the underdetermination of theory by fact; and in the exploration of the ways

in which all description and observation are theory-impregnated, we
find claims and arguments that are consonant with those that have been
at the very heart of hermeneutics. (Bernstein, 1983, p. 301)

In nearly all these more recent references, hermeneutic philosophy is cited as a philosophy that provides us with an alternative view
of science itself and with a different understanding of inquiry in
general.

Discussions like these, which have identified the relevance of
hermeneutics in the philosophy of science, have been matched in
individual disciplines, where methodologists have also identified
the relevance of the hermeneutic philosophy for research activity
within their respective fields. For example, in their critique of positivism, educators Lincoln and Guba (1985, p. 7) identified hermeneutics (along with other philosophies) as an alternative paradigm that
is changing contemporary understandings of science.

This book describes an alternative paradigm that . . . is now traveling
under the name "naturalistic." It has other aliases as well, for example:
the postpositivistic, ethnographic, phenomenological, subjective, case
study, qualitative, hermeneutic, humanistic.

And in her feminist critique of gender and science, Ruth Bleier
(1984, p. 202) referred to hermeneutics in a similar way when she
noted that

other philosophies and methods—Hegelian dialectics, Marxist dialectical materialism, phenomenology, hermeneutics—also appreciate the realities of change, interconnectedness, and contextuality, but they are not
modes of thought that are part of mainstream biological and social
science. . . . women's experiences of life generally engender such modes
of thought.

In recent years, several nurses have also identified the relevance
of hermeneutics as a philosophy that has important implications for
nursing research (Allen, Diekelmann, & Benner, 1986; Benner, 1984a,
1985; Leonard, 1989; Reeder, 1989; Thompson, 1985). The progression
to hermeneutics in nursing has occurred through a steady development of philosophical work within the discipline, where nurses have
continued to reflect about the nature of practice and the kind of
inquiry that is appropriately linked to practice in this postempiricist
era. Over the last two decades, this work has produced a growing

self-consciousness within the discipline. Nurses now critically reflect about their role in corporate structures, about their contributions in formulating and evaluating health policy, about the nature of their work and the kind of practical knowledge it requires, and about the kind of research that can adequately inform and transform practice. In this reflexivity, and through this historical development, nurses have joined others in critiquing the politics of prevailing worldviews and exploring alternative perspectives as guides for research and practice.

The Relevance of Hermeneutics for Nursing Research

A discussion of hermeneutics is an appropriate part of nursing research texts, because, in recent years, hermeneutics has emerged as a contemporary philosophy that has significant methodological implications for any field of inquiry (Hekman, 1986). In nursing, the turn to hermeneutics and other philosophies has been part of a larger interest in alternative viewpoints and alternative research methods (Moccia, 1986; Morse, 1989; Munnhall & Oiler-Boyd, 1986). For example, one of the most well-known research applications of hermeneutic philosophy has appeared in the work of Patricia Benner (1984a), who draws on hermeneutic philosophy in her investigations of expert practice. In nursing education, Nancy Diekelmann (1988) has also drawn on hermeneutic philosophy in her discussion of curriculum reform.

The emergence of hermeneutic discourse in nursing research is a natural consequence of academic and social processes. Increasingly, insights from hermeneutic philosophy and other Continental schools of thought have found their way into many fields of inquiry. As nurses participate in academic settings, we have been and will continue to be exposed to discussions of hermeneutics in topics as diverse as the development of social theory, the philosophy of science, methods of criticism, and practical competence or skill acquisition. In the last 15 years, hermeneutics has emerged as a postmodern philosophy that speaks to or informs a broad range of existential issues. It is, therefore, understandable that hermeneutic philosophy would have found recent applications in nursing research.

Although hermeneutics did not begin as a philosophy of science, in recent years, scholars have drawn on hermeneutic insights in discussions that are beginning to alter our understanding of the philosophy of science (Bernstein, 1983; Hekman, 1986; Hesse, 1980). These applications show that hermeneutic philosophy is an important contributor in the postmodern critique of logical empiricism. Like recent feminist criticism (Bleier, 1986; Harding, 1986) and like American historicist and neopragmatic accounts of science (Kuhn, 1977; Lauden, 1984; Rorty, 1979, 1982), hermeneutic philosophy emphasizes the social and historical nature of inquiry and argues that understanding cannot be separated from the social interests and standpoints we assume. This is why hermeneutic philosophy has maintained its link with practical philosophy and with Aristotle's notions of *praxis* and *phronesis* (Arendt, 1958; Gadamer, 1975; Lobkowicz, 1967). These schools of thought, like the sociology of knowledge, maintain that knowledge and understanding cannot be separated from application (Bernstein, 1983, p. 38) or from the interests and standpoints we assume as a result of being cultural agents. Our interests are always showing up in the questions we ask, in the concepts we use, in the methods we choose. The development of knowledge and understanding then cannot be reduced to the accumulation of technical expertise through facts. Rather, the hermeneutic account of inquiry reminds us of the ways in which inquiry is affected by the political and ethical standpoints we internalize as a result of being cultural agents. This insight links the hermeneutic account of inquiry to practice disciplines (Polkinghorne, 1988) and shows why hermeneutics has been appropriated by fields other than the humanities.

In nursing, the study of hermeneutics is an important addition to the socialization of researchers for many reasons. Like any good philosophy, hermeneutics helps us to better understand ourselves. It is a good philosophy for nurses because it avoids many of the patriarchal biases inherent in Western philosophies. It avoids Cartesian dualism. It shows us that human understanding is limited and conditioned by our social interests, our values, our language and concepts, and our time in history. It helps us to understand research not so much as a "logocentric" activity but as an extension of the ways we live or have our being in the world. Hermeneutics is also an important background for nurse-researchers because it helps us to better understand the decisions we make in the process of doing research as value laden and interest bound. It emphasizes the social, political, and ethical dimensions of each and every step of the research process, and, therefore, it can lead to more insightful, more reflective, and, hopefully, more liberating kinds of research (Lather, 1986; Wolff, 1975).

Hermeneutic philosophy has long informed many interpretive approaches in research, including grounded theory, symbolic interactionism, ethnography, ethnomethodology, historical research, and phenomenology. It is, therefore, an important background for nurse-researchers who maintain methodological commitments to interpretive research methods. And, finally, hermeneutic philosophy has in recent years paralleled some feminist scholarship in its critique of scientism and its explication of patriarchal bias in scientific method (Bowles, 1984). Reading in hermeneutic philosophy can help nurse-researchers deal with the linkages between one's philosophy of science, one's methodological commitments, and the actual practice of doing research (Harding, 1986). In the experience of many nurses, it may be important to discover that hermeneutics is a philosophical tradition that is consistent with alternative points of view and with alternative research methods. Hermeneutics may then be seen as an important successor to empiricism as a philosophy that informs different understandings of the research process in nursing.

In recent years, several texts have appeared that trace important developments in the history of hermeneutic philosophy (Bleicher, 1980; Howard, 1982; Palmer, 1969; Wachterhauser, 1986). These works and others are important reading for nurses who are interested in hermeneutics. References at the end of this chapter list sources that may be helpful in understanding the hermeneutic tradition.

Background and Evolution of Hermeneutics

The term *hermeneutics* has historically been associated with the theory and practice of interpretation. As an academic discipline, hermeneutics first developed within the field of theology during the Renaissance and Reformation. During these centuries, *hermeneutics* referred to the theory and practice of biblical exegesis, especially to the principles and methods used by Protestant theologians to interpret biblical texts (Mueller-Vollmer, 1985, p. 2).

Formerly, "hermeneutics" referred to theory and practice of interpretation. It was a skill one acquired by learning how to use the instruments of history, philology, manuscriptology, and so on. The skill was typically deployed against texts rendered problematic by the ravages of time, by cultural differences or by the accidents of history. As such, hermeneutics was a regional and occasional necessity—a subdiscipline in theology, archaeology, literary studies, the history of art and so forth. (Howard, 1982, p. xiii)

The word *hermeneutics*, however, has a more ancient origin, having been derived from the Greek verb, *hermeneueuein*, "to interpret," and from the noun, *hermeneia*, or "interpretation." Both words were in turn derived from Hermes, the wing-footed messenger-god, who was associated with the Delphic oracle. Hermes was responsible for changing the unknowable into a form that humans could comprehend or understand. He accomplished this through the discovery and use of language and writing.

The Greek origins of the word *hermeneutic* are still relevant, for, in contemporary usage, *hermeneutics* now refers to a broad range of theoretical and practical approaches that are concerned with interpretation. In its focus on the philosophy, theory, and practice of interpretation, hermeneutics still emphasizes the importance of language and the way that language functions to "make something foreign, strange, separated in time, space or experience familiar, present, or comprehensible" (Palmer, 1969, p. 13).

Although hermeneutics was a more specialized subdiscipline in its early history, located in theology and limited to the study of interpretive canon, during the nineteenth and twentieth centuries, the scope of hermeneutics expanded greatly, and hermeneutic practice found applications in many fields. In contemporary times, the nature and scope of hermeneutics has continued to expand until, today, hermeneutics has served as a philosophical and methodological foundation in such diverse fields as comparative religion, cultural anthropology, literary criticism, history, and linguistics.

During the twentieth century, hermeneutic philosophy has increasingly moved away from questions regarding specific interpretive method and now focuses more on existential-ontological questions of how, in general, people come to understand. Today, hermeneutics is known as a contemporary philosophy that emphasizes the human experiences of understanding and interpretation. Hermeneutics focuses on acts of interpretation and understanding not only as experiences that are found in academic disciplines but as experiences that are fundamental to human life. The work of the German philosopher Hans-Georg Gadamer (1900-) has been recognized as central to the evolution of contemporary hermeneutic philosophy.

It is vital at the outset to understand the distinction between Gadamer's philosophical hermeneutics and the kind of hermeneutics oriented to methods and methodology. Gadamer is not directly concerned with the practical problems of formulating right principles for interpretation; he wishes rather to bring the phenomenon of understanding itself to light. This does not mean that he denies the importance of formulating such principles; on the contrary, such principles are necessary in the interpretive disciplines. What it means is that Gadamer is working on a preliminary and more fundamental question: How is understanding possible, not only in the humanities, but in the whole of man's [sic] experiences of the world. (Palmer, 1969, p. 163)

Contemporary hermeneutic philosophy is usually characterized as a Continental school of thought, with historical roots in other European philosophies. But philosophical hermeneutics has much in common with the American school of philosophy of pragmatism and with such thinkers as Charles Saunders Peirce, William James, and James Dewey. The similarities between neopragmatism and contemporary hermeneutic philosophy may be noted in the work of Bernstein (1971, 1976, 1983, 1986) and Rorty (1979, 1982). These similarities between pragmatism and hermeneutics may also be noted in nursing in discussions by Fry (1987) and Thompson (1987).

Within the last decade then, hermeneutics has emerged as a broadly based philosophy that focuses on the experience of understanding and on the act of interpretation as general features of human life (Howard, 1982). Like other postmodern schools of thought, philosophical hermeneutics is perhaps best known for its emphasis on the social and historical character of human understanding.

Hermeneutical thinkers can be characterized quite generally by their concern to resist the idea of the human intellect as a wordless and timeless source of insight . . . hermeneutical theories of understanding argue that all human understanding is never "without words" and never "outside of time." On the contrary, what is distinctive about human understanding is that it is always in terms of some evolving linguistic framework that has been worked out over time in terms of some historically conditioned set of concerns and practices. In short, hermeneutical thinkers argue that language and history are always both conditions and limits of understanding. (Wachterhauser, 1986, pp. 5-6)

Hermeneutics then joins other contemporary philosophies in reminding nurses of the social and historical grounding of all research.

This has implications for the way we understand research, and for the ways we understand ourselves and our activity in the research process.

Phenomenology and Hermeneutics

During the twentieth century, the development of hermeneutic philosophy was greatly influenced by two important schools of thought in Continental philosophy: phenomenology and existentialism. The close association between hermeneutics and phenomenology is evident in some recent discussions that have referred to hermeneutics as "Heideggerian phenomenology" (Allen, Diekelmann, & Benner, 1986). The influence of phenomenology is also apparent in works that trace the history of the phenomenological movement and identify hermeneutics as "hermeneutic phenomenology" (Ihde, 1971; Spiegelberg, 1982).

The association between hermeneutics and phenomenology is important, although it may be confusing for students to see the terms "hermeneutics" and "phenomenology" used interchangeably. In general, when authors use the term "hermeneutic philosophy" or "Heideggerian phenomenology," they are distinguishing hermeneutics from a philosophical forerunner, Husserlian or transcendental phenomenology. The distinction between hermeneutic phenomenology and Husserlian phenomenology is one that deserves some emphasis, because there are important differences between these two influential schools of thought.

The founding of phenomenology as a school of thought is usually attributed to the work of the German philosopher Edmund Husserl. While the historical evolution of phenomenology is very complex (Spiegelberg, 1982), it is possible to sketch a brief description of phenomenology as a philosophical movement. Husserl's investigations began as a search for the philosophical foundations of logic and evolved into a study of the logical structure of consciousness. For Husserl, it was the logical (as opposed to psychological) structure of consciousness that is transcendental, lying at the base of our experiences, the medium through which objects are constituted. In the course of Husserl's career, phenomenology then came to mean the study of phenomena, as-phenomena-appear-through-consciousness.

Today, many nurses still equate the phenomenological tradition with Husserl. Nurses who have been influenced by the Husserlian or transcendental school of phenomenology continue to emphasize the concepts and ideas of early phenomenology. These include

(1) an analysis of the subject and object-as-the-object-appears-through-consciousness,

(2) an emphasis on bracketing or epoche as a method for suspending naive realist awareness,

(3) and an emphasis on describing the full appearance of the object of inquiry.

During the last few years, several works in nursing literature have discussed Husserlian phenomenology as a philosophy and as a method with significant implications for nursing research (Knaack, 1984; Morse, 1989; Munhall & Oiler-Boyd, 1986; Oiler, 1983, 1986; Omery, 1983). One important insight from this work in nursing is our awareness that there is not a single phenomenological method but, instead, several techniques that apply Husserlian principles.

While these discussions were important ways of bringing phenomenology into the awareness of nurses, they did not present the evolution in Continental philosophy that resulted in Heideggerian phenomenology. The evolution of the phenomenological movement produced several theoretical and methodological extensions such as Schutzian phenomenology, symbolic interactionism, and grounded theory in sociology. Each of these interpretive approaches illustrates the historical development of the phenomenological movement. In these later applications, emphasis shifted from an earlier transcendental concern with consciousness as the medium through which we know objects to an emphasis on ordinary language as the ground of intersubjectivity, as the medium through which meaning is established.

The transcendental, or Husserlian, version of phenomenology has been more widely discussed in nursing literature, perhaps because nurses were more frequently exposed to this version of phenomenology in graduate study and also because this school of thought somehow appeals to nurses' professional interests in methods and techniques of knowledge development. But hermeneutic philosophy differs from this version of phenomenology in important ways. Hermeneutic philosophy owes much of its contemporary evolution to the work of Martin Heidegger, who literally redefined phenomenology (Palmer, 1969). It is this Heideggerian turn that should be understood when nurses study hermeneutics, for Heidegger and many contemporary hermeneutic thinkers moved away from Husserlian phenomenology.

Hermeneutic philosophy is best understood as a historical revision or extension of Husserlian phenomenology. The progression from Husserlian phenomenology to hermeneutic phenomenology can be illustrated by naming the line of philosophers in this tradition. Edmund Husserl, the father of the phenomenological movement, was Martin Heidegger's teacher. Heideggerian phenomenology resulted then from extensions and revisions that Heidegger made in his work with Husserl. Most accounts of these revisions note that Heidegger radically altered Husserlian phenomenology. But his work nevertheless demonstrates the influence of his teacher, Husserl. Similarly Martin Heidegger was Hans-Georg Gadamer's teacher, and although the contemporary work of Gadamer resolves some problems in Heidegger's thought, Gadamer's philosophical hermeneutics clearly demonstrates the influence of Heidegger's work. This historical progression from Husserl to Heidegger to Gadamer produced the transition from Husserlian phenomenology to hermeneutic phenomenology, or from transcendental phenomenology to philosophical hermeneutics.

Heideggerian phenomenology resists most of the epistemological assumptions of Husserlian phenomenology. It rejects the notion of subject and object and thus does not begin from a position that needs to show how we can know an object. Philosophical hermeneutics argues that experience is not primarily a "knowledge affair" (Bernstein, 1971). This means that our experiences in the world are not characterized by this separation of subject and object, at least they are not characterized by this separation as we are experiencing them before we stop to reflect about them. Instead, we have our experiences, or, rather, they have us, prereflectively, without any falling away of subject and object. In this way, we live or have our being in the world; we live our lives by experiencing the world and not primarily by "knowing" it.

Heideggerian phenomenology, therefore, does not emphasize the epistemological questions of knowing. Instead, it emphasizes the ontological-existential questions of experiencing. Whereas Husserlian phenomenology focuses on consciousness and knowing as a medium of uniting subject and object, Heideggerian phenomenology focuses on language and temporality, or historicity, as the medium through which we experience the world or have our being.

This distinction between Husserlian and Heideggerian phenomenology was also echoed in existentialism, a school of thought that greatly influenced the phenomenological movement. The work of the existentialist philosopher M. Merleau-Ponty has been identified in nursing as a phenomenological perspective that is consistent with nursing's concern for people as embodied beings (Oiler, 1986). Existentialism argued that, when we stop to reflect about an experience, to question what we know and how we know it, we have already altered the experience in so much as we remove the quality of immediacy from our experience. Existentialism was, therefore, somewhat skeptical about the phenomenological project of locating the constitution of objects and meaning in consciousness.

> Reflection does not withdraw from the world towards the unity of consciousness as the world's basis; it steps back to watch the form of transcendence fly up like sparks from a fire; it slakens the intentional threads which attach us to the world and thus brings them to our notice . . . [From this epoche] we can learn nothing but the unmotivated upsurge of the world. The most important lesson which the reduction teaches us is the impossibility of a complete reduction . . . since we are in the world, since indeed our reflections are carried out in the temporal flux on to which we are trying to seize, there is no thought which embraces all our thought . . . radical reflection amounts to a consciousness of its own dependence on an unreflective life. (Merleau-Ponty, 1962, pp. xiii-xiv)

The turn from consciousness to existence was, therefore, a crucial part of the development of hermeneutic phenomenology. The hermeneutic turn in phenomenology is one that literally reframed the *problematic* of the phenomenological movement. Concern shifted from questions of knowing to questions of being or experiencing the world. The distinction between knowledge and experience, between knowing and being, is typical of Western thought in general, and it has played itself out in philosophy, in nursing, and in many disciplines.

In philosophy, questions of knowing are central to epistemology, while questions of being and existence are central to ontology. In nursing, this distinction may be seen in works that focus on conditions of knowledge, or nursing epistemology (Carper, 1978), versus works that focus on nursing ontology, on the existential reality or "being" of nursing (Watson, 1988). In Continental philosophy, Husserl's work was concerned primarily with epistemological issues, while Heidegger's hermeneutic revisions were more concerned with questions of ontology and existence.

Because nurses, as people, have participated in social and historical developments during the last few decades, it is not surprising to find that the history of ideas in Western thought has influenced the history of ideas in nursing. The evolution of ideas in phenomenology has been paralleled in nursing by a movement that now shows the influence of both Husserlian and Heideggerian phenomenology. In asking scientific questions, nurses have sometimes borrowed from the tradition of epistemology and transcendental phenomenology. We have constructed our research activity to include ourselves (as subject) and others (as objects of investigation). In epistemological work in nursing, we have asked questions about knowing: How is it that we can come to know the experience of another? Certainly, most academic fields of study in Western culture experience this analytic posture. But, on the other hand, to take this posture is to alter the experience, for, when we reflect, we are one step removed from living or having the experience.

Hermeneutic philosophy emphasizes the prereflective quality of experience and maintains that knowing or knowledge is very much in the background, a tacit part of most of our experiences. This is why Patricia Benner's work, for example, refers to the tacit knowledge of nurses by eliciting stories about their clinical practice in natural contexts. The emphasis on the experiences of nurses is very much consistent with existentialism's focus on everyday lived reality and demonstrates the application of hermeneutic phenomenology in nursing research.

Three Conversations in Hermeneutics

Although hermeneutic philosophy has taken these existentialist/ontological turns, contemporary hermeneutic discourse is very diverse and includes many differing assumptions. Not all hermeneutic thinkers have followed Heidegger and Gadamer into the more broadly based philosophical hermeneutics discussed above. The hermeneutic tradition has undergone a complex evolution, with many important internal divisions and differing assumptions. Paul Ricouer (1970, pp. 26-27), for example, has suggested that "there is no general hermeneutics, no universal canon for exegesis, but only disparate and opposed theories concerning the rules of interpretation. The hermeneutic field . . . is internally at variance with itself."

While contemporary hermeneutic discourse does reflect this level of complexity, it is still possible to characterize different hermeneutic perspectives based on the way hermeneutic thinkers discuss interpretation and understanding. There are at least three conversations in contemporary hermeneutics that address different interpretive questions and begin from different assumptions.

Hermeneutics and Existentialist Ontology

As indicated earlier, hermeneutic thinkers who have been most influenced by Heidegger's work speak about interpretation and understanding ontologically. This hermeneutic conversation emphasizes understanding as a broad category of life, as a way of being or as an activity that is fundamental to life at the cultural level. This conversation has been labeled "philosophical hermeneutics" (Hoy, 1982) and its most well-known living thinker is Hans-Georg Gadamer. When hermeneutic thinkers in this conversation link the act of interpretation with being, they argue for the universality of interpretation, claiming that interpretation is the activity that enables us to experience the world. For these thinkers, everything that exists in the world exists for people through acts of interpretation and understanding. This account of hermeneutics maintains that we cannot have a world, cannot have life at the cultural level, except through acts of interpretation. Contemporary parallels of this strand in hermeneutic philosophy may be found in nursing in the work of Watson (1988) and Benner (1984a), who discuss transpersonal and practical features of being in nursing.

Hermeneutics and Epistemology

For other hermeneutic thinkers, interpretation is considered epistemologically. For these thinkers, there is a more important juncture to be explored in the connection between epistemology and interpretation, and, in some cases, these hermeneutic thinkers are openly skeptical of ontological discourse. "Hermeneuts" in this conversation are concerned about conditions of knowledge. They ask questions regarding the extension of "forestructures" of understanding in different forms of knowledge. They sometimes argue that the sciences and the human studies are characterized by different logics of inquiry or by different kinds of knowledge claims. In this conversation, hermeneutic thinkers are concerned with social and historical conditions of knowledge in the human species. Because they link the act of interpretation with conditions of knowledge, they maintain that everything in the world that can be *known* is known by people through acts of interpretation. Interpretation is presented again as a broad human activity, as the way we have access to the world or the way we apprehend reality.

Hermeneutics and Methodology

Still other hermeneutic thinkers discuss interpretation in a more restricted or less philosophical sense as a methodological foundation for humanistic disciplines. During the nineteenth and early twentieth centuries, many hermeneutic thinkers argued that interpretive methods and practices were the unique, distinguishing feature of the human studies. Remnants of this conversation remain today in discourse about the use of qualitative and quantitative methods in the social sciences. In this conversation, hermeneutics is examined as philosophy that guides methods and forms of analysis found in the humanities and the social sciences. Here, hermeneutics opposes empiricism as a methodological foundation for humanistic disciplines. This is a more specialized conversation, which examines questions of proper research methods and analytic techniques for those working with academic fields and research contexts. Hermeneutic thinkers in this conversation frequently investigate criteria of adequacy or truth as standards that can guide interpretive methods.

While these three conversations may be separated for the purpose of discussion, nurses usually experience them as connected and interrelated. All three conversations in hermeneutic discourse may speak to nurses and all three may find applications in nursing research. The thesis of this chapter is that a thorough understanding of all three conversations helps nurses to make clearer and more productive applications of hermeneutic discourse. Additionally, this chapter maintains that specific applications of hermeneutic philosophy in nursing reflect the interests and commitments of the scholar.

The evolution of contemporary hermeneutics contains several important insights that can lead to a different understanding of the research process. The following sections of this chapter briefly review some of these insights from hermeneutic philosophy and discuss their implications for nursing research.

The Hermeneutic Account of Language

To understand the hermeneutic tradition, it is important to see a shift that occurred in common conceptions of language and understanding. These two notions, language and understanding, are central in contemporary hermeneutic philosophy, and they lead to a very different account of inquiry and method.

In Hans-Georg Gadamer's work *Truth and Method* (1975), there appeared a major turn in hermeneutic philosophy, one that has important implications for our understanding of the research process. While Gadamer's discussions of language and understanding demonstrate the influence of Heidegger, he avoids ontologizing and so presents a more socially and historically grounded philosophy. His account of language is a central and crucial feature of his philosophical hermeneutics.

> Ultimately, the one issue that is important, the one that must be understood because it is the key to understanding others, is language. This issue overshadows all subsidiary issues that Gadamer discusses and provides a perspective by which those other issues must be approached. Thus for example instead of trying to discover Gadamer's position on ontology, it would be more fruitful to ask how language reveals Being; the question of language supercedes that of ontology and dictates how the question must be approached. (Hekman, 1986, p. 95)

Gadamer followed Heidegger in rejecting conventional notions about language. It is commonplace in modern times to think of language in instrumental ways. That is, most people think of language as an instrument or a tool that is used to refer, to describe, to make clear, and so on. This way of using language is basic to science, "with its ideal of exact designation and unambiguous concepts."

But Gadamer (and many other thinkers influenced by ordinary language philosophy) rejects this notion of language and, in so doing, asks us to follow him in a very difficult turn. "It requires a feat of mental gymnastics to remember that outside of the scientific ideal of unambiguous designation, the life of language itself goes its way unaffected" (Palmer, 1969, p. 202). The alternative description of language that Gadamer presents is crucial to an understanding of contemporary hermeneutics.

If language is neither sign nor symbolic form created by [an individual], what is it? In the first place, words are not something that belong to [a person], but to the situation. One searches for words, the words that belong to the situation. . . . The maker of the assertion did not invent any of the words; he/she learned them. The process of learning the language came only gradually, through immersion in the stream of the heritage. [A person] does not make a word and "endow" it with a meaning; the imagining of such a procedure is pure correction of linguistic theory. . . . in formulating an assertion one only uses the words already belonging to the situation. . . . the early Greeks had no word or concept for language itself; like being and understanding, language is medium, not tool. . . . world and language both are transpersonal matters. (Palmer, 1969, pp. 203-205)

This account of language has extremely important implications for research and for the philosophy of science. It is a reiteration of the existentialist insight that language and cultural practices [or language and being] are inextricably linked, that we only have a world through language.

Gadamer amplifies this by stating that language carries everything with it, not only "culture" but "everything (in the world and out of it) is included in the realm of 'understanding' and understandability in which we move." . . . Thus language is not simply a tool that, like many others, human beings put to use. When we take a word in our mouth, we are "fixed in a direction of thought." Words themselves prescribe the only way we can use them; we cannot use them arbitrarily as we might a tool. We become acquainted with the world and even ourselves through language because language is the universal mode of being and knowledge . . . it is more correct to say that language speaks us rather than we speak it. (Hekman, 1986, pp. 110-111)

This account of language reminds us that, even in scientific discourse, we are only entering a "language game" that has already been established and that prescribes, predefines, or prejudges the ways in which we orient ourselves to given phenomena. This view of language brings the hermeneutic tradition more in line with neopragmatic accounts of truth, where the emphasis is on concepts as a way of fixing belief, as a way of orienting ourselves. Hermeneutics then differs significantly from more familiar positions in nursing, such as realism, which view concepts as a lens that can be used to accurately mirror reality (Rorty, 1979). Instead, on this hermeneutic account of language, we are born into linguistic communities, and the language(s) we speak are at once the conditions of new knowledge, opening us to new understandings, and the limits of what we can know or understand in the future.

Hermeneutic discussions of language emphasize the historicity and the value-laden quality of human understanding. They remind us, for example, that concepts are not just value neutral, ahistorical entities that more or less accurately mirror our worlds. Rather, concepts are conditioned by our historical era and by our social interests. For some hermeneutic thinkers then, theories, concepts, theoretical terms, observations, and acts of interpretation are more ideological than realism or empiricism would allow.

Gadamer's accounts of language also suggests that, within any given historical and social context, scholars come to their work with an already established background of preunderstanding. These preunderstandings are linguistically conveyed; they are produced, reproduced, and transformed in the course of cultural evolution. Gadamer refers to this background of linguistically mediated preunderstanding by using the term "prejudice." It is a "forestructure" or a condition of knowledge in that it determines what we may find intelligible in any given situation. Arguably, such forestructures reflect social reference groups; they are a product of culture, gender, race, and class. In contrast to common usage, Gadamer argues that prejudice is not something that is negative or something that we should try to eliminate. In fact, he argues that we can only have access to the world through our prejudices. "[Gadamer] replaces the opposition between truth and prejudice with the assertion that prejudice—our situatedness in history and time—is the precondition of truth, not an obstacle to it" (Hekman, 1986, p. 117).

Hermeneutics: Philosophy of Human Understanding

The hermeneutic account of language leads to a different perspective about understanding. Since the nineteenth century, there have been lengthy and continuous discussions that describe the phenomenon of understanding and differentiate it from scientific knowledge. For centuries, hermeneutic philosophers maintained that understanding occurs for us or happens to us because we are born into a cultural-linguistic community; we have a world and understand our world through our language(s). Hermeneutic thinkers, therefore, emphasize the linguistic and historical nature of understanding.

Understanding then is not to be confused with knowledge and with the explanations that science provides.

For years, many hermeneutic thinkers also maintained that the natural sciences and human studies could be separated based on different logics of inquiry or different objects of inquiry. Early hermeneutic philosophy argued, for example, that the natural sciences provide explanations while the human studies yield understanding of the human condition. Some, like Dilthey, maintained that the essential difference between the natural sciences and human studies lies "in the context within which the perceived object is understood. The human studies will sometimes make use of the same objects or 'facts' as the natural sciences, but in a different context of relationships, one which includes or refers to inner experience" (Palmer, 1969, p. 105).

Some hermeneutic thinkers still maintain that the sciences and human studies operate according to different logics of inquiry. Habermas (1971, 1988) extended insights from ordinary language philosophy by proposing that natural sciences place their objects (scientific facts) within the context of the human interest of predicting and manipulating the natural environment. The hermeneutic disciplines, in contrast, place the object of inquiry, human beings, within the context of social relationships and, therefore, include and refer to subjectivity and intersubjectivity. Other hermeneutic thinkers, like Ricoeur (1981) and Hesse (1980), have argued that, in both the natural sciences and the human studies, understanding and explanation are part of the same interpretive arc and they should not be separated and dichotomized as functions that occur independently in different fields of study.

Throughout this lengthy debate, hermeneutic philosophy has produced a massive description of human understanding (Howard, 1982). As a result of this discourse, hermeneutics presents us with a description of human understanding as a more complicated operation than explanation. "We explain by means of purely intellectual processes, but we understand by means of the combined activity of all the mental powers in apprehending" (Palmer, 1969, p. 115).

This emphasis on the experience of understanding has led hermeneutic thinkers to discuss several metaphors of understanding. In the hermeneutic tradition, the experience of understanding has been compared with at least three recurring metaphors or analogies. These are the hermeneutic circle, the fusion of the horizons, and the act of dialogue.

The Hermeneutic Circle

Many hermeneutic thinkers have contended that understanding occurs through a complex experience labeled the "hermeneutic circle." In the United States and Great Britain, there has been a tendency to misunderstand what Europeans mean by the term "hermeneutic circle." We have a tendency to reduce this concept to some mysterious kind of intuition (Outhwaite, 1985, p. 24). But hermeneutic thinkers have not described understanding in this way; it is not primarily a psychic event. Because of its early emphasis on language, hermeneutic philosophy described understanding as a cognitive, affective, and practical process *that is based on a sphere of shared meanings and shared experiences within a common linguistic community.* For hermeneutic thinkers, it is language and history that supply this shared sphere.

In the work of Dilthey, hermeneutic philosophy first began to reject psychic or psychologistic descriptions of understanding. An emphasis on shared language and a shared background of meaning was identified as part of the hermeneutic circle.

> Every word or sentence, every gesture or form of politeness, every work of art and every historical deed are only understandable because the person expressing [her- or] himself and the person who understands [her or] him are connected by something they have in common; the individual always experiences, thinks, acts and also understands, in this common sphere. (Dilthey, 1988, cited in Outhwaite, 1985, p. 24)

In the hermeneutic tradition, understanding is described as a process of moving dialectically between a background of shared meaning and a more finite, focused experience within it. The *hermeneutic circle* is a metaphor used to describe the experience of moving dialectically between part and whole. Nearly all hermeneutic thinkers have relied on this metaphor as a way of expressing what occurs in "understanding." For example, in his description of understanding, Palmer (1969, p. 87) noted that

> understanding is a basically referential operation; we understand something by comparing it to something we already know. What we understand forms itself into systematic unities, or circles made up of parts. The circle as a whole defines the individual part, and the parts together form the circle. A whole sentence, for instance, is a unity. We understand the meaning of an individual word by seeing it in reference to the whole

of the sentence; and reciprocally, the sentence's meaning as a whole is dependent on the meaning of individual words. By extension, an individual concept derives its meaning from a context or horizon within which it stands; yet the horizon is made up of the very elements to which it gives meaning. By dialectical interaction between the whole and the part, each gives the other meaning; understanding is circular, then. Because within the "circle" the meaning comes to stand, we call this the "hermeneutic circle."

This account of the hermeneutic circle suggests that understanding is really a universal experience, one that is prior to scientific inquiry or scholarship of any kind. One of Gadamer's most important contributions to hermeneutic philosophy is his claim of universality for the hermeneutic experience. He argues that the hermeneutic experience, the interpretation of our world in light of our preunderstandings, is a universal feature of human life and that these interpretive practices are only extended in our scholarship.

> The circularity of understanding has another consequence of greatest importance to hermeneutics; there is really no true starting point for understanding, since every part presupposes the others. This means that there can be no "presuppositionless" understanding. Every act of understanding is in a given context or horizon, even in science one explains only "in terms of" a frame of reference. . . . An interpretive approach which ignores the historicality of lived experience and applies atemporal categories to historical objects can only with irony claim to be "objective," for it has from the outset distorted the phenomenon. (Palmer, 1969, p. 120)

From hermeneutics, we learn that preunderstandings (and the theories that are connected with them) are pragmatic. They have the potential of showing us something about ourselves and our preferred actions and something about the object of our inquiry. Hermeneutic investigations, unlike empiricist ones, are reflective; they show us glimpses of ourselves, for, in the act of interpretation, one must be ever conscious of one's prejudices and must examine them reflectively so that the object of investigation can speak.

The connection between language, preconceptions, theory, and research then is very different given the insights from hermeneutic philosophy. For the hermeneutic account of understanding and interpretation suggests that our theories, our methodological commitments, our ethical commitments, and, in a more preliminary and holistic sense, our cosmology provide us with conditions of knowledge. In a larger cultural sense, the hermeneutic account of under-standing indicates that our human interests cannot be eliminated or neutralized, as argued in positivist accounts of science.

Understanding as the Fusion of Horizons

While many hermeneutic thinkers have emphasized the herme-neutic circle as a metaphor for human understanding, Gadamer is perhaps best known for his description of understanding as the "fusion of horizons." This metaphor of understanding draws on the hermeneutic tradition, extending the notion of the hermeneutic cir-cle and avoiding both subjectivist and objectivist objects of under-standing. In Gadamer's notion of the fusion of horizons, meaning is neither located in the subjective intentions of the author or actor nor produced by the interpretive methods and preconceptions of the scholar. Rather, understanding happens when the horizons of the scholar intersect or fuse with the horizon, context, or standpoint of the object of inquiry. "Understanding is not a mysterious commu-nion of souls in which the interpreter grasps the subjective intention of the author. Rather it is a fusion of the text's horizon with that of the interpreter" (Hekman, 1986, p. 111).

Gadamer defines *horizon,* consistent with Nietzsche and Husserl, as "the range of vision that includes everything that can be seen from a particular vantage point" (1975, p. 269). Horizons then encompass what we find intelligible given our specific cultural perspectives and our place in history. The notion of horizon might then be seen as the background or frame of reference one adopts as a result, for example, of being a white middle-class professional woman. It is the back-ground of meanings that are acquired by living in a linguistic com-munity, by internalizing the culture in which we live (Dreyfus, 1980). Gadamer (1975, p. 288) again asserts that horizons are temporal, historically changing features of life that have limits but that, never-theless, are open.

> The historical movement of human life consists in the fact that it is never utterly bound to any one standpoint, and hence can never have a truly closed horizon. The horizon is, rather something into which we move and that moves with us. Horizons change for a person who is moving. Thus the horizon of the past, out of which all human life lives and which exists in the form of tradition, is always in motion.

Gadamer describes understanding as the fusion of these stand-points, as the intersection, coming together, or merging of different vantage points. The term "fusion" implies that one does not eliminate one's own horizon, or ever leave it entirely behind. Neither does Gadamer suggest that all differences are collapsed and smoothed over, but rather that one's horizon's can change. This description also suggests that understanding cannot be reduced to an experience in which we see things empathically through another's perspective or entirely from their vantage point. Instead, the fusion of horizons resembles the "I-Thou" relationship.

> In the I-Thou relationship, I am open myself to the other; I am dominated by the will to hear rather than to master, and I am willing to be modified by the other. Analogously, in understanding I open myself to tradition, that is I let it speak to me allowing the meaning hidden it in to become clear. . . . The I-Thou relationship . . . involves a dialogic relationship. (Hekman, 1986, p. 104)

By drawing this analogy, hermeneutics suggests that the fusion of horizons is more like a posture, a style, a way of living, or a way of conducting oneself than it is a way of knowing. It involves the willingness to open oneself to the standpoint of another in such a way that we genuinely let the standpoint of another speak to us, and in such a way that we are willing to be influenced by the perspective of another.

For Gadamer, the ambiguity in this description is not a weakness, rather it is a positive structure of understanding. Specifically, in order to experience the fusion of horizons, one must be able to tolerate the ambiguity of relaxing (not eliminating) one's own preconceptions.

> A consciousness informed by the authentic hermeneutic attitude will be receptive to the origins and entirely foreign features of that which comes to it from outside it's own horizons. Yet this receptivity is not acquired with an objectivist "neutrality": it is neither possible, necessary, nor desirable that we put ourselves within brackets. The hermeneutic attitude supposes only that we self-consciously designate our opinions and prejudices and qualify them as such, and in so doing strip them of their extreme character. In keeping to this attitude we grant the text the opportunity to appear as an authentically different being and to manifest its own truth, over and against our own preconceived notions. (Gadamer, 1979, p. 152)

An important outcome of Gadamer's insights regarding the fusion of horizons is that understanding has a practical and moral orientation. This is why so much of hermeneutic philosophy has retraced insights from practical philosophy, arguing that the act of understanding is similar to the ancient Greek description of practical wisdom *phronesis*. Understanding is like wisdom; it grasps particular situations and, when wisdom understands, it also has a moral sense of what should be done. For Gadamer, and most hermeneutic thinkers, there has been a serious deformation in contemporary times that obscures the difference between knowledge and wisdom. Science may provide experts with knowledge, but it cannot provide them wisdom; wisdom and understanding are complex experiences in which we encounter our own preconceptions in the act of understanding something that is foreign or unfamiliar. This fusion of horizons usually results in greater self-understanding, a greater moral awareness, and an appreciation for other vantage points.

A final outcome of the fusion of horizons then is that understanding results in ever-increasing openness, for hermeneutic experiences always enlarge and enrich our understanding of the human condition. Hermeneutic philosophy again reminds us of the difference between explanation and understanding. The kind of practical wisdom that accompanies understanding is different from the accumulation of technical, problem-solving knowledge attributed to science and to experts. Rather, understanding leaves one open to future experiences and able to encounter the foreign and unfamiliar with this openness.

> The truly experienced person, one who has wisdom and not just knowledge, has learned the limitations, the finitude of all expectation. Experience teaches him [or her] not so much a storehouse of facts that will enable [her or] him to solve the same problem better next time, but how to expect the unexpected, to be open to new experience. It teaches him [sic], in short, the poverty of knowledge in comparison with experience. (Palmer, 1969, p. 232)

Understanding as Dialogue:
The Logic of Question and Answer

Gadamer's insights about language, understanding, and the fusion of horizons reveal his ontological perspective. He argues that understanding is a mode of being and not a way of knowing. It is crucial to recognize this distinction, for, when Gadamer describes understanding, he is talking about existence and about ways of living, which may or may not find their extension in ways of knowing. In his most famous work, *Truth and Method* (1975), Gadamer effectively demonstrated that understanding is not produced by scholars who rely exclusively on proper method, neither is it produced in fields of study where experts are socialized to produce knowledge through sophisticated research techniques. Technique and method, in general, can yield factual knowledge, like the knowledge of science, but method cannot produce truths. This is why the title of Gadamer's book is a paradox, for he argues that truth is something that happens to us, above and beyond any method or specific technique, in the experience of understanding.

Gadamer's insights regarding understanding lead him to formulate a third metaphor for understanding. He compares hermeneutic understanding to the act of dialogue and to the experience that happens between two partners in dialogue. This emphasis on the dialogic relationship is not surprising, given the centrality of language in hermeneutic philosophy.

The emphasis on dialogue owes some of its origin to the rhetorical and humanist tradition (in which Gadamer is an important participant). In this tradition, the center of discourse includes questions from philosophical anthropology, questions about what it means to be a human being, and questions about our relationship to our world. This is a reflective tradition that asks moral and ethical questions in a nonobjectivist way, a tradition that thus produces self-understanding, a deeper understanding of oneself and of others (Schrag, 1980).

Gadamer draws on this tradition when he equates understanding with the metaphor of dialogue. He draws out the analogy of question and answer and suggests that human understanding can be compared with the logic of question and answer or to the play of conversation that occurs between two partners in a dialogue. The metaphor of dialogue is a complex one and not all conversations would count for Gadamer as true examples of dialogue. A lot depends on the type of question that is asked.

Beginning with Socrates, hermeneutics has recognized three different types of questions. A rhetorical question is one that gives its own answer. A pedagogical question is one that implies the direction of its answer but leaves room for the student to cross in order to reach the answer. And a genuine question, while it is not infinitely open, leads in several possible directions to several possible answers

(Weinscheimer, 1985, pp. 206-209). In the hermeneutic tradition, the logic of *genuine* questions defines true dialogue.

When Gadamer compares the act of understanding with the metaphor of dialogue, he is suggesting that, when we understand, it is usually because we have opened ourselves to the logic of question and answer, where the questions asked are genuine questions.

> Gadamer asserts that hermeneutic experience is characterized by . . . the logical structure of openness. This structure is found in the dialectic of question and answer. The hermeneutic phenomenon contains within itself the original meaning of the structure of question and answer, and thus it follows that the logic of human sciences . . . is coincident with the logic of the question. For a text to become an object of interpretation it must ask a question of the interpreter. This is not an arbitrary procedure because a question is always related to the answer that is expected in the text. An examination of the dialectic of question and answer reveals, furthermore, that understanding, like conversation, is always related to the answer that is expected in the text. An examination of the dialectic of question and answer reveals, furthermore, that understanding, like conversation, is always a reciprocal relationship. (Hekman, 1986, p. 108)

Gadamer asserts that, in dialogue (and analogously in hermeneutic experiences), understanding occurs when we surrender to the movement of question and answer. It is important to note the reciprocity involved in this account. It is not just that scholars ask a question of a text or of a participant. It is that scholars open themselves to the question that the material or the participants ask of them. This feature of hermeneutic philosophy is perhaps most at odds with an empiricist account of science and with the kind of socialization that most contemporary researchers experience. In most situations, scholars and researchers undergo intense socialization that prepares them to derive and refine their own research questions and then apply these questions by matching them with appropriate techniques. This approach to inquiry is at odds with the hermeneutic experience.

> The scientist, in many cases looks at the object with one or more hypotheses and with the purpose of the research in mind, and thus 'uses' the object to corroborate or disprove a hypothesis, but does not encounter the object as such in its own fullness. . . . In their (scientists') attempt . . . to fit some object or phenomenon into some system, preconception, or hypothesis, one can often observe a blinding of themselves toward the full being of the object itself. (Schachtel, 1959, p. 171)

In contrast, the hermeneutic tradition would encourage scholars to remain open to questions that emerge from the object of inquiry. In the hermeneutic experience, the locus of inquiry and of understanding is found in the perspective of neither one or the other participant but in the free movement that occurs between them, in the fusion of horizons that occurs in the process of dialogue.

Hermeneutic philosophy then presents understanding and the act of dialogue as "transpersonal" affairs, as events that are more than the summation of subjective intentions or perspectives of the participants. Rather, dialogue (and, analogously, understanding and hermeneutic inquiry) is an event or experience that happens to the participants. But this does not mean that those who experience hermeneutic understanding do so with naive passivity. For Gadamer also insists that the hermeneutic experience contains an active element, which has been termed "negativity."

Gadamer maintains that to engage in a dialogue with the object of our inquiry is neither to interrogate nor to passively surrender to it. Instead, dialogue and genuine questions contain an element of negativity, which brings one to the point of fused horizons.

> The creative negativity of true questioning, which is essentially the negativity in experience that teaches and transforms, is the heart of the hermeneutical experience. For to experience is to understand not better but differently; experience does not tell one what s/he expected, but tends to transcend and negate expectations. A "deep" experience teaches us not to understand better what is already partially understood so much as that we were understanding wrongly.... Analysis and methodical questioning, however, tend not to call into question their own guiding presuppositions but rather to operate within a system, so that the answer is always potentially present and expected within the system. Thus they are not so much forms of true questioning as of testing. But experience does not follow the model of solving a problem within a system.... When any truly great work of art or literature is encountered, it transforms one's understanding; it is a fresh way of seeing life. (Palmer, 1969, p. 233)

Like dialogue, understanding is an experience that takes us out of ourselves and the context of our ordinary lives and conceptions and relates us to a discovery, to discovering something new, which we had not recognized before. This element of negativity in the hermeneutic experience comes from the willingness to risk our preconceptions, to open ourselves to the material we question and to allow it to speak.

Theories of Interpretation and
Their Methodological Implications

While Gadamer's metaphors of understanding show us some important features of hermeneutic philosophy, they represent only one face of contemporary hermeneutics (Howard, 1982). As indicated earlier, not all hermeneutic thinkers agree with these revisions and many have resisted the turn that occurred with Heideggerian phenomenology. Contemporary hermeneutic discourse is an exceedingly complex field, consisting of many competing theories of interpretation. But many methodological and philosophical issues in hermeneutics can be examined by focusing on three major branches of hermeneutic theory. Each theoretical position carries with it major differences in terms of methodological implications. It is these methodological implications that are most relevant for contemporary researchers in nursing.

Objective Hermeneutics

A theoretical position that has consistently resisted Gadamerian and Heideggerian insights is one that maintains some of the objectivist assumptions associated with the earlier classical hermeneutic tradition. These hermeneutic thinkers share a common standard that determines the validity and objectivity of interpretive work.

> Theoretical objectivism insists that *in principle* there is an unchanging meaning that must be presupposed as the goal of every interpretation, if it is to be believed that some interpretations are more true or correct than others. . . . [this position argues that] while the *importance* of a work may vary with time and within different interpretive contexts, the one underlying meaning of the work does not change. The meaning of the text, which, on this account, is the author's willed meaning—is said to be self-identical, determinate, and reproducible (that is, shareable rather than private). The understanding that grasps this determinate and unchanging meaning is totally neutral and unsullied by the interpreter's own normative goals or views of the work's importance. Only on such grounds, is it possible to speak of the validity of interpretation. (Hoy, 1982, pp. 13-14)

Within this kind of objective hermeneutics, theorists of interpretation have argued that texts have a more or less determinate meaning and that authors and historical actors have fairly fixed intentions that can be determined by adequate methods. This interpretive position defends the validity or objectivity of interpretation against the passion, self-interest, or prejudice of the scholar.

This hermeneutic theory has been labeled objectivist because it is most concerned with identifying standards of objectivity that apply to interpretive work and that guarantee the validity of interpretations, irrespective of historical changes or cultural bias. In most instances, scholars who work from this theoretical perspective are skeptical of the "radical relativism" they see in Heideggerian or Gadamerian notions of historicity and understanding.

Within objectivism, some scholars also maintain intentionalist positions. Intentionalism is frequently associated with early phenomenology and argues that the subjective intentions of an author or a social actor should be reconstructed in interpretive work. The term *intention*, or *intentionality*, is a very important one that has specific meanings within the phenomenological movement. Sometimes, the term *intention* has carried with it a psychologistic meaning, referring to the private mental events or processes of authors and historical figures. In this usage, scholars have sometimes argued that the validity of interpretive work comes from the ability to empathically understand the intentions of the historical figures or social actors they study. In other instances, *intentionalism* can have a more linguistic and less psychologistic meaning, focusing more on the expressions contained in a text or uttered by social actors (Hoy, 1982, p. 29).

Both versions of intentionalism carry important methodological implications. These positions are objectivist in the sense that they carry an injunction against the bias of the researcher or scholar. On this account, interpretive methods are adequate if they "bracket," or suspend, the bias of the scholar and disclose the original meaning of the object of inquiry. In this sense, the objectivist perspective bears a clear resemblance to both positivist and phenomenological notions of value neutrality and presuppositionless approaches in research. It resembles positivism in its search for ahistorical principles of objectivity and its emphasis on value neutrality. And it resembles phenomenology in its injunction to "bracket" the presuppositions of the scholar and focus exclusively on the object of inquiry.

While this position has been seriously challenged during the last decade, it is a viewpoint that continues to inform a great deal of work in the humanities, in the social sciences, and in nursing. An emphasis on the actor's intentions, or "emic" perspectives, is the hallmark of interpretive approaches in the social sciences and in nursing.

It is a common characteristic of Wittgensteinian social science, Schutzian phenomenology and ethnomethodology to insist that the meaning of an action is determined by the meaning bestowed on it by the actor. Interpretive social scientists . . . argue that the actors' understanding of their actions, that is, their subjective meaning, not only establishes the meaning of the action but must be the point of departure of all social scientific analysis. . . . Although most interpretive social scientists now argue that "subjective meaning" is not established by probing the internal mental events of the social actor but, rather is established by the intersubjective meanings of the social context, they nevertheless assert that this meaning is the fundamental unit of social scientific analysis. (Hekman, 1986, p. 145)

This discussion has important methodological implications for nursing research. Most descriptions of qualitative research in nursing have been influenced by the methodology of interpretive social science and most demonstrate this objectivist bias. In nursing, this approach to interpretation is found in qualitative methods that are employed to render an accurate reconstruction of the meaning expressed by social actors. The use of ethnomethod, ethnography, or other qualitative field methods, the use of some feminist methodology and, even phenomenological research, can be objectivist, if the researcher holds this theory of interpretation. Among many qualitative researchers, this approach involves the use of various techniques, such as participant observation, ethnographic interviewing, and qualitative analysis, to reconstruct the "emic" reality of research participants. Among historical researchers, objectivism is demonstrated in the use of internal and external criticism to yield an accurate reconstruction of a period in the life of a historical figure.

Qualitative research in nursing then can be identified as objectivist if it focuses primarily or exclusively on the meanings expressed by participants as the fundamental unit of analysis. But the way that nurse-researchers understand this interpretive process is also important. Most nurses have been strongly influenced by the humanistic tradition and by a socialization process that encourages the use of empathy or intuitive understanding. This may lead some nurse-researchers to view what they do in research as an expression of empathy, as a process of "seeing things through the native's eyes." But this approach to qualitative research is not consistent with contemporary insights in the hermeneutic tradition.

Because of developments in the philosophy of mind and in the philosophy of language, it is generally not acceptable to attribute the interpretive process to empathy or intuitive connections with others. As a result of recent advances, there is now a growing awareness that we cannot have direct access to the mental processes of others. Rather, it is now generally accepted that we only have access to the way mind is expressed through language and through action. This has led to a much stronger emphasis on language and the role it plays when we are trying to understand the inner experience and actions of others. As a result, most interpretive research focuses on the expressions of participants in a context and what these expressions and participants' actions mean in that context.

When nurse-researchers study meaning in context by interviewing, participating with, or observing others, they usually present findings that identify recurrent themes or meanings that have been expressed by participants (Wolf, 1988). Such research demonstrates an objectivist approach to interpretation if the exclusive focus of the researcher has been on the expressions, message, or actions of historical actors in context. Here, inquiry is judged valid, or "objective," because the researcher has used methods that yield an accurate or appropriate reconstruction of the phenomenon. It may be argued that researchers influenced by this theory of interpretation generally adopt a definition of objectivity that differs only slightly from a positivistic account of objectivity. Here, the "facts" recovered in interpretive work demonstrate "validity" and "objectivity" if the researcher is "bracketed" and if the interpretation provides an accurate reconstruction of original meaning or meaning in context.

In nursing, as in most social scientific work, this methodological approach is one that does not incorporate Heideggerian insights or methodological implications from critical social theory.

Gadamerian Hermeneutics

A second major theory of interpretation is one that appropriates the revisions in classical hermeneutic theory made by Heidegger and Gadamer. While this theory of interpretation has been identified in nursing by the label "Heideggerian phenomenology" (Allen, Diekelmann, & Benner, 1986), some methodologists in the social sciences would not identify with Heidegger and would emphasize Gadamer's philosophy of interpretation instead (Hekman, 1986).

Gadamer's theoretical position emphasizes the fusion of horizons and dialogue as metaphors for interpretive work. The methodological implications of this metaphor are quite different from those found in objectivism and in most interpretive social science. While there is still very little literature that deals explicitly with the methodological implications of Gadamer's hermeneutic philosophy, recent years have seen some beginning discussions of methodological implications for the social sciences. In her work, for example, Hekman (1986) lays careful groundwork by presenting a thorough analysis of Gadamer's position and then poses the question of methods in the social sciences.

> Although Gadamer is most definitely not offering a methodology for the social sciences in his work, his position has profound implications for the social sciences. He defines a philosophical perspective that so revolutionizes the way the social sciences are conceived that it calls into question our very notion of method. It follows that his position on language and the human sciences and the anti-foundational thrust of that insight necessarily dictate a methodology that is radically different from that conceived by most social scientists. (Hekman, 1986, pp. 92-95)

Because Gadamer maintains that interpretation always occurs through the fusion of horizons, his work suggests that researchers cannot grant epistemological priority either to the "emic" reality of research participants nor to their own conceptual lenses. Rather, hermeneutic investigations would, on this account, demonstrate a dialectic, an interplay between the expressions of those that are studied and the interpretive scheme used by the scholar. Most important, hermeneutic research would show *explicitly* how the horizon of the researcher fused with the horizon of the researched.

> The first task of the interpreter is to understand the "horizon" of the action, that is, what the action meant to the participants. But for Gadamer, understanding action in the actor's terms does not involve probing subjective intentions or "getting inside the actor's mind", . . . for accomplished action has a meaning that is detached from the actor's subjective intentions. What it means thus becomes what it means in the social context in which it occurred. For Gadamer, however, understanding the action in the actor's terms is only the first movement in the dialectic of interpretation. . . . By continuing to insist on the epistemological primacy of the actor's meaning, [social scientists] misunderstand . . . the dialectic of interpretation. . . . the task of understanding is to explain how the horizon of interpreter and interpreted are fused. (Hekman, 1986, pp. 148-149)

From these methodological discussions, Hekman goes on to pose specific guidelines for hermeneutic researchers.

How then would a Gadamerian social scientist approach the analysis of a concrete event? First, the Gadamerian, like the interpretive social scientist, would seek to define the historical and cultural horizon of the actors involved in the event. This would entail understanding the action in terms of the social actors. Secondly, the Gadamerian would be aware that in the course of the interpretation a different horizon of meaning would necessarily be imposed on the actor's horizon, that of the interpreter. The horizon of the interpreter is defined jointly by the historical perspective of the interpreter *and a specific ideological perspective.* . . . Awareness of this imposition of the "prejudice" of the interpreter is the result of the self-reflection that occurs in interpretation; in his words, I understand myself "in front of the text." Thirdly, the Gadamerian, unlike the interpretive social scientist, would be aware of the effect of the analyzed event to subsequent history. . . . This consciousness enhances interpretation because the interpreter is aware that the effect of the event influences the interpretation. (Hekman, 1986, p. 151; emphasis added)

Hekman here identifies three methodological implications that result from Gadamer's hermeneutics. These implications apply equally to historical research and to interpretive studies. As in any interpretive work, the first task of the researcher is to describe the historical and cultural horizon of participants involved in the research. The researcher does this by describing actions and what these actions mean in context. The second task of the researcher is to show how, in the course of analysis/interpretation, the researcher employs a different horizon of meaning, so that the actions of participants are understood differently. "The horizon of the interpreter is defined jointly by the historical perspective of the interpreter and a specific ideological perspective" (Hekman, 1986, p. 151). This means that hermeneutic researchers deal *explicitly* with their own interpretive theories and understand that the use of these theories provides one with a specific ideological perspective. For example, in historical research, hermeneutic scholars who study the history of professionalization in nursing (Melosh, 1982) may use the theory of professionalization as an interpretive background that provides a specific orientation to the "facts": the point for the hermeneutic scholar is to demonstrate how this horizon has operated in the choice of a question and in interpretive work during the course of the research.

A third methodological implication of Gadamer's hermeneutics has to do with the self-consciousness of the researcher. For the Gadamerian researcher, there is an awareness that one has chosen a research question or a situation or phenomenon because of its perceived effect on history. This effect is discernible to the researcher because of the interpretive scheme that informs the researcher and because of one's standpoint in history. Hermeneutic researchers must, therefore, be self-conscious, must be aware that they have chosen an action or an event because of the effect they believe the event or phenomenon will have on history. In this sense, Gadamerian—unlike a Schutzian—interpretive work is not concerned with "bracketing" the perspective of the researcher. Rather, the point is to *explicate* how and why the interpretations (horizon) of the researcher have informed the choice of the research question and the research process.

One outcome of this theoretical and methodological position is that there is not a single, accurate privileged perspective in hermeneutic scholarship (Leonard, 1989). Rather, interpretations necessarily change with interpreters and with the questions, historical standpoints, and theoretical schemes or conceptual leanings that inform their research. Cultural anthropologist Clifford Geertz (1979) discussed this methodological issue when he argued that interpretation is a dialectical process of moving back and forth between the "experience near" concepts of informants and the "experience distant" concepts of researcher. Both are a necessary part of interpretive work.

This hermeneutic approach suggests important dilemmas for nursing researchers. As with all social scientists, there is the immediate question of how one deals with the differences that arise between the researcher's interpretation of an event and the participants' interpretations of those events. Hermeneutic philosophy takes up this dilemma where the grounded theory movement left off (Hekman, 1986). For hermeneutics helps the scholar to know that there is no such thing as uninterpreted observations and that the "theory" or interpretations that emerge from the data are influenced by the conceptual leanings and interpretive background used, consciously or unconsciously, by the scholar.

Practical strategies for dealing with this dilemma depend, to a large extent, on the politics and consciousness of the researcher. For some, differences between the "emic" expressions of participants and the "etic" descriptions of the researcher can be addressed by keeping a journal in which the researcher documents personal reactions, noticing that his or her own horizon is operating in the way interpretations are made, and documenting differences in the way the researcher analyzes events versus the meaning those events have in their natural context. Wilson (1985) argues for the use of several different forms of field notes, such as personal, theoretical, observational, and methodological, as a way of documenting interpretive work. Lincoln and Guba (1985) presented another strategy for dealing with this dilemma in their notion of an audit trail, in which the researcher documents methodological decisions and theoretical moves during the course of the research.

Another strategy that extends this concept would be to design opportunities for dialogue with participants into the research plan (Connors, 1988), so that the researcher provides explicitly for the "fusion" of horizons, allowing time for participants to hear how the researcher is proceeding in the analysis of data and documenting the effects of these discussions on the researcher and the participants. In this way, the hermeneutic researcher deals actively and explicitly with the dilemma of allowing one's own theoretical or conceptual leanings to assume a privileged position.

Critical Hermeneutics

A final branch of interpretive theory has been identified as "critical" hermeneutics (Bleicher, 1980), or radical hermeneutics (Caputo, 1987). Like objective hermeneutics, critical hermeneutics begins from an assumption that not all interpretations are equally valid or true and that it is important for people to discern better from worse interpretation. But unlike objectivist hermeneutics, this critical strand of hermeneutics rejects the notion of a single, univocal meaning in any interpretive act. Like other postmodern acts of interpretation, critical hermeneutics maintains that texts or messages have a history of the development of meaning and that, with each successive interpretation, meanings are constituted. Critical hermeneutics further operates explicitly on the assumption that not all social actors are heard; that tradition contains many socially accepted meanings that are hegemonic, that represent the interests of a few; and that it is important to demystify socially oppressive meanings that may be unnoticed by participants themselves.

Paul Ricouer (1981) identified an important difference between critical hermeneutics and other forms of interpretive theory in his analysis of phenomenology and psychoanalysis. Ricouer would have characterized the difference between objective hermeneutics, Gadamerian hermeneutics, and critical hermeneutics by emphasizing the difference between faith and suspicion. He argued that, in most traditional forms of hermeneutics, interpretive method is characterized by positive belief or faith in the hidden meaning of the symbol or the text or the message. Traditional hermeneutics is generally motivated by the aim of restoring lost meaning, and it rests on the interpreter's faith that such meaning can be restored.

> [Objective] hermeneutics is first a listening, a "belief." This presupposition is one which grants the symbol a certain "truth" from the beginning. This "truth" may be merely that of the possibility of a signifying intention which may then be classified among other types of intentionality. But it is only through the willingness to "believe" that the symbolic dimension may be so described . . . the "belief" that the symbol has something to say and that the [scholar] may learn from the symbol finally presupposed a degree of active participation on the part of the [scholar] which belies the presumed disinterestedness of a transcendental consciousness. . . . Hermeneutics in this version of restoration of (lost) meaning is motivated by the will-to-hear. (Ihde, 1971, p. 141)

If objective hermeneutics is characterized by a belief or faith in the meaning of the text or message, critical hermeneutics may be characterized by what Ricouer termed "suspicion." Critical hermeneutic theory emphasizes the need to demystify, to go behind given meanings that are illusory to meanings that actors themselves cannot see. According to Ricoeur, Marx, Nietzsche, and Freud were practitioners of this critical hermeneutics, and the methodological styles found in psychoanalysis and the critique of ideology are ideal-type examples of critical hermeneutic practice.

> The countermotivations of a hermeneutics of suspicion are those which begin from the demystification of the symbol. A hermeneutics of suspicion takes as its aim the removal of illusions. Its hypothesis is one which begins with the positing of a "false consciousness" which is deceived (either by its situation or in self-deception). . . . It is a motivation which opposes the decision to "believe." . . . [In] the implied iconoclasm of a "suspicious" hermeneutics . . . all immediacy of meaning is questioned. (Ihde, 1971, p. 152)

Ricouer then identified an important difference between critical hermeneutics and objectivist hermeneutics. This is a distinction that leads to significant differences in the theoretical and methodological commitments of most interpretive researchers and critical social theorists.

> According to one view, hermeneutics is construed as the restoration of a meaning addressed to the interpreter in the form of a message. This type of hermeneutics is animated by faith, by a willingness to listen, and

it is characterized by a respect for the symbol as a revelation of the sacred. According to another view, however, hermeneutics is regarded as the demystification of a meaning presented to the interpreter in the form of a disguise. This type of hermeneutics is animated by suspicion, by a skepticism towards the given, and it is characterized by a distrust of the symbol as a dissimulation of the real. (J. B. Thompson, 1981, p. 6)

The critical impulse in this strand of hermeneutics is an intellectual remnant of the Enlightenment. In contemporary social theory, this influence appears in the work of the Frankfurt School, also known as Critical Theory. The most well-known living representative of the Frankfurt School is Jürgen Habermas, whose social theory (1979, 1985, 1987) has found recent applications in nursing (Allen, 1985; Hedin, 1986; Stevens, 1989; Thompson, 1987). Critical theorists are best known for their critique of ideology and their continuation of the contemporary neo-Marxist tradition (Held, 1980; McCarthy, 1979; O'Neill, 1976). Critical scholars maintain that human interests are not always served by a hermeneutics of faith, by noncritically interpreting the human condition. The existence of ideological structures, of half-truths and propaganda, of manipulation and oppression of thought, these are all conditions that may remain hidden from people. The suspicion that motivates critical hermeneutics aims at demystifying such structures by uncovering meanings that may be hidden from social actors themselves.

The tension between faith and suspicion is an interesting part of contemporary hermeneutic discourse. While objectivist hermeneutics is characterized more by faith, and critical hermeneutics more by suspicion, both impulses may be found within the work of a single thinker.

Within the more secularized variants of modern German hermeneutics, it is possible to see the effects of both tendencies (faith and suspicion), often in uneasy tension within the same thinker's work. In two recent traditions particularly, that of *Existenzphilosophie* and Critical Theory, both impulses have been operative. . . . The tensions between the two impulses are in part responsible for the continued fecundity of the two traditions. Indeed, it might be said that the cutting edge of contemporary German hermeneutics is precisely where *Existenzphilosophie* and Critical Theory intersect, for it is here that the implications of the two types of hermeneutics have been most profoundly exposed. (Jay, 1982, pp. 91-92)

The tension between suspicion and faith is present in the works of both Gadamer and Habermas. The debate between them has produced an enormous amount of commentary and still generates important insights regarding central controversies in hermeneutic theory (Bleicher, 1980; Hoy, 1982; Jay, 1982). Habermas has been especially critical of philosophical hermeneutics and what he sees as a politically conservative tendency in Heideggerian thought in general.

For Habermas, as with Gadamer, the hermeneutic experience does include the horizon of the interpreter, the historical conditions that are brought to the interpretive project. But for Habermas, the whole notion of a fusion of horizons threatens the very possibility of scholarship as a critical activity, as a use of reason. Habermas maintains that the critique of texts, of meanings, and of participants' understandings of their world is an important way of showing us systematically distorted power relations, relations that are institutionally produced and reproduced, from generation to generation, because people do not see through them. He maintains that, as the critical theorist/scholar remains somewhat distanced, skeptical, and able to critique taken-for-granted meanings, the social world can be transformed, can move toward greater freedom.

In response, Gadamer argues that it is not possible to remove or distance oneself to a vantage point that is outside cultural, linguistic traditions and that critique cannot occur outside of the hermeneutic circle. Gadamer's influence on Habermas has been real. Critical social theory no longer maintains transcendental, "Eurocentric" perspectives about the critique of practice and action (Bernstein, 1983; Habermas, 1987). Instead, critical hermeneutics maintains that, within the symbolic dimension of the life-world, it is possible to slacken commitments to tradition and critically examine one's cultural practices. Language itself contains this critical function. The debate between Heideggerian scholars and critical social theorists then frequently centers on the extent to which people can go beyond their context-dependent understandings of a situation and leave behind meanings that are accepted because of uncritically internalizing the authority of tradition.

This controversy in the hermeneutic tradition is important for nursing, because issues that are raised in this debate may influence the theoretical and methodological perspectives held by nurse-researchers. One way to understand these issues is to look more closely at the ontology that is implied in Gadamer's hermeneutics, and in Heideggerian thought in general, and to see why Habermas is so skeptical of these philosophical leanings.

On one hand, hermeneutic philosophy grasps some important insights from postmodern philosophy. Gadamer and Heidegger both deal with what has been termed "the metaphysics of presence." During the twentieth century, this phrase has emerged in Western thought as we have become more reflexive and aware of the function of language in the construction of meaning. Insights from ordinary language philosophy have helped us to recognize that language always functions in ordinary life as a medium of meaning making. In language, things and the meaning of things in our world become present to us. This function of language to make things present to us is captured in the phrase "metaphysics of presence." Things become present for us in and through language. For some postmodern thinkers, this insight has led to nihilistic conclusions, to an emphasis on the function of language as a dissimulation, as an act of violence that imposes meaning.

Heidegger and Gadamer, however, hold a view of language that does not lead to this kind of nihilism. The hermeneutic act of language and history maintains that it is in and through our traditions, our practices, our preconceptions, our historical perspectives and worldviews, and our specific concepts and ideas that we are able to constitute the world and objects in it. Tradition gives us a world, makes it present to us. Hermeneutic philosophy also acknowledges that most of our naive, natural attitudes are characterized by pre-reflexive efforts to "fill in," to constitute objects and meanings. We do this frequently in un-self-conscious ways, without stopping to reflect, because we are already socialized as competent speakers.

But hermeneutic philosophy, as other postmodern schools of thought, is skeptical of this "foundation" of presence. Gadamer's work is especially antifoundational in that he emphasizes the social and historical nature of our understandings. Gadamer does not suggest that we should remain naive and comfortable within our traditions, in our ideas and in our ways of constituting the world. Like Heidegger, he holds absence and presence in an uneasy tension. For Gadamer, the hermeneutic experience is one in which the presence of the subject can be eclipsed, can be called into question because it is recognized as prejudice. With this recognition, we can see our attempts at making things present, and, in this moment, presence recedes, or withdraws, leaving mystery and letting things be (Caputo, 1985). The dialectic of absence and presence is reflected in Gadamer's notion of the fusion of horizons, because the fusion for Gadamer does not mean that all differences are collapsed, rather that one is opened up to different understanding. In this way, Gadamer's hermeneutic holds some opening for traditions to be transformed, to change.

This aspect of hermeneutic discourse is a precursor of other postmodern accounts of interpretation, where greater emphasis has been placed on this notion of eclipsing the perspective of the subject, on questioning the view or vantage point of the knower. In postmodernism, the uneasy tension between presence and absence is shifted, and there is a major emphasis on critique that decenters, that questions the perspective of the knowing subject as the seat of meaning making, and that, therefore, challenges the entire tradition of humanism, questioning the notion that humans are the center or the seat of meaning making. Postmodernism helps us to notice that only certain privileged voices have been heard in the construction of meaning and that these voices, which usually have belonged to white, privileged, heterosexual men, have held a monopoly on the establishment of meaning. Hermeneutics falls short of deconstruction here, however, in that it resists the tendency to equate human attempts to establish meaning with acts of violence that impose significance. In the evolution of Continental philosophy then, Gadamer's hermeneutics assumes a moderate position, "taking one to the abyss, but maintaining that there are things to be done" (Caputo, 1987).

The critical dimensions of hermeneutics are more skeptical of the ways in which meaning is constituted. In critical hermeneutics, there is an explicit focus on uncovering or deconstructing the role of tradition and the way tradition operates to establish meaning. There is a more explicit concern with questioning the authority of given meanings and of noticing that not all speakers' meanings count. Critical hermeneutics then does not thematize trust and notices that meanings that endure are largely the meanings of winners (Caputo, 1987).

The tension between Gadamerian hermeneutics and critical hermeneutics is one that appears increasingly in nursing research literature (Allen, Diekelmann, & Benner, 1986; Diekelmann, Allen, & Tanner, 1989; Leonard, 1989; Stevens, 1989; Thompson, 1985). In social scientific literature, recent discussions suggest that the debate between Gadamer and Habermas was more an issue of degree (Hekman, 1986; Jay, 1982), that hermeneutics may be more or less radical, depending on the extent to which one emphasizes the importance of critique and decentering. The debate between Habermas and Gadamer was important, however, because, as a result of it, Habermas (1987) modified an earlier transcendental leaning in his work and, following Gadamer, located the possibility of critique within the functions of language and the life-world.

These issues of critique and tradition are important for researchers in nursing because they help us to understand our role in the social production of knowledge, in the development or the transformation of cultural traditions. For this reason, the movement between Gadamer, Habermas, and others' notions of deconstruction (Dzurec, 1989) is one that holds important implications for theory, method, and practice in nursing.

For many critical theorists, the language of being that is so characteristic of Heideggerian thought is problematic. Critical theorists will want to know who is speaking about being and how this speaker is situated in relation to other, more marginal discourse. Furthermore, an ontology of presence is problematic when it obscures context, remaining open to the moral presence of being but not dealing with the politics that are ever present in the social construction of our world. In so doing, Heideggerian thought may be criticized for contributing to the deformation of the world and of being, of helping to preserve a world in which the traditions, interests, and constructions of a few prevail. Critical hermeneutics, in contrast, is "constantly drawing our attention to those systematic features of contemporary society that inhibit, distort, or prevent dialogue from being concretely embodied in our everyday practices" (Bernstein, 1983, p. 224).

These differences in the theoretical leanings of hermeneutic scholars may also lead to differences in methodological commitments. Some recent discussions in the social sciences have identified methodological differences between critical hermeneutics and Gadamerian hermeneutics. These are methodological implications that also hold for nursing researchers, because they derive from differences in the theory of interpretation held by the researcher.

In her analysis of research informed by critical theory, Lather (1986) noted that critical inquiry is implied in at least three contemporary paradigms: feminist research, neo-Marxist critical ethnography, and Freirian "empowering," or participatory educational research. While there are several sources of examples of critical hermeneutic work in research, these have remained somewhat isolated, and the methodological implications of critical hermeneutics have been largely unexplored.

Like Gadamerian hermeneutics, critical hermeneutics maintains that there are no neutral, objective interpretations. Critical hermeneutics argues, however, that there are many instances when researchers believe that "because they are unconscious of any bias or political agenda, they are neutral and objective, when in fact they are only unconscious" (Namenwirth, 1986). Unlike objective hermeneutics, which maintains that the interests of the scholar can be bracketed, critical hermeneutics argues that the vantage point and interests of the scholar are always involved in interpretation and that they should be explicit rather than hidden. In contrast to other interpretive approaches, critical inquiry is openly conscious of its interests and is committed to critiquing distorted power relations and to building a more just society. Critical hermeneutics leads to a kind of research that "allows us not only to understand the maldistribution of power and resources underlying our society but also to change that maldistribution to help create a more equal world . . . [it is] research as praxis" (Lather, 1986, p. 258).

One feature of critical scholarship then is its function as an intervention, as a practice that can lead to greater understandings of injustice and through these understandings to transformations of the social world. Because critique, or "suspicion," is a feature of critical hermeneutic theory, researchers influenced by this tradition usually deal with the phenomenon of "false consciousness" or "consciousness-raising."

The critique of "false consciousness," or the critique of ideologies, then is a hallmark of critical hermeneutics, and while there is much controversy surrounding these notions, in general, they suggest that people may not always be aware of oppressive features of their situations. Critical hermeneutics maintains that we are frequently unaware of oppressive conditions because social and personal beliefs operate, as any ideology does, to convince us of the truth or authority of a situation. Such beliefs or ideologies may be critiqued as "false" if people have not had the opportunity to see through them or if such a "false" consciousness functions to legitimize a reprehensible situation (Guess, 1981). The "suspicion" behind critical hermeneutics then is intended to go behind "commonsense," socially acceptable meanings and to uncover hidden meanings that may be unnoticed by social actors themselves but that, nevertheless, function to sustain and reproduce inequities and injustices.

Like consciousness-raising, critical or emancipatory research has an effect. The insights that are generated from self-reflection in critical hermeneutics intervene in people's lives and, subsequently, affect their realities.

Emancipatory social research calls for empowering approaches to research. For researchers with emancipatory aspirations, doing empirical research offers a powerful opportunity for praxis to the extent that the research process enables people to change by encouraging self-reflection and a deeper understanding of their particular situations. (Lather, 1986, p. 258-262)

Lather identified five characteristics of emancipatory research that illustrate the methodological implications of critical hermeneutics. While there are some similarities between this methodology and that found in Gadamerian hermeneutics, one important difference is the extent to which researchers explicitly situate themselves in relation to cultural practices. Critical researchers are committed to the critique of false consciousness and to an active, nonelitist engagement with participants to address social injustices.

First, critical inquiry is a response to the experiences, desires, and needs of oppressed people. Its initial step is to develop an understanding of the world view of research participants. Central to establishing such understanding is a dialogic research design where respondents are actively involved in the construction and validation of meaning. The purpose of this phase of inquiry is to provide accounts that are a basis for further analysis and a corrective to the "investigator's preconceptions regarding the subjects' life-world and experiences." Second, critical inquiry inspires and guides the dispossessed in the process of cultural transformation. At the core of the transformation is a "reciprocal relationship in which every teacher is always a student and every pupil a teacher." [In the critique of "false consciousness"] . . . the present is cast against the historical backdrop while at the same time the "naturalness" of social arrangements is challenged so that social actors can see both the constraints and the potential for change in their situations. Third, critical inquiry focuses on fundamental contradictions which help dispossessed people see how poorly their "ideologically frozen understandings" serve their interests. Fourth, the validity of a critical account can be found, in part, in the participants' responses. . . . The point is to provide an environment that invites participants' critical reaction to the researcher's accounts of their worlds. Fifth, critical inquiry stimulates a "self-sustaining process of critical analysis and enlightened action." . . . The researcher joins the participants in a theoretically guided program of action extended over a period of time. (Lather, 1986, p. 268)

Box 7.1. The Need for Reciprocity

SOURCE: Adapted from Lather (1986).

Interviews are conducted in an interactive, dialogic manner, that requires self-disclosure on the part of the researcher.

There are sequential interviews of both individuals and small groups to facilitate collaboration and a deeper probing of research issues.

Negotiation of meaning. At a minimum, this entails recycling description, emerging analysis, and conclusions to at least a subsample of respondents. A more maximal approach to reciprocity would involve research participants in a collaborative effort to build empirically rooted theory.

Interviews involve discussions of false consciousness that go beyond the researcher simply dismissing participants' "resistance."

Triangulation is critical in establishing data trustworthiness . . . and includes multiple data sources, methods, and theoretical schemes.

These methodological commitments have a significant impact on issues of validity in critical research. In effect, they "raise the stakes," or increase the need for rigor, because researchers must demonstrate that their interpretations are "valid" and that they have done such work in a nonelitist and nonmanipulative manner, "meaning that one wants to be not a 'one-way propagandist' " (Lather, 1986).

The summaries in Box 7.1 and Box 7.2 present methodological suggestions that guide interpretive work in emancipatory or critical research. Lather notes that these approaches explicitly address issues of validity and trustworthiness in data collection and interpretation.

Recent literature demonstrates the influence of critical hermeneutics in nursing research. Examples of this approach may be found in the work of Hedin (1986), who studied the socialization of nurses in German training programs, and in Allen and Peterson (1986), who studied shared governance in bureaucratic settings. In nursing education, the work of Diekelmann (1988) demonstrates the impact of critical research and empowering approaches in the curriculum. While this approach to research is clearly grounded in contemporary hermeneutic scholarship, an important issue for nurse-researchers influenced by this tradition is the extent to which prevailing institutions will support and remain open to critical interpretive work.

Box 7.2. Establishing Validity: Dialectical Theory-Building versus
          Theoretical Imposition

SOURCE: Adapted from Lather (1986).

Construct validity must be dealt with . . . [It] requires a ceaseless confron-
tation with and respect for the experience of people in their daily lives to
guard against theoretical imposition. A systematized reflexivity which
reveals how a priori theory has been changed by the logic of the data
becomes essential in establishing construct validity.

Face validity needs to be reconsidered. "Research with face validity provides a 'click of recognition' and a 'yes, of course' instead of 'yes, but'
experience." Face validity is operationalized by recycling description,
emerging analysis and conclusion back through at least a subsample of
respondents . . . refining in light of the participants' reactions. One caution . . . the possibility of encountering false consciousness creates a limit
[for face validity] . . . most people to some extent identify with and/or
accept ideologies which do not serve their best interests. . . .

Catalytic validity represents the degree to which the research process
reorients, focuses, and energizes participants toward knowing reality in
order to transform it, a process termed conscientization.

Hermeneutic Research in Nursing:
The Research Program of Patricia Benner

One of the most well-known applications of hermeneutics in nursing research has occurred in the work of Patricia Benner (1982, 1984a,
1985; Benner & Wrubel, 1989), who developed the paradigm of
expert practice in nursing. Benner's research program is a clear
example of hermeneutic applications in nursing research, although
it will be argued here that it is difficult to locate this work within any
one of the three theories of interpretation discussed in this chapter.
Benner identifies her research as an example of "Heideggerian phenomenology" (Benner, 1985). The influence of Heidegger is clearly
expressed in Benner's theoretical leanings, in her research questions,
and in her assumptions about the importance of situated meaning.

While Benner's application of hermeneutics has made a significant
contribution by helping nursing better understand the features of
skilled practice, it will be argued here that the influence of Heidegger
results in both theoretical and methodological ambiguities that have
important implications for nursing research and for practice.

While Benner (1985) acknowledges the influence of Heidegger in her intellectual development, there is less evidence that she has been influenced by Gadamer's interpretive work and by the social and historical implications of his philosophy of interpretation. The absence of Gadamer's influence can be seen in a methodological ambiguity that places Benner's research somewhere between objective hermeneutics and Gadamerian hermeneutics. This ambiguity is an important one because, in dealing with it, one can anticipate future directions in the development of Benner's research program.

The study of expert practice in nursing was first discussed in 1982 (Benner, 1982a) and continued as a line of research that drew interest throughout the 1980s. Benner's research design uses "exemplars," which she defines as "an example that conveys more than one intent, meaning, function or outcome and [that] can easily be compared or translated to other clinical situations whose objective characteristics might be quite different" (Benner, 1984a, p. 293). The methodology involves interviews with highly skilled and experienced nurses who are encouraged to relate critical incidents from their practice in which they feel their interventions have made a difference in the patient's outcome. The exemplar interviews are then analyzed for themes that demonstrate common meanings and intentions. Benner also conducted interviews with pairs of nurses consisting of preceptors and newly graduated nurses to determine differences in practice between beginner and experienced nurses.

As a result of this research, Benner identified five levels of proficiency in clinical nursing practice. These levels of proficiency were labeled as follows: novice, advanced beginner, competent, proficient, and expert. In Benner's research, the movement from novice to expert involves changes in nurses' perceptions and use of past experience and movement from detachment to involvement. In addition to levels of proficiency, Benner also identified domains of competency in nursing practice, which include functions such as teaching-coaching, helping, diagnosing and monitoring, and managing rapidly changing situations.

The interpretation of data and identification of these competencies and levels of proficiency involved the use of a model of skill acquisition developed by Stuart Dreyfus, a mathematician, and Hubert Dreyfus, a philosopher. The Dreyfus model, in turn, was developed while studying the performance of airplane pilots responding to emergency situations (Dreyfus & Dreyfus, 1986).

In the design of her research program and in the theoretical influence apparent in her work, Benner clearly demonstrates the application of hermeneutic thought in nursing. For example, throughout her work, there are repeated references to the importance of meaning and the ways in which context determines meaning.

> Meaning resides not solely within the individual or solely within the situation but is a transaction between the two so that the individual both constitutes and is constituted by the situation. (Benner, 1985, p. 7)

The idea of situated meaning is a predominant part of Benner's work, as indicated in another statement, where she argues that the notion of skill acquisition used and developed in her research was a "situational model," where "the characteristics of the situation have as much influence on successful performance as does knowledge of procedural steps for performing the task" (Benner, 1982b, p. 304).

These references to situated meaning are a hallmark of Heideggerian discourse and in Benner's later work they are extended in a grand theory of what it means to be a person (Benner & Wrubel, 1989). Benner's theoretical leanings are reflected in her notions about people being nonmechanistic and more than the sum of behaviors and cognitions. There is a clear emphasis on the primacy of being situated, of always interpreting one's situation and constituting its meaning. This use of hermeneutics is consistent with Heideggerian phenomenology and with Heidegger's claims about the primacy of interpretation and his insistence that interpreting is the ground of Being. But Benner's work also demonstrates a tendency to ontologize in ways that obscure the politics of situated meaning. Her use of hermeneutics is then not as socially and as historically grounded as it might be if influenced by different strands in the hermeneutic tradition. This influence can be discussed both at the level of theory and at the level of methodology.

First, at the level of theoretical influence, Benner's familiarity with Heideggerian scholarship has allowed her to break away from prior theories of nursing. Her approach to nursing practice emphasizes the holistic quality of actions. She maintains, along with most Heideggerians, that Western culture has for too long neglected the primacy of being embodied and already situated in social contexts. She, therefore, begins from a vantage point that is more interested in people's experiencing of the world and less in how we know what we know. Such an interest is a natural application of the hermeneutic tradition, especially because this vantage point enables Benner to focus on skilled actions and the kind of interpretations that are involved in the practice of expert nurses.

In taking this theoretical approach to nursing practice, Benner extended the Dreyfus model of skill acquisition. The research developed by Dreyfus and Dreyfus was part of a trend labeled "applied Heidegger" that occurred during the 1960s, 1970s, and 1980s. In philosophy, some of this impulse was translated into efforts to distinguish between artificial intelligence and human skill acquisition and it emerged in the work of Dreyfus and Dreyfus in their notions of skilled activity and embodied intelligence. These ideas emphasize the ways in which human decision making and expertise are holistic, experiential, and contextual.

The theory of skill acquisition implied in Benner's work shows how she has taken up a conversation that is central in hermeneutic discourse. The hermeneutic tradition has a long history of reconstructing ancient Greek distinctions between skilled technical knowledge and other forms of knowledge and wisdom. Many hermeneutic thinkers have explored the differences and similarities between wisdom, knowledge, and technical proficiency. Most scholars in this tradition refuse to reduce practical knowledge to the accumulation of technical experience. They have been part of an important conversation in hermeneutic discourse that recollects Aristotle's distinction between *techne* and *praxis* (Arendt, 1958; Bellah, 1982; Bernstein, 1983; Gadamer, 1975; Habermas, 1971; Lobkowicz, 1967; Parekh, 1981). For Aristotle, *techne* (poeisis) was the kind of technical knowledge one acquired as a result of repeated experiences in doing or making. In contrast, *praxis* (phronesis) was the kind of wisdom one acquired as a result of living in moral and political communities (Gadamer, 1975).

While Benner's work elevates the kind of knowledge found in skilled bodily activity, and this should be recognized as an important contribution to nursing, her research also deals with the wisdom, the ethics, and the politics of nursing practice. Benner's research retains a tie with hermeneutic discourse and with practical philosophy because she does not collapse the distinction between wisdom and knowledge. Specifically, she does not equate the knowledge of the expert nurse with technical proficiency. Underlying her descriptions of the expert nurse are descriptions of wisdom, of the ethics of knowing what should be done in specific clinical situations. Thus the technical proficiency, or the "knowledge" one acquires in the course of becoming an expert nurse, also includes wisdom, the ethics and politics of understanding, a prudent grasp of the situation with a moral sense of what should be done (Benner, 1989). For Benner, the wisdom of nursing is expressed in the term "care," or "concern"

(Benner & Wrubel, 1989), an ethical expertise that is expressed in nursing practice.

An important theoretical issue in Benner's research stems from an ambiguity regarding this dimension of expert practice. For many hermeneutic thinkers, the wisdom of practice is derived from context, specifically from cultural practices that define the good and the virtuous. Many hermeneutic scholars notice that, in the transition from communal societies to capitalist ones, we have lost the cultural categories that made praxis a real activity, as opposed to an ideal (Bernstein, 1983; Heller, 1978). Other hermeneutic scholars have noted that, in the transition from communal societies to individualistic ones, contexts no longer bring diverse people together in ways that define, at the cultural level, what is good and virtuous (MacIntyre, 1981).

It is this cultural frame of reference that is muted or missing from Benner's research program. Most critical scholars would ask how the contexts of nursing practice influence the wisdom of nursing. Critical scholars might notice that, in many instances, nurses are losing the context of care (Moccia, 1988), and that the wisdom of nursing is gradually being eclipsed by the politics of hierarchical bureaucracies. The things that have significance or meaning for nurses, the way of being that is involved in caring, happens in a context, and we know that, in the modern world, these contexts do not always support the concerns of nurses or other marginal people.

Although Benner indicates that she is aware of the importance of context, her research does not sufficiently address the social and political contexts in which nurses practice. She does not show us, as a critical ethnographer would (Todd, 1989), how the context—both the macro and micro levels of the social world—set up meanings, how the culture of bureaucracies influences the wisdom, the ethics, and the politics of practice. A critical emphasis on the contexts in which nurses practice would help this research program not only describe the nature of "being" in nursing but show us how the social and political contexts in which we practice require our attention.

Additionally, Benner's theoretical ties to Heidegger become problematic when ontology is discussed in universalizing ways. It is important to notice who is speaking about "being" or whose narratives are being considered. Postmodernism would remind us that the existential reality of white, middle-class women is not the same existential reality shared by working-class women or men of color. The "being" of a critical care nurse, if generalized to all categories of nursing practice, becomes another example of a privileged standpoint developing into a discourse that is unconscious of its own hidden dimensions of power. It is, therefore, important to notice that the expert practice of nursing does not constitute a single standpoint, rather, expert practice in nursing derives from the experiences of nurses who share different standpoints in terms of gender, race, class, and sexual preference.

These theoretical issues are matched by another concern, which occurs at the level of methodology. Again, Benner's work is more clearly influenced by Heidegger than by Gadamer, and it is this influence that may be responsible for an ambiguity in methodology. Benner's research occupies a somewhat ambiguous position that cannot be easily identified as objectivist, Gadamerian, or critical hermeneutic. On one hand, her methodology emphasizes the "emic" reality of nurses, recounting the stories of expert nurses as these are told in their natural settings. She uses three related interpretive processes in data analysis: thematic analysis, analysis of exemplars, and the search for paradigm cases (Benner, 1985).

This methodological strategy is of concern in that the analysis of themes and the development of coding schemes is presented without situating the researcher in relation to the practices. In her published work, there is not an explicit position that identifies Benner's interest in these practices as part of a larger cultural scene.[1] There is very little analysis or discussion that locates her interests "in front of" the texts so that the reader understands how and why Benner has chosen these practices as having an effect on history. The failure to situate herself in relation to the material suggests that this methodology is more consistent with objective hermeneutics.

But Benner's research program has also included many public appearances in which she discusses exemplars with nurses and consultation that addresses the development of expert practice in institutional settings. This strategy could be consistent with Gadamer's theory of interpretation, if it were used as a way to discuss the "fusion of horizons" that has occurred in Benner's research. Such discussions would presumably situate Benner in relation to the texts and the practices of nurses, explicating her interests in expert practice and her choice of this topic or subject as having a potential effect on history. This research strategy needs to be explicit and readily available to the reader so that Benner's audience can determine the ways in which the researcher understands the nurses' stories in light of her conceptual background, an interpretive scheme involving practical ethics, embodied intelligence, and her own ideological perspective. If resolved, this methodological ambiguity will clearly locate Benner's research program within one of the following approaches to research: an objective hermeneutic, a Gadamer hermeneutic, or a critical hermeneutic.

The last possibility, that of Benner's research occupying a clear position as critical hermeneutic research, seems unlikely. On one hand, Benner is a strong advocate of nurses, sees her work as informed by feminist commitments, and presents her work with the insight that "a lack of adequate description of clinical expertise has contributed to a lag in adequate recognition and reward in nursing" (Benner, 1984a, p. 11). But on the other hand, her methodological commitments do not include an active, *explicit* engagement with participants in the critique of oppressive social conditions, in the critique of ideology, or in the explicit transformation of the injustices in nursing.

Ironically, these criticisms are especially relevant for Benner's research. While she adamantly resists the use of her research to certify novice, proficient, or expert nurses (1984), her work has, in fact, been used to develop clinical ladders and has contributed to increased tendencies toward hierarchy and stratification in nursing. This leaves Benner's work open to a common criticism from feminist and critical social theorists.

A work that does not explicitly situate itself in relation to the cultural issues of its time does not help people to make cultural transformations. A work that does not address the politics of context does not succeed in being neutral or apolitical. It merely obscures impediments to cultural transformation. In hermeneutic research in nursing, theoretical and methodological ambiguities are important because they may contribute, albeit unknowingly, to the superficial use of a work in support of the status quo in nursing.

Closing Thoughts

This chapter provides an introduction to the hermeneutic tradition and explores issues and questions that are raised in the application of hermeneutics in nursing research. Patricia Benner's work has been explored as a well-known example of hermeneutic scholarship in nursing. The strengths and limits of Benner's research program may be summarized from several vantage points. On one hand, Benner's work has clearly moved nursing discourse into a postempiricist era. Her views about science, research, and knowledge are some of the first indications that nursing is moving away from an empiricist perspective about science and theory and into a historical hermeneutic understanding of knowledge, wisdom, research, and practice.

Her work should also be recognized as an important practical intervention. She successfully locates the potential in nursing and in the practice of communities of nurses to believe in the significance of our contributions to the health and well-being of people. She elevates the "knowledge" of nursing at a time when the social world has consistently devalued it, and she does this not by appropriating an empiricist paradigm for knowledge development but by affirming the knowledge and wisdom that are embedded in the practice of nurses. This aspect of her research program brings to mind insights from practical philosophy.

> One of the great needs of the modern democratic polity is to recover a sense of significant differentiation, so that partial communities, be they geographical, or cultural, or occupational, can become again important centres of concern and activity for their members *in a way which connects them to the whole.* (Taylor, 1975, pp. 441-416; emphasis added)

Because Benner's hermeneutic fosters self-understanding and a sense of community in nursing, her work is an important empowering postmodern voice in nursing. But, from the perspective of critical social theory, this work needs also to show how the contexts in which we practice inhibit the development of a wider community, close off the possibility of free, unconstrained dialogue, and, while they may be empowering for the few, may also reduce the practices of many to a one-dimensional sphere of technical reason and purposive-rational action.

Why? Because the threat of power and domination is ever present in modernity and it cannot be resisted if we obscure it. Critique is an important moment in the hermeneutic experience, and nurses as well as others can benefit from the incorporation of a critical hermeneutic voice in nursing research. Critical hermeneutics is not a totalizing nihilistic critique. It is rather a voice that is ever alert to the systematic deformation of the social world, showing us concretely what needs to be overcome so that the wisdom and knowledge of *all* people can flourish.

> For what is characteristic of our contemporary situation is not just the playing out of powerful forces that are always beyond our control, or the spread of disciplinary techniques that always elude our grasp, but a paradoxical situation where power creates counter-power (resistance)

and reveals the vulnerability of power, where the very forces that undermine and inhibit communal life also create new, and frequently unpredictable, forms of solidarity. (Bernstein, 1983, p. 228)

By showing us how nurses resist systematically distorted communication and the power relations embedded in hierarchical contexts, and by showing us different models of community in bureaucracy, critical hermeneutics in nursing sketches the contours of a different social world. This form of scholarship not only is consistent with nursing's heritage and its tradition of care but is also an intervention that is urgently needed, a sketching, a spinning of metaphor that keeps alive the prospect of a genuinely human(e) world.

Note

1. In a personal communication (October, 1989), Benner argues that her dissertation (1984b) illustrates the differences between her research program and one informed by grounded theory.

References

Allen, D. (1985). Nursing research and social control: Alternative models of science that emphasize understanding and emancipation. *Image, 17*(2), 58-64.

Allen, D., Diekelmann, N., & Benner, P. (1986). Three paradigms for nursing research. In P. Chinn (Ed.), *Nursing research methodology.* Rockville, MD: Aspen.

Allen, D., & Peterson, M. (1986). Shared governance: A strategy for transforming organizations, Part 1 and 2. *Journal of Nursing Administration, 16*(1/2), 9-12, 11-16.

Arendt, H. (1958). *The human condition.* Chicago: University of Chicago Press.

Bauman, Z. (1978). *Hermeneutics and social science.* London: Hutchinson.

Bellah, R. (1982). Social science as practical reason. *Hastings Center Report, 12*(5), 32-39.

Benner, P. (1982a). From novice to expert. *American Journal of Nursing, 82*(3), 402-407.

Benner, P. (1982b). Issues in competency based testing. *Nursing Outlook, 30*(5), 303-309.

Benner, P. (1984a). *From novice to expert.* Menlo Park, CA: Addison-Wesley.

Benner, P. (1984b). *Stress and satisfaction on the job: Work meanings and coping of mid career men.* New York: Praeger.

Benner, P. (1985). Quality of life: A phenomenological perspective on explanation, prediction and understanding in nursing science. *Advances in Nursing Science, 8*(1), 1-14.

Benner, P. (1989). *The primacy of caring, the role of experience, narrative and community in skilled ethical comportment.* Paper for the Task Force on the Experiential Turn in Ethics, University of California, San Francisco.

Benner, P., & Tanner, C. (1987). How expert nurses use intuition. *American Journal of Nursing, 87*(1), 23-32.

Benner, P., & Wrubel, J. (1989). *The primacy of caring.* Menlo Park, CA: Addison-Wesley.

Bernstein, R. (1971). *Praxis and action: Contemporary philosophies of human activity.* Philadelphia: University of Pennsylvania Press.

Bernstein, R. (1976). *The restructuring of social and political theory.* New York: Harcourt Brace Jovanovich.

Bernstein, R. (1983). *Beyond objectivism and relativism: Science, hermeneutics and praxis.* Philadelphia: University of Pennsylvania Press.

Bernstein, R. (1986). *Philosophical profiles.* Philadelphia: University of Pennsylvania Press.

Bleicher, J. (1980). *Contemporary hermeneutics: Hermeneutics as method, philosophy and critique.* London: Routledge & Kegan Paul.

Bleier, R. (1984). *Science and gender: A critique of biology and its theories of women.* New York: Pergamon.

Bleier, R. (1986). *Feminist approaches to science.* New York: Pergamon.

Bowles, G. (1984). The uses of hermeneutics for feminist scholarship. *Women's Studies International Forum, 7*(3), 185-188.

Caputo, J. (1985). From the primordiality of absence to the absence of primordiality. In H. Silverman & D. Ihde (Eds.), *Hermeneutics and deconstruction* (pp. 191-200). Albany: State University of New York Press.

Caputo, J. (1987). *Radical hermeneutics: Repetition, deconstruction and the hermeneutic project.* Indiana University Press.

Carper, B. (1978). Fundamental patterns of knowing in nursing. *Advances in Nursing Science, 1*(1), 13-23.

Connors, D. (1988). A continuum of researcher-participant relationships: An analysis and critique. *Advances in Nursing Science, 10*(4), 32-42.

Diekelmann, N. (1988). Curriculum revolution: A theoretical and philosophical mandate for change. In *Curriculum revolution: Mandate for change.* New York: National League for Nursing.

Diekelmann, N., Allen, D., & Tanner, C. (1989). *The NLN criteria for appraisal of baccalaureate programs: A critical hermeneutic analysis.* New York: National League for Nursing.

Dreyfus, H. (1980). Holism and hermeneutics. *Review of Metaphysics, 34,* 3-24.

Dreyfus, H., & Dreyfus, S. (1986). *Mind over machine.* New York: Free Press.

Dzurec, L. (1989). The necessity for and evolution of multiple paradigms for nursing research. *Advances in Nursing Science, 11*(4), 69-77.

Fry, S. (1987). Pragmatism, the aims of science and nursing science. In *Proceedings of Fourth National Nursing Science Colloquium.* Boston: Boston University, School of Nursing.

Gadamer, H. G. (1975). *Truth and method.* New York: Seabury.

Gadamer, H. G. (1979). The problem of historical consciousness. In P. Rabinow & W. Sullivan (Eds.), *Interpretive social science: A reader.* Berkeley: University of California Press.

Geertz, C. (1979). From the native's point of view: On the nature of anthropological understanding. In P. Rabinow & W. Sullivan (Eds.), *Interpretive social science: A reader.* Berkeley: University of California Press.

Geuss, R. (1981). *The idea of critical theory.* Cambridge: Cambridge University Press.

Habermas, J. (1971). *Knowledge and human interests.* Boston: Beacon.

Habermas, J. (1979). *Communication and the evolution of society* (T. McCarthy, Trans.). Boston: Beacon.

Habermas, J. (1985). *The theory of communicative action: Vol. 1. Reason and the rationalization of society.* Boston: Beacon.

Habermas, J. (1987). *The theory of communicative action: Vol. 2. Lifeworld and system: A critique of functional reason.* Boston: Beacon.

Habermas, J. (1988). *On the logic of the social sciences* (S. Nicholson & J. Stark, Trans.). Cambridge: MIT Press.

Harding, S. (1986). *The science question in feminism.* Ithaca, NY: Cornell University Press.

Hedin, B. (1986). Nursing, education and emancipation: Applying the critical theoretical approach to nursing research. In P. Chinn (Ed.), *Nursing research methodology: Issues and implementation.* Rockville, MD: Aspen.

Hekman, S. (1986). *Hermeneutics and the sociology of knowledge.* Notre Dame, IN: University of Notre Dame Press.

Held, D. (1980). *Introduction to critical theory.* Berkeley: University of California Press.

Heller, A. (1978). *Renaissance man.* New York: Macmillan.

Hesse, M. (1980). *Revolutions and reconstructions in the philosophy of science.* Brighton, England: Harvester.

Howard, R. (1982). *Three faces of hermeneutics: An introduction to current theories of understanding.* Berkeley: University of California Press.

Hoy, D. (1982). *The critical circle: Literature, history and philosophical hermeneutics.* Berkeley: University of California Press.

Ihde, D. (1971). *Hermeneutic phenomenology: The philosophy of Paul Ricoeur.* Evanston, IL: Northwestern University Press.

Jay, R. (1982). Should intellectual history take a linguistic turn? In D. LaCapra & S. Kaplan (Eds.), *Modern European intellectual history.* Ithaca, NY: Cornell University Press.

Keller, E. F. (1985). *Reflections on gender and science.* New Haven, CT: Yale University Press.

Knaack, P. (1984). Phenomenological research. *Western Journal of Nursing Research, 6*(1), 107-114.

Kuhn, T. (1977). *The essential tension: Selected studies in scientific tradition and change.* Chicago: University of Chicago Press.

Lather, P. (1986). Research as praxis. *Harvard Educational Review, 56*(3), 257-277.

Lauden, L. (1984). *Science and values: The aims of science and their role in scientific debate.* Berkeley: University of California Press.

Leonard, V. (1989). A Heideggerian phenomenologic perspective on the concept of the person. *Advances in Nursing Science, 11*(4), 40-55.

Lincoln, Y., & Guba, E. (1985). *Naturalistic inquiry.* Beverly Hills, CA: Sage.

Lobkowicz, N. (1967). *Theory and practice: The history of a concept from Aristotle to Marx.* Notre Dame, IN: University of Notre Dame Press.

MacIntyre, A. (1981). *After virtue: A study in moral theory.* Notre Dame, IN: University of Notre Dame Press.

McCarthy, T. (1979). *The critical theory of Jurgen Habermas.* Cambridge: MIT Press.

Melosh, B. (1982). *The physician's hand: Work, culture and conflict in American nursing.* Philadelphia: Temple University Press.

Merleau-Ponty, M. (1962). *The phenomenology of perception.* London: Routledge & Kegan Paul.

Mischler, E. (1979). Meaning in context: Is there any other kind? *Harvard Educational Review, 49,* 1-19.

Moccia, P. (1986). *New approaches to theory development.* New York: National League for Nursing.

Moccia, P. (1988). At the faultline: Social activism and caring. *Nursing Outlook, 36*(1), 30-33.

Morse, J. (1989). *Qualitative nursing research: A contemporary dialogue.* Rockville, MD: Aspen.

Mueller-Vollmer, K. (1985). *The hermeneutics reader: Texts in the German tradition from the Enlightenment to the present.* New York: Continuum.

Munhall, P., & Oiler-Boyd, C. (1986). *Nursing research: A qualitative perspective.* New York: Appleton-Lange.

Namenwirth, M. (1986). Science through a feminist prism. In R. Bleier (Ed.), *Feminist approaches to science.* New York: Pergamon.

Oiler, C. (1983). Phenomenological approach in nursing research. *Nursing Research, 31,* 178-181.

Oiler, C. (1986). Qualitative methods: Phenomenology. In P. Moccia (Ed.), *New approaches to theory development.* New York: National League for Nursing.

Omery, A. (1983). Phenomenology: A method for nursing research. *Advances in Nursing Science, 5,* 49-63.

O'Neill, J. (1976). *On critical theory.* New York: Seabury.

Outhwaite, W. (1985). Hans-Georg Gadamer. In Q. Skinner (Ed.), *The return of grand theory in the human sciences.* Cambridge: Cambridge University Press.

Palmer, R. (1969). *Hermeneutics: Interpretation theory in Scheiermacher, Dilthey, Heidegger and Gadamer.* Evanston, IL: Northwestern University Press.

Parekh, B. (1981). *Hannah Arendt and the search for a new political philosophy.* London: Macmillan.

Polkinghorne, D. (1983). *Methodology for the human sciences.* Albany: State University of New York.

Polkinghorne, D. (1988). *Narrative knowing and the human sciences.* Albany: State University of New York.

Reeder, R. (1989). Hermeneutics. In B. Sarter (Ed.), *Paths to knowledge: Innovative research methods in nursing.* New York: National League for Nursing.

Ricoeur, P. (1970). *Freud and philosophy: An essay on interpretation* (D. Savage, Trans.). New Haven, CT: Yale University Press.

Ricoeur, P. (1981). *Hermeneutics and the human sciences* (J. B. Thompson, Ed. and Trans.). Cambridge: Cambridge University Press.

Rorty, R. (1979). *Philosophy and the mirror of nature.* Princeton, NJ: Princeton University Press.

Rorty, R. (1982). *Consequences of pragmatism.* Minneapolis: University of Minnesota Press.

Schachtel, E. (1959). *Metamorphosis.* New York: Basic Books.

Schrag, C. (1980). *Radical reflection and the origin of the human sciences.* West Lafayette, IN: Purdue University Press.

Spiegelberg, H. (1982). *The phenomenological movement* (3rd ed.). The Hague, the Netherlands: Martinus Nijhoff.

Stevens, P. (1989). A critical social reconceptualization of environment in nursing: Implications for methodology. *Advances in Nursing Science, 11*(4), 56-68.

Taylor, C. (1975). *Hegel* (pp. 414-416). Cambridge, England: Cambridge University Press.

Thompson, J. B. (Ed. & Trans.). (1981). Editor's introduction. In P. Ricoeur, *Hermeneutics and the human sciences.* Cambridge: Cambridge University Press.

Thompson, J. L. (1985). Practical discourse in nursing: Going beyond empiricism and historicism. *Advances in Nursing Science, 7*(4), 59-71.

Thompson, J. L. (1987a). Critical scholarship: The critique of domination in nursing. *Advances in Nursing Science, 10*(1), 27-38.

Thompson, J. L. (1987b). Effective historical consciousness in nursing. In *Proceedings of Fourth National Nursing Science Colloquium*. Boston: Boston University, School of Nursing.

Todd, A. (1989). *Intimate adversaries: Cultural conflict between doctors and women patients*. Philadelphia: University of Pennsylvania Press.

Wachterhauser, B. (1986). *Hermeneutics and modern philosophy*. Albany: State University of New York Press.

Watson, J. (1988). *Nursing: Human science and human care*. New York: National league for Nursing.

Weinscheimer, J. (1985). *Gadamer's hermeneutics*. New Haven, CT: Yale University Press.

Wilson, H. (1985). *Research in nursing*. Menlo Park, CA: Addison-Wesley.

Wolf, Z. (1988). *Nurses' work: The sacred and the profane*. Philadelphia: University of Pennsylvania Press.

Wolff, J. (1975). Hermeneutics and the critique of ideology. *Sociological Review, 23*, 811-823.

Response to Hermeneutic Inquiry

PATRICIA E. BENNER

While there is much I agree with in Janice Thompson's chapter, I will respond critically to the assertions: (1) that interpretive hermeneutics fails to provide a critique; (2) that according to Gadamer and a three way classification scheme, my work is methodologically ambiguous; (3) that the practical applications of *From Novice to Expert* to the development of clinical promotion programs create divisive hierarchies; and (4) finally, I argue for pluralism in critical methods rather than giving one critical method privilege.

Critique from an Interpretive Hermeneutical Perspective

Janice Thompson introduces the reader to the issues in the post modern critique of logical positivism and relevant philosophy of science issues that distinguish the natural sciences and the human sciences. Those who do interpretive research begin with notions of the person that differ from the Cartesian assumptions inherent in logical positivism (Benner and Wrubel, 1989; Leonard, 1989; Taylor, 1989). I agree with Thompson that critical theory is an important method for critiquing false consciousness and oppressive ideologies, but do not agree that it is the only critical approach. Thompson, like other critical theorists, fails to see the possibility of critique that is not procedural or based upon the ethics of rights and justice.

Interpretive hermeneutics augments critical theory because in order to set up the rational discourse about justice, one needs a substantive set of goods that one wants to conserve and preserve. Critical theory provides a procedural approach (a *freedom from* dialogue, and a rights and justice dialogue) but does not provide a coherent statement of substantive notions of good (a positive freedom to do and be). Interpretive phenomenology of nursing practice and stress and coping in health and illness gives voice to the substantive good. Critical theorists might be called the pinnacle of Enlightenment thinking in which the focus of the critique is on *freedom from* rather than a substantive positive project of what to do with the freedom. This blind spot is what makes Thompson overlook the critical project in *From Novice to Expert* and *The Primacy of Caring*. Both of these works focus on the positive project of nursing, as Thompson notes, without focusing on the structural constraints of the practice. But Thompson fails to notice that the narratives of excellence (the freedom to or positive project) and nurses' own critiques of constraints are used in both works to critique dominant cultural and organizational constraints to these nurses' practice, e.g., a technological self-understanding and discourses of power that overlook everyday skillful ethical comportment and the ethics of care and responsibility.

Thus Thompson overlooks the ways that enlightened expert practice can be a source of liberation. Theory (critical or otherwise) is not the *only* source of liberation. In *From Novice to Expert*, and *Primacy of Caring*, excellent practice is used to critique the constraints of the practice, as well as to critique Cartesian dualism, techno-cure, a technological self-understanding and a strictly procedural approach to liberation. Both works critique the cultural crisis in caring practices. With a technological self-understanding comes a quest for control and a freedom from vulnerability that devalues caring practices and systematically overlooks many in the society who are vulnerable and require care. This is a central fault with the grand dream of freedom from the burdens of care that Enlightenment thinkers *purchased* by their liberation and freedom through the work of many supporting caregivers. This, in fact, is a blind spot in the discourse ethics proposed by Habermas (1989a; 1989b) and critical theorists, where the communicative context is based upon rational discourse among equals (see Fraser, 1987; Benhabib, 1987; 1989; Murphy & Gilligan, 1980).

I suspect attention to the procedural approach to critique used by critical theorists causes Thompson to overlook the critical passages in both works, perhaps because the definition of the problem is different in critical theory and interpretive phenomenology. The following excerpts are cited as evidence of this oversight, for example, in *From Novice to Expert*:

> The disparagement of feminine perspectives on power is based upon the misguided assumption that feminine values have kept women and nursing subservient, rather than recognizing that society's devaluing of and discrimination against women are the sources of the problem. The former view—the misguided assumption—blames the victim and promises that discrimination will stop when women abandon what they value and learn to play the power games like men do . . . Adopting coercive, dominating notions of power or strictly public-relations approaches abandons the values and commitments required for powerful caring and excellence; it adopts the pathologies inherent in a unipolar view (Benner, 1984a, p. 208).

And in *The Primacy of Caring*:

> The rational-technical model of management has no language or strategies for determining what are worthy goals (MacIntyre, 1981; March, 1976). The rational-technical model is limited to the assumption that we know what are the appropriate ends and that the only problem is how to be more efficient in reaching them. To go beyond the rational-technical model we need to develop a discourse on worthy ends. We need to examine our caring practices and augment the rational-technical model of management with narrative forms about what is required to support and facilitate excellence in caring practices. . . . If nurses are to liberate caring practices, organizations will have to be redesigned to facilitate and sponsor caring practices (Benner & Wrubel, 1989, p. 399).

Both books provide commentary on the constraints in practice identified by the nurses. I conclude that Thompson does not recognize the form of critique that my work takes. This conclusion is sensible since these works critique critical theory's only critical strategies for liberation, i.e., rational discourse and abstract principled ethics. In fact this form of liberation overlooks notions of good unamenable to adjudication. Critical theory is limited to epistemological and power issues, it cannot offer new webs and new metaphors. It *can* help us clear the way for the new metaphors, and that is a significant contribution.

Methodological Ambiguity

I disagree that my work is methodologically ambiguous because it "does not show the influence of Gadamer." Gadamer's methodological insights stem from Heidegger and Kierkegaard, and indeed I too have been influenced by Gadamer's cogent arguments about the impossibility of separating theory and method as is referenced in most of my work (Benner & Benner, 1979; Benner, 1984b; Benner & Wrubel, 1989). Thompson is correct, my work does not fit the three categories: an objective hermeneutic, a Gadamerian hermeneutic, or a critical hermeneutic approach to research. My work is based upon the writings of Kierkegaard (1846, 1967; 1842, 1968), Heidegger (1962; 1982), Dreyfus (1990), Rubin (In press), and Taylor (1985, 1989), where the goal is to study naturalistically the habits, skills, practices and meanings of people. The interview and observation data provide a text analogue. The goal is to get beyond "subjectivism" and "objectivism" by critiquing the Cartesian view of the person as private, disconnected, subject standing over against an objective world. The assumption is that common language, habits, skills, practices, situations, meanings, and embodiment make it possible to understand others, not as private subjects but as embodied participants and members of a common humanity, language and culture group. The common taken for granted meanings and practices do not ensure agreement. Indeed they provide enough commensurability for disagreement and for different voices to be heard. Complete incommensurability would not allow for meaningful differences to show up (Gadamer, 1975; Kuhn, 1970). As noted above, interpretive phenomenology seeks to elucidate the meanings, knowledge, skill, and notions of good embedded in divergent practices and human activity, in order to provide the substantive alternatives and to provide a critical perspective based upon the substantive content and notions of good embedded in the practices. In this way it contains a positive project (a hermeneutics of understanding, or faith, i.e., giving voice to the observed practices) and a critical project of identifying the voice embedded in the practice as well as the conflicts, constraints and blocks to this voice and practice in its most liberated form. The focus tends to be on content, context, function, and process and less on structure. Interpretive phenomenology is well suited to the study of habits, skills, and practices that are not limited to language, and therefore it is well suited to study embodiment. Interpretive phenomenology is not the best method for studying structures.

Divisive Hierarchies or Qualitative Distinctions?

Thompson states that my "work has in fact been used to develop clinical ladders and has contributed to increased tendencies and stratification in nursing." This is critical theory at its *freedom from* worst. Is the unstated critical theory alternative a non-stratified, non-hierarchical, completely classless, egalitarian system that recognizes no distinctions between knowledge, function and skill levels? It is hard to imagine what such an arrangement would be other than chaotic and nihilistic. I interpret clinical promotion programs as a valid way to develop the practice (knowledge, skill, and notions of good), an approach that gives credit and empowerment to nurses fairly and appropriately. I would not like for the only hierarchy and reward system to be administrative. I believe that strategies that attend to the focus on the actual knowledge and skill embedded in the practice are the best approach to develop the practice, and to promote and reward excellent practice. The Dreyfus model of skill acquisition is not a trait or talent approach, it is based upon actual performance in practice and is judged by peers. When done well it can provide sound, just distinctions that help nurses provide the best health care.

Pluralism in Theories and Methods

Finally, I do not think that it is possible for one method or one paradigm to make *all* voices or all aspects of our human world visible. In the human sciences, the existence of one normal paradigm or choosing only one critical method would create totalitarianism or totalism, not diversity, not increased possibility. We need critical theory, but it is not the only critical method. We need interpretive phenomenology because it has both a critical and a positive project, but it too is not the only interpretive approach. It is less suited for structural analysis and like any method cannot be adequately evaluated by examining one study or one researcher.

References

Benhabib, S. (1987). In the shadow of Aristotle and Hegel: Communicative ethics and current controversies in practical philosophy. *The Philosophical Forum, Vol. XXI* (1-2), 1-31.

Benner, P. & Benner, R. (1979). *New nurses work entry, a troubled sponsorship*. New York: Tiresias.

Benner, P. (1984a). *From novice to expert*. Reading, MA: Addison-Wesley.

Benner, P. (1984b). *Satisfaction on the job: Work meanings and stress coping of mid-career men*. New York: Praeger.

Benner, P. & Wrubel, J. (1989). *The primacy of caring, stress and coping in health and illness*. Reading, MA: Addison-Wesley.

Dreyfus, H. L. (1990). *A Commentary on Being and Time, Division I*, Cambridge, MA: MIT Press.

Fraser, N. (1987). What's critical about critical theory? The case of Habermas and gender. *Feminism as critique, on the politics of gender*. Minneapolis: University of Minnesota Press.

Gadamer, H. (1975). *Truth and Method*. New York: Seabury.

Habermas, J. (1989a). Mortality and ethical life: Does Hegel's critique of Kant apply to discourse ethics? *Northwestern University Law Review, Vol. 53* (1&2), 38-53.

Habermas, J. (1989b). Justice and solidarity: On the discussion concerning "stage 6." *The philosophical forum, a quarterly, Vol. XXI*, 32-52.

Heidegger, M. (1962). *Being and time*. J. Macquarrie & E. Robinson (Trans.). New York: Harper & Row.

Heidegger, M. (1977, transl.). The question concerning technology. In *Martin Heidegger, Basic Writings*. D. F. Krell (Ed.), New York: Harper & Row.

Heidegger, M. (1982). *The basic problems of phenomenology* (rev. ed.) (A. Hofstadter, Trans.). Bloomington: Indiana University Press.

Kierkegaard, S. (1843, 1968). *Fear and trembling* (W. L. Lowrie, Trans.). Princeton, NJ: Princeton University Press.

Kierkegaard, S. (1846; 1967). *Philosophical Fragments* (D. Swenson, N. Thulstrup, & H. V. Hong, Trans.). Princeton, NJ: Princeton University Press.

Kuhn T. (1970). *The structure of scientific revolutions* (2nd ed.). Chicago: University of Chicago Press.

Leonard, V. (1989). Heideggerian phenomenological perspective on the concept of the person. *Advances in Nursing Science, Vol. II*, 4.

Murphy, J. M., & Gilligan, C. (1980). Moral development in late adolescence and adulthood: A critique and reconstruction of Kohlberg's theory. *Human Development, 23*, 77-104.

Rubin, J. (In press). *Too much of nothing: Modern culture and the self in Kierkegaard's thought*. Cambridge: Harvard University Press.

Taylor, C. (1985). *Philosophical papers, Vols. I & II*. Cambridge: Cambridge University Press.

Taylor, C. (1989). *Sources of the self*. Cambridge: Harvard University Press.

8

Sociolinguistic Inquiry

MARY LOU VANCOTT

... the process of communication always involves a mutual exchange of impressions between the patient and the care provider.

The achievement of goals in health care often hinges on the professional health care provider's ability to interpret as a coherent whole the very diverse needs and perceptions of individual patients or clients. Among a number of factors that may influence the patterns of communication in health care settings are the individuals themselves, interacting in a specific situation. The patient's perspective may influence the outcome of care, may affect the quality of the intervention experience, or may contribute to the degree of adherence to the treatment plan (Brink, 1986). An analysis that deals with both the interaction process between patients and health care providers and the social and perceptual processes that affect the interaction has the potential to increase understanding substantively, methodologically, and theoretically by adding new dimensions to our understanding of the patient's social environment and reactions to that environment. From such analysis, it is possible to build a theoretical link that connects social interaction with the context within which it occurs. The focus of this chapter will be on the use of sociolinguistic analysis as a method of inquiry to advance knowledge for nursing interventions in areas where language, communication, and the interaction process are the focus of study.

Theoretical Assumptions

Cassell, Skopek, and Fraser (1976) state that language is one of the most important tools that health care professionals employ. Speech is the primary manner by which patients inform health care providers of their history, symptoms, and concerns and by which health care professionals respond to the patient's needs.

One cannot assume that all persons in a situation perceive events in the same manner. Not only are individuals endowed with different skills, but, when taking part in an interaction, each defines the situation based on how the information that others provide is perceived. Communication cannot be understood without reference to how individuals receive and interpret, or fail to receive and misinterpret, the information made available in the situation. Further, the process of communication always involves a mutual exchange of impressions. In nurse-patient interactions, the nurse's perceptions of the patient are as important as the patient's perceptions of the nurse. The need to give attention to individual perceptions in health care interactions derives from communication theory, which states that what nurses and patients perceive as happening will influence their behavior regardless of what is actually happening in a situation. This is why there is a need for research that provides a more comprehensive understanding of the processes and skills health care providers use in thinking about and understanding patients and in interpreting the situations health care providers confront in the process of planning and giving care (Kasch, 1986).

Human contact invariably results in information being exchanged, and information may be transmitted verbally by the use of speech or nonverbally by use of facial expressions, eye contact, touch, body movements, posture, appearance, and so on (Ashworth, 1985). The use of time also conveys messages; time spent with a patient when no procedure is performed may communicate interest and caring (Blondis & Jackson, 1982). Nonverbal signals not only convey messages but may also be used deliberately or unconsciously to reinforce verbal messages, to convey emotions, and to regulate interaction.

Usually people are simultaneously both sending messages and receiving feedback; the reception of information about how others are responding to one's communication is important. Lack of feedback is often so disconcerting that it may lead to disruption of verbal communication. Other factors such as role relationships and the physical and social environment also affect interpersonal interaction (Ashworth, 1985).

When any two people interact, many reasons may cause them to misunderstand or misinterpret each other. For instance, a person may not hear all of what the other person has said; or, if he or she hears it, he or she may not recognize or interpret the words the way the speaker intended. The underlying thoughts, meanings, ideas, and feelings may differ from what was intended to be communicated to what was actually understood by the recipient of the message (Cassell, Skopek, & Fraser, 1976). In addition, messages may not be understood in certain social situations because participants are afraid or embarrassed to acknowledge their confusion, or because certain forms of speech are used with which recipients are unfamiliar (for example, jargon or complex sentence structure). Cassell, Skopek, and Fraser (1976, p. 10) state, "It is of vital importance to distinguish these different factors if we want to understand the processes which lead to successful communication between patient and health care provider."

Nurses find it difficult to identify what types of communicative relationships seem effective in helping the patient. Therefore, nurses might benefit from a better understanding of the communication-interaction process so that its components can be identified, repeated, taught, and made standard in nursing practice (Daubenmire, 1976).

The area of communication and interpersonal skills in nursing has been explored for at least two decades with a variety of methods and approaches (Clark, 1985). Recently, there has been an increasing recognition of the central role of communication in nursing practice, and an important part of research in nursing practice is concerned with what goes on between the nurse and the patient and the consequences this has for the patient. Researchers have investigated, either directly or indirectly, the extent to which patients are satisfied with the care they receive. According to Clark, it has been generally shown that patients are satisfied neither with communication in general nor with the amount of information they receive. A common thread between these studies is the finding that patients are frequently more critical about poor communication between hospital personnel and patients than about any other aspect of their experience in hospitals (Clark, 1985; Maguire, 1985; Skipper, 1965).

Little research has been conducted on communication as a process and on its effect on nurses and patients in a health care setting. Most communication studies have dealt with a single or limited number of variables, the frequency or occurrence of those variables, cause-effect relationships, and controlled or experimental environments. Incorporating findings from these studies into nursing practice is difficult because the findings are not readily adaptable and applicable to a natural health care setting.

Of the studies conducted on communication in patient care settings, most were done prior to 1980. These nurse-patient interaction studies predate demographic changes, such as the graying of America. The changing status of women, the patient consumer rights movement, and changes in health professional roles are new social developments that may have an effect on interaction processes. Updated research is needed to uncover and analyze the impact of these changes.

Sociolinguistics: An Analytical
Method for the Study of Interaction

Information is exchanged between individuals in a variety of ways. Fisher (1982) states that the work of sociolinguists, ethnomethodologists, and discourse analysts suggests that language is a social production in which different linguistic arrangements are visible in different situations. They propose that there is a relationship between the words spoken, the actions performed, and the structure of the discourse.

Sociolinguistics was originally influenced philosophically by social anthropology and sociology (Svejcer, 1986). Since the 1980s, various sociolinguistic research methods have been principally aimed at improving linguistic theory and acquiring a better understanding of the nature of language variation and the sources of linguistic change (Trudgill, 1983).

Fishman (1971, p. 4) defines sociolinguistics as "the study of the characteristics of language varieties, the characteristics of their functions, and the characteristics of their speakers as these three constantly interact, change and change one another within a speech community." Sociolinguistics is that part of linguistics that is concerned with language as a social and cultural phenomenon. It investigates the field of language and society and has close connections with the social sciences, especially psychology, anthropology, human geography, and sociology (Trudgill, 1983). The study of the way in which language is used in conversations is an important part of sociolinguistics. Because much of human interaction is actually verbal interaction, sociolinguists have focused much of their attention on how people use language in their relationships with one another.

Box 8.1.   Analyzing Nursing Communicative Competence with the Hospitalized Elderly

SOURCE: VanCott, M. L., & Moody, L. E. (1989, November). Paper presented at the Sigma Theta Tau International's 30th Biennial Convention, Indianapolis, IN.

The purposes of this study were to explore and describe communication patterns between nurses and elderly patients during nursing admission interviews in hospital settings and to apply a sociolinguistic model to identify factors related to communicative competence during admission interviews with the elderly. These research questions were addressed: (1) What kind of communication problems typically occur in nurse-elderly patient interactions during admission interviews in hospital settings when the patient is over 65 years of age. (2) How do nurses respond to these communication problems?

The methodological framework was sociolinguistic microanalysis that included analysis of recorded interactions in a natural setting and a replay of key segments during interviews with participants. The sociolinguistic model for analyzing communicative competence included six dimensions: acoustics, phonology and syntax, lexicon, conceptions, intent, and credence. The sample consisted of 20 hospitalized elderly and 20 registered nurses who conducted the nursing admission interviews and consented to audio and video recording. Verbatim transcripts of these dyad interactions and transcripts of investigator-conducted individual interviews with each participant of the admission interview, and review of nurse subject documentation material in the patient record were analyzed.

Results indicated instances of both effective communication and miscommunication in the dyad interactions in all six areas of communicative competence. Findings indicated that elderly individuals typically do not express needs and concerns overtly; disclosure tends to be through long, narrative discourse. The elderly were often vague in describing health history and symptoms, which created problems when direct responses were needed for the initial data base for nursing care. Factors that contributed to miscommunication occurred in all six areas: acoustics (hearing deficits and environmental noise), phonology and syntax (vague, ambiguous statements), lexicon (abbreviated words), conceptions (vague statements, inattentive listening), intent (lack of explanation of purpose, indirect manner of expressing emotions), and credence (inaccurate messages). Misperception of speech events represented an important source of conflict in the dyad relationship. Task-oriented communication approaches most often resulted in failure to explore and identify psychosocial needs of elderly subjects. Communicative competence during the admission interview is essential to the provision of effective health care of the elderly.

A presupposition in sociolinguistic analysis is that any social relationship or event tends to develop an organization of verbal means specific to itself (Hymes, 1971). Sociolinguistics seeks to discover the societal rules or norms that explain and constrain language behavior and the behavior toward language in speech communities (Fishman, 1971).

An example of a nursing sociolinguistic study is depicted in Box 8.1. The purposes of this nursing study were particularly well suited for sociolinguistic inquiry. Sociolinguistic analysis offered a means of studying communication patterns between nurses in acute health care settings and elderly patients being admitted for care in those settings while also offering a means for analyzing the entire situation through the insights of those actually involved in the situation. This added an important dimension to the data obtained for the purposes of the study and thus helped provide a more complete analysis of the factors involved in the nurse-patient interaction.

An approach that is in line with sociolinguistics is the interactionist approach exhibited in the writings of Garfinkel (1967) and Cicourel (1970). These authors point out that information on social categories is obtainable only through language and that sociological measurement, therefore, involves both the informant's and the investigator's perceptions of the categories that are being measured. According to Gumperz and Cook-Gumperz (1982), communication cannot be studied in isolation; it must be analyzed in terms of its effect on people's lives. The focus must be on what communication does—how it constrains evaluation and decision making—not merely how it is structured. The interpretation of speech is impossible without due regard for the previous experience of the individual participants in the communication event or without taking into account their knowledge of the social institutions and norms of their environments (Saville-Troike, 1982; Svejcer, 1986). Gumperz (1977) has proposed the following general processes through which meaning is conveyed in the process of conversational interaction:

(1) Meaning and intelligibility of ways of speaking are at least partially determined by the situation and the prior experience of the speakers.
(2) Meaning is negotiated during the process of interaction and is dependent on the intent and interpretation of previous utterances.
(3) A participant in conversation is always committed to some kind of interpretation.
(4) An interpretation of what happens now is always reversible in the light of what happens later.

Gumperz and Tannen (1979, p. 308) explain that "by studying what has gone wrong when communication breaks down, we seek to understand a process that goes unnoticed when it is successful."

Measurement Issues

One of the strengths of a qualitative approach to knowledge development, such as sociolinguistic inquiry, is recognition of the relationship between the knower and the known (Benner, 1986; Lincoln & Guba, 1985). The phenomenon under study cannot be known straight from the knower. Even the choice of a method for exploration of a phenomenon is value laden in that the investigator's worldview and the phenomenon of study guide the selection. In a sociolinguistic approach, an explication of the investigator's view of the phenomenon is undertaken to enable the investigator to be cognizant of his or her own personal perspective and to take care that, during the investigation, that perspective does not interfere in the analysis. The explication also enables those who read the research to determine for themselves how the investigator's views might confound the analysis and, therefore, how they may interpret and use the findings.

Validity and Reliability in Sociolinguistic Inquiry

A primary concern in qualitative field research, including sociolinguistics, concerns the truth value and accurate impression of the phenomenon under study (Kirk & Miller, 1986; Leininger, 1985). Verification needs to be done by clarifying what specific incidents mean and by comparison of data throughout the study. In sociolinguistic inquiry, methodological triangulation is a means by which validity of data is supported. *Triangulation* refers to the use of multiple referents to draw conclusions about what constitutes the "truth" (Denzin, 1978; Polit & Hungler, 1987; Shaffer, Stebbins, & Turowitz, 1980). For example, a combination of data collection sources—such as transcripts of communication interaction from audiotape recording and/or videotape recording, written documentation materials, and investigator-conducted interviews with interaction participants and other informants—may be used by the investigator for data analysis. This allows the investigator to view the phenomenon under study in a variety of different ways. The purpose of using triangulation is to provide a basis for convergence on truth.

The sociolinguistic method of inquiry also deals with the validity and reliability problem through participant validation. The actual participants in the interaction included in the study sample are involved in clarifying and validating what occurred during the interaction process and include their own personal insights into and perceptions of the meaning of individual speech events in the situation.

Reliability concerns the replicability of observations. According to Kirk and Miller (1986, p. 41), reliability in qualitative research "depends essentially on explicitly described observational procedure." Sociolinguistic research, like other forms of qualitative research, must deal with problems related to data getting and the actual field setting, which include (a) effects of the observer's presence on the phenomenon being observed, (b) limitations of the observer to witness all relevant activities of the phenomenon under study, and (c) effects of observer perception and interpretation on the observed activities during observation and analysis.

Lincoln and Guba (1985) describe a method of triangulation that assists the sociolinguistic researcher in dealing with the reliability issue. The triangulation method Lincoln and Guba offer is called "inquiry audit," in which the process of the inquiry is assessed for dependability and the products of the inquiry (data, findings, interpretations, and recommendations) are examined to establish confirmability. This can be accomplished by the use of external review of interpretation transcripts, compiled investigator field notes, follow-up participant interview transcripts, and written documentation materials.

Reactive effects are behavioral responses that subjects make because they are aware the investigator is observing in the setting. These responses may be atypical in the situation during routine circumstances. For instance, the subject may react by striving to "make a good impression" by performing beyond the typical performance level when he or she is aware the investigator is present and collecting data. Reactive effects could alter the quality of the collected data.

Investigators can employ methods to limit reactive effects such as prolonging the period of entry into the situation by the investigator or observer. This entails a period of nonparticipant observation and/or participant observation without data collection to allow the investigator or observer time to acclimate to the setting and permit time for rapport and trust between observer and subject to begin. The entry period also offers the investigator the opportunity to view the situation for relevant aspects of the social situation, thus enabling the investigator to view the interaction situation from a variety of angles (the principle of methodological triangulation).

Protection of Human Subjects

While all field researchers are faced with ethical decisions in the course of their work, literature on fieldwork research similar to sociolinguistic analysis reveals that there is no shared consensus concerning the researcher's responsibilities either to those who participated in the study or to the discipline itself (Shaffer, Stebbins, & Turowitz, 1980). The protection of human subjects poses unique questions in sociolinguistics research. Sociolinguistic inquiry raises the issue of who in the field situation must be informed that a study is in process, the extent of the original implied consent, and disposition of information obtained through the data collection process. The investigator must be guided by his or her professional judgment in protecting the rights of the individual subjects and collection sites while maintaining the integrity of the research. Sociolinguistic research, like all other forms of research, must be explicated in accordance with local institutional requirements and include contracts and/or consent forms for interviews.

Data Analysis Approaches

A qualitative approach is selected for expanding knowledge related to the many human responses in health care provider-patient social interactions (Aamodt, 1982; Benoliel, 1984). The selection of research methodology originates in assumptions regarding the nature of the phenomena under investigation, the appropriate means of inquiry regarding the phenomena, and the subject matter and end results sought (Fawcett, 1984; Gortner, 1975; Smith, 1984). Data selection for sociolinguistic studies focuses on descriptions of feelings and perceptions from the participants in communication interactions and thus requires a qualitative research approach for data collection and analysis. Sample selection for sociolinguistic inquiry uses the technique called "judgment sampling," or "purposive sampling," in which the nature of the study will determine the characteristics of the sample and sample size. Informants or participants in the interaction are specifically selected with specific criteria in mind. The aim of the analysis of the discourse is to discover and describe social and

environmental variables that have an effect on the interaction between the health care provider and the patient or between health care
providers in the clinical health care setting. Schatzman and Strauss
(1973) suggest "casing," or "mapping," a data collection site as a way
to begin identifying a sample. This generally involves a period of
participant and/or nonparticipant observation at the field site prior
to actual collection of data.

Prior to data collection in sociolinguistic inquiry, the investigator
needs to establish what the procedures for data collection will be,
including the instrumentation that needs to be developed and the
actual methods of data collection. Multiple avenues for collection of
data are important in sociolinguistic inquiry due to the importance
of acquiring accurate and complete recording of the discourse between the interaction participants for eventual transcription. Field
notes are crucial to the data collection phase. The notes should be
transcribed at the earliest opportunity and categorized and coded for
easy retrieval throughout the data collection and analysis period.
Data collection methods can include audiotape recording, videotape
recording, and on-the-spot observation, depending on the situation.

In sociolinguistic inquiry, the speech event is the focus for data
collection. Any two participants in a speech event, such as a nursing
admission interview, must recognize the role relationship that exists
between them at any particular time. Such recognition is part of the
commonality or norms and behaviors upon which the existence of
speech communities depend (Fishman, 1971). According to Fishman
(1971), role relationships are implicitly recognized and accepted sets
of mutual rights and obligations between members of the same
sociocultural system. Three ingredients taken together constitute a
construct in sociolinguistics, which is the social situation. The three
ingredients are (a) the implementation of the rights and duties of a
particular role relationship, (b) the place most typical for that relationship, and (c) the time societally defined as appropriate for that
relationship. An example of the social situation in a nursing sociolinguistic study is depicted in Box 8.2.

Sociolinguistic variables constitute the basic operational unit for
the sociolinguistic analysis of language and speech variation. Revealing the mechanism of selecting sociolinguistic variables is essential to distinguish between the status of participants in communicative events and their role relations. Role relationships are implicitly
recognized and accepted sets of mutual rights and obligations between members of the same sociocultural system. The participants'
status is determined by their social characteristics and place in the

Box 8.2. The Social Situation	
SITUATION: Acute Care Hospital, Medical-Surgical Clinical Unit	TIME: Admission to the Clinical Unit
SPACE: Patient room (private or semiprivate)	ROLES: Nurse Patient Teacher Student Interviewer Interviewee

social structure of the social situation (Svejcer, 1986). Box 8.3 depicts an example of a conceptual map of a sociolinguistic analysis for a nursing study concerned with the analysis of the interaction that occurs between nurse and patient during the nursing admission interview in an acute health care setting.

The smallest sociolinguistic unit is a speech act, which is a segment of talk that is also societally recognizable and recurring. Speech acts are normally parts of somewhat larger speech events, such as conversations, lectures, arguments, and, as in the case of the study depicted in Box 8.2, an interview (Fishman, 1971).

Sociolinguistics is necessarily of interest to those investigators who are concerned with determining the functionally different role relationships that exist within a given community. Microsociolinguistics is concerned with validation of such relationships, via the demonstration of different role access, role range, and role fluidity as well as via the demonstration of differential proportions of interaction through the data of "talk" (Fishman, 1971; Saville-Troike, 1982). Because the nursing care process involves the nurse in direct interaction with patients, it seems logical that communication theory, in combination with linguistic theory, may be synthesized into a conceptual framework of health care provider-patient interaction that may be viewed as a sociolinguistic process.

A field approach to research permits the examination of an immediate interaction situation in a manner that is more than purely descriptive. It allows recognition of some factors that may influence the participant's choice of behavior, even though the actual motivation may not have been evident (Byerly, 1969). According to Byerly, this type of process involves "a sensitive awareness of the behaviors of the persons being observed, similar insight into the investigator's

Box 8.3. Conceptual Map for Sociolinguistic Analysis for a Study
Concerned with Analysis of Nurse-Patient Interaction in an
Acute Health Care Situation

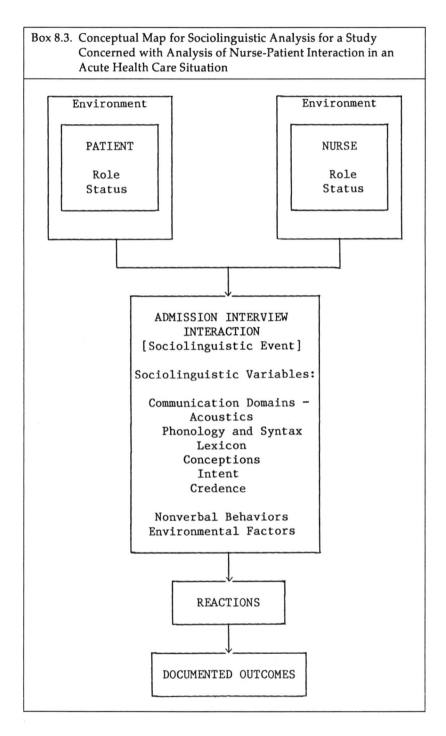

own actions and reaction, a careful and complete recording of these events and retrospective evaluation and analysis of data" (Byerly, 1969, p. 235). It is a combination of inductive and deductive approaches in which the investigator focuses the research according to a conscious selective process. Rather than following a series of linear steps, the investigator works within a matrix in which several research processes are in operation at once. The investigator examines data as they arrive and begins to code, categorize, conceptualize, and write the first few thoughts concerning the research report almost from the beginning of the study (Stern, 1980). This method aims to generate theoretical constructs that explain the action in the social context under study. According to Benoliel (1984), qualitative approaches in science are distinct modes of inquiry oriented toward understanding the unique nature of human thoughts, approximate behaviors, negotiations, and institutions under different sets of historical and environmental circumstances. These approaches to inquiry are built on a paradigm that considers the symbol-producing nature of the human species, the act of interpretation as a basic human characteristic, and intentional or goal-directed behavior as a complicated human activity affecting individual and group endeavors.

The procedure for data analysis for sociolinguistic inquiry includes five interrelated steps:

(1) The researcher prepares and reads the entire interaction speech upon event transcription and reviews, if available, the audiotape and/or videotape recording of the event. Additional data sources such as written records and field notes are included in the initial overview to obtain a sense of the whole.

(2) The researcher reads the transcription more slowly and deliberately, identifying transitions or units in the interaction that apply to the units of analysis identified in the analysis model.

(3) The perceptions of the participants involved in the interaction are then taken into account to add to the meaning of the analysis. This is a particularly important step in the analysis process in sociolinguistic inquiry because it is during this stage that the meaning of the speech events are clarified and validated by the actual participants in the speech event interaction. Any other data from other sources, such as written records and investigator field notes, are also reviewed to add richness of meaning to the analysis of the interaction transcription.

(4) The researcher reflects on the given units of analysis and transforms the concrete language from context into the language or

Box 8.4. Map of Miscommunication Occurrences in Dyad Interactions in a Sociolinguistic Analysis Concerning Nurse-Patient Interaction During a Nursing Admission Interview in an Acute Health Care Setting

		Area of Miscommunication				
Dyad	Acoustics	Phonology & Syntax	Lexicon	Conceptions	Intent	Credence
1		N^a/E	N^a/E	N	N^a	
2	N	E				
3		N^a/E^a	N^a	N/E	N^a/E	N^a
4						
5	N	N^a/E^a			E	
6	E^a		E^a			N^a
7				N		N
8	N^a/E	N^a		N^a/E	N	
9	E^a	N		N	E^a	
10	N/E			N		N^a
11	E	E^a	N/E^a	N^a/E	N^a/E	N^a/E^a
12						
13	E^a	N				N^a
14	N^a/E^a	N^a		N/E	N^a	N^a
15		N/E				
16					E	N^a
17	E^a					
18	N/E^a	N/E	N/E^a	N^a/E^a	N^a/E	N^a
19		E				
20	E	N^a	E^a	N	N	

N = Nurse Subject experienced a problem with communication during the speech event.
E = Elderly Subject experienced a problem with communication during the speech event.
a. Indicates more than one occurrence during the dyad.

concepts of science. Examples of how the data were transformed for analysis in the study are depicted in Box 8.1 and Boxes 8.4 to 8.6. Box 8.4 depicts a map of miscommunication occurrences identified through analysis of the dyad interactions using the sociolinguistic model. This map indicates how data can be displayed to assist the researcher in identifying trends within the analysis model.

Box 8.5 demonstrates how speech acts, from data collected in the sociolinguistic study depicted in Box 8.1, were categorized into the

Box 8.5. Model of Communication Competence in Nursing Admission
          Interview

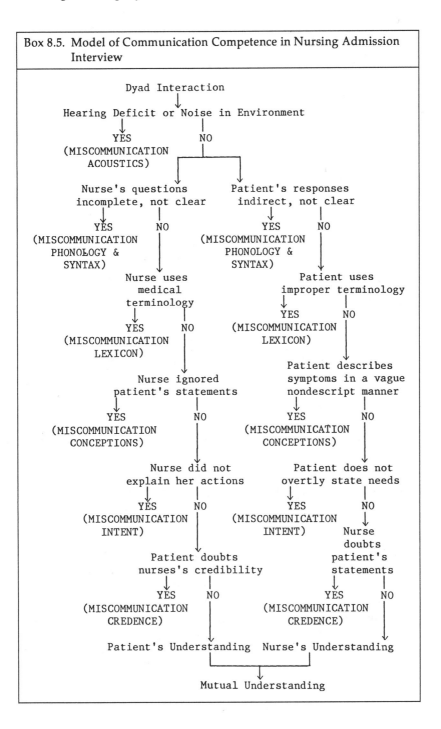

Dyad Interaction

Hearing Deficit or Noise in Environment

YES   NO
(MISCOMMUNICATION
ACOUSTICS)

Nurse's questions   Patient's responses
incomplete, not clear   indirect, not clear

YES   NO   YES   NO
(MISCOMMUNICATION   (MISCOMMUNICATION
PHONOLOGY &   PHONOLOGY &
SYNTAX)   SYNTAX)

Nurse uses   Patient uses
medical   improper terminology
terminology
                         YES   NO
YES   NO   (MISCOMMUNICATION
(MISCOMMUNICATION   LEXICON)
LEXICON)
                         Patient describes
Nurse ignored   symptoms in a vague
patient's statements nondescript manner

YES   NO   YES   NO
(MISCOMMUNICATION   (MISCOMMUNICATION
CONCEPTIONS)   CONCEPTIONS)

Nurse did not   Patient does not
explain her actions   overtly state needs

YES   NO   YES   NO
(MISCOMMUNICATION   (MISCOMMUNICATION   Nurse
INTENT)   INTENT)   doubts
                                                 patient's
Patient doubts   statements
nurses's credibility

YES   NO   YES   NO
(MISCOMMUNICATION   (MISCOMMUNICATION
CREDENCE)   CREDENCE)

Patient's Understanding   Nurse's Understanding

Mutual Understanding

Box 8.6. Themes Regarding Perceptions of Nurses Toward the Nursing Interview and the Patient During Investigator Interviews		
Purpose of an admission interview	Nurse:	Obtaining information Obtaining past history Get to know the patient Find out what problems patient is experiencing Development of plan of care based on patient needs
	Patient:	To see who I am For me to see who the nurses are
Characteristics of patient that interferes with the interview process and purposes		Wasn't real specific Didn't seem to know much about her condition Tended to go off the subject Wouldn't give a direct answer to a question Poor historian
Environmental factors that interfered with interview process		Hectic time period More than one patient admitted to the unit at the same time End of shift Interruptions to interview: x-ray transporter staff member asking question

six areas of communicative competence indicated in the sociolinguistic analysis model. Each dyad interaction between a nurse subject and an elderly patient subject were analyzed according to the sociolinguistic model and coded by area of communicative competence in the model. Categories of occurrences were then identified from the data codes. This allowed the researcher to view the data conceptually.

The data analysis shown in Box 8.6 demonstrates how themes are generated from content from investigator-subject interviews. The themes can then be applied to the interaction transcript analysis to assist the investigator in gaining insight into the perceptions of those who were involved in the interactions being studied.

(5) The researcher then integrates the insights gained from the data analysis and synthesizes them into a descriptive structure of the meaning of the interaction in the life experience of those involved in

Box 8.7. Model of Nurse Actions to Achieve Communicative
Competence in the Area of Credence From a Sociolinguistic
Study Concerned with Analysis of Nurse-Elderly Patient
Interaction During Nursing Admission Interview to Acute
Health Care Settings

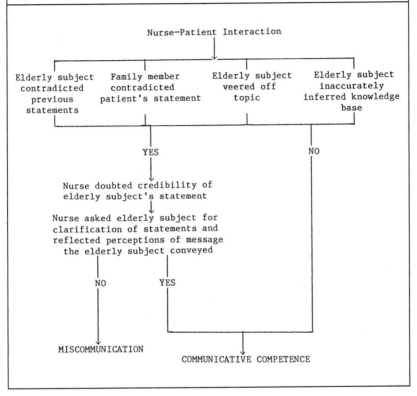

the setting. The final product is then communicated to those in the area of clinical practice and to other researchers for critique.

An example of a model format for data display is presented in Box 8.7, which demonstrates how the synthesis of the data analysis was displayed from the sociolinguistic study depicted in Box 8.1. The model in Box 8.7 indicates the potential pathways an elderly patient can take related to one particular area of communicative competence during an admission interview of an elderly patient entering an acute health care nursing unit. This model concerns the communicative competence area of credence. The potential blocks to communicative competence that the elderly patient exhibits are indicated along with the nurse's response to the elderly patient's interaction. Whether the nurse seeks clarification or not determines whether communicative competence has been gained on whether a miscommunication event occurred in the interaction.

The synthesis of the analysis can also be present inside a descriptive or narrative form such as the analysis display depicted in Box 8.8. The analysis display in Box 8.8 identifies the sociolinguistic variables analyzed in the study depicted in Box 8.1. For this study, problems in communicative competence were identified within the speech acts of the nursing admission interviews according to the sociolinguistic variable areas of the model. The speech acts were then categorized and the results of the dyad interactions were analyzed.

The sociolinguistic variables can also be displayed narratively by presentation of examples of actual discourse from the interactions under study. For instance, data from the sociolinguistic study depicted in Box 8.1 included the following excerpt from a nurse-patient interaction:

Nurse Subject: Ah, then they'll take you into the operating room. By this time they'll put a mask on you. Most times people don't know er or else, you know, if nobody says somethin and, and it's scary.

Elderly Subject: [well let me tell you what happened, this doctor was a scrub in surgeon, he's a surgeon but he scrubbed in with my doctor.

Nurse Subject: [Okay

Elderly Subject: He came up to me and I was in, I wan on, if I'm not mistaken, I was still in BED! All right now

Nurse Subject: [Yeah sometimes they do things differently.

Elderly Subject: [all right, Okay, now he come up to me and he said, they had that thing in my wrist or my palm of the

Nurse Subject: [right

Elderly Subject: back of my hand, but he says "are you scared?" I said, "You're [expletive] right I, he ways well, Okay, he says "when I shoot you with this" he says "you're gonna know nothin." He says you know, a real

Nurse Subject: [right

Elderly Subject: nice guy, just scrubbin so I said "well, I can count to five." He says, "no that's a lot of Hollywood crap. He says "when I hit you with this needle you

---

Box 8.8. Causes of Miscommunication for Elderly Subjects

Area of Miscommunication	*Results on Dyad Interaction*
Acoustics	
Hearing deficit	Prolonged interview time
	Inaccurate message from nurse
Noise in environment	to elderly subject
Phonology and Syntax	
Nurse's statements not clear, vague	Inaccurate message from nurse to elderly subject
	Insufficient or inaccurate
Nurse's statements ambiguous or incomplete	feedback from elderly subject to nurse
Lexicon	
Nurse used initials, abbreviations instead of whole names (ICU, EKG, GI)	Prolonged interview time Inaccurate feedback from elderly subject to nurse
Conceptions	
Nurse used value-laden adjectives	Increased anxiety level in elderly subject
Nurse ignored elderly subject's statements	Incomplete message from elderly subject to nurse
Intent	
Nurse failed to explain purpose behind actions	Nurse perception of uncooperativeness in elderly subject Prolonged interview time
Credence	
Elderly subject questioned nurse's information based on elderly subject's past hospitalizations	Prolonged interview time

Nurse Subject.   [(laughter)
Elderly Subject: ain't gonna know nothin."
Nurse Subject: No cause it works that quick.
Elderly Subject: Oh, my [expletive]! I was out in a flash!

Nurse Subject:　Right, and that's probably what they'll be going to you
　　　　　　　　again this time. They'll put a needle in your

Elderly Subject:　　　　　　　　　[well I guess so

Nurse Subject:　hand.

Elderly Subject:　[yeah

Nurse Subject:　Usually they put em in the left hands. But that's

Elderly Subject:　　　　　　　　　　　　　　　　[right

Nurse Subject:　just because how they sit behind you. Okay?

Elderly Subject:　　　　　　　　　[yeah　　　　[yeah

Elderly Subject:　Well the needle was there. I didn't know it. The needle
　　　　　　　　was there, he shot me and went bonk.

Nurse Subject:　　[right

Nurse Subject:　That's right. It's the same thing that's gonna go on

Elderly Subject:　　　　　　　　[Oh it is

Nurse Subject:　this time also. It's gonna be the same thing.

Elderly Subject:　　　　　　　　　　[tomorrow morn. . .

This excerpt represents an example of a miscommunication occurring in a nurse-patient interaction in the communication area of
intent, which served as one of the six areas of communication competence in the sociolinguistic analytic model depicted in Box 8.2. In
this speech event, the true message that the elderly subject was
expressing was his fear. The elderly subject found it difficult to
express his fear at the time of the interaction but could easily relate
what he was feeling during his last hospitalization. He expressed
himself during the interaction in a rapid, loud volume with frequent
points of intonation. The nurse stated later in her interview with the
investigator that she was impressed with this elderly subject's understanding of his surgical procedure and what his pre- and postoperative care would entail, and she felt that he would "do very well
after surgery." She did not indicate that she felt he was overly
anxious about the surgery based on her perceptions of the interaction. The elderly subject, however, stated to the investigator, after
direct questioning regarding his feelings about his upcoming surgery, "You're [expletive] right I'm scared! Anybody who tells you
they're not are lying!" As a result of the miscommunication of intent,
the nurse was unable to establish a plan of nursing care based on the
patient's true emotional needs. Through the use of excerpts from the
actual discourse, the researcher can more fully describe the processes
and themes acquired through sociolinguistic analysis.

Summary

A major strength of sociolinguistic analysis is the consistency of the method with the nature of the phenomenon of interest. A sociolinguistic method aims at uncovering the status and role relationships of participants in communication events. Data are obtained in the actual situation in which interaction occurs. Subjects are permitted to be active participants in identifying their own perceptions regarding the interaction and the environment in which the interaction takes place. The data obtained are enriched with the advantage of including the perceptions of the actual participants.

Suggestions for Further Study

The limited research in the areas of nurse-patient interaction and communication between health care providers creates many possibilities for future research utilizing the sociolinguistic method of inquiry. Research related to communication techniques used by nurses when interacting with patients, the public, and other health care providers will assist the profession of nursing in examining the functions of the nurse in relation to the role of communicator. Studies related to how skills such as interview technique, active listening, and assessment of the individual, especially regarding psychosocial needs, will assist in furthering our understanding of how communication and interpersonal skills should be introduced into nursing curricula. Findings from sociolinguistic inquiry into nursing communication interaction will provide a more comprehensive understanding of the processes and skills nurses and their interactive partners use in dealing with communication in a variety of clinical settings. The analysis that deals with the process that affects the interactions adds new dimensions to our understanding of the nurse and others' social reactions in a variety of clinical health care situations and settings. Nurses must be critically aware of their essential role as communicator—of receiver and/or transmitter of thoughts, feelings, desires, and fears. The establishment of effective relationships between nurses and other individuals in the health care setting depends heavily on the nurse's ability and willingness to be an open listener and communicator. Sociolinguistic inquiry offers the nursing profession a unique opportunity to examine a critical area of clinical practice that is not amenable to other types of research inquiry.

Point-Counterpoint

(1) What ethical ramifications can you identify that would need to be considered when planning a clinical sociolinguistic analysis in health care settings such as acute health care hospitals, clinics, and home/community health care settings? What can the researcher do in these settings to minimize these ethical issues?

(2) Propose nursing situations that could be appropriately analyzed using a sociolinguistic approach. Develop a proposal for one of these situations focusing on what specific data collection procedures would be most beneficial.

(3) Identify research studies published in the last three years in a nursing research journal, such as *Nursing Research* or *Western Journal of Nursing Research*, that could have been conducted using a sociolinguistic analytic approach. How would you redesign the studies using a sociolinguistic approach?

(4) Review the nursing sociolinguistic study displayed in Box 8.1. Identify the validity and reliability concerns in the study and suggest how the investigator could have dealt with these issues.

(5) Based on the results of your analysis for the item 3 above, project a budget for the proposed study that you have designed. Include all resources: tape recorders, tape cassettes, video-equipment, staff, and all other needed supplies.

References

Aamodt, A. M. (1982). Examining ethnography for nurse researchers. *Western Journal of Nursing Research, 4*(2), 209-221.

Ashworth, P. (1985). Interpersonal skill issues arising from intensive care nursing contexts. In C. M. Kagan (Ed.), *Interpersonal skills in nursing: Research and application.* London: Croom Helm.

Benner, P. (1985). Quality of life: A phenomenological perspective on explanation, prediction, and understanding in nursing science. *Advances in Nursing Science, 8*(1), 1-14.

Benoliel, J. Q. (1984). *Advancing nursing science: Qualitative approaches.* Boulder, CO: WICHEN Research Program Committee.

Blondis, M. N., & Jackson, B. E. (1982). *Nonverbal communication with patients* (2nd ed.). New York: John Wiley.

Brink, P. J. (1986). The patient's perspective. *Western Journal of Nursing Research, 8*(2), 133-134.

Byerly, E. L. (1969). The nurse researcher as participant-observer in a nursing setting. *Nursing Research, 18*(3), 230-236.

Cassell, E. J., Skopek, L., & Fraser, B. (1976, December). A preliminary model for the examination of doctor-patient communication. *Language Sciences, 43,* 10-13.

Cicourel, A. (1970). The acquisition of social structure: Towards a developmental sociology of language and meaning. In J. Douglas (Ed.), *Existential society*. New York: Appleton-Century-Crofts.

Clark, J. M. (1985). The development of research in interpersonal skills in nursing. In C. Kagan (Ed.), *Interpersonal skills in nursing, research and applications* (pp. 9-21). London: Croom Helm.

Daubenmire, M. J. (1976). Nurse-patient-physician communicative interaction process. In H. H. Werley, A. Zuzich, M. Zajkowski, & A. D. Zagornick (Eds.), *Health research: The systems approach* (pp. 139-154). New York: Springer.

Denzin, N. K. (1978). *Sociological methods*. New York: McGraw-Hill.

Fawcett, J. (1984). Another look at utilization of nursing research. *Image: The Journal of Nursing Scholarship, 16*, 59-62.

Fisher, S. (1982). The decision-making context: How doctors and patients communicate. In R. J. Di Pietro (Ed.), *Linguistics and the professions: Proceedings of the Second Annual Delaware Symposium on Language Studies* (pp. 51-81). Norwood, NJ: Ablex.

Fishman, J. A. (1971). *Sociolinguistics: A brief introduction*. Rowley, MA: Newbury.

Garfinkel, H. (1967). *Studies in ethnomethodology*. Englewood Cliffs, NJ: Prentice-Hall.

Gortner, S. R. (1975). Research for a practice profession. *Nursing Research, 24*, 193-197.

Gumperz, J. J. (1977). Sociocultural knowledge in conversational inference. In M. Saville-Troike (Ed.), *Linguistics and anthropology* (pp. 191-212). Washington, DC: Georgetown University Press.

Gumperz, J. J., & Cook-Gumperz, J. (1982). Introduction: Language and the communication of social identity. In J. J. Gumperz (Ed.), *Language and social identity* (pp. 1-21). New York: Cambridge University Press.

Gumperz, J. J., & Tannen, D. (1979). Individual and social differences in language use. In C. Fillmore, D. Kempler, & W. Wang (Eds.), *Individual differences in language ability and language behavior*. New York: Academic Press.

Hymes, D. (1971). Sociolinguistics and the ethnography of speaking. In E. Ardener (Ed.), *Social anthropology and linguistics* (pp. 47-93). London: Tavistock.

Kasch, C. R. (1986). Toward a theory of nursing action: Skills and competency in nurse-patient interaction. *Nursing Research, 35*(4), 226-230.

Kirk, J., & Miller, M. L. (1986). *Reliability and validity in qualitative research*. Beverly Hills, CA: Sage.

Leininger, M. M. (1985). Ethnography and ethnonursing: Models and modes of qualitative data analysis. In M. M. Leininger (Ed.), *Qualitative research methods in nursing* (pp. 33-71). Orlando, FL: Grune & Stratton.

Lincoln, Y. S., & Guba, E. G. (1985). *Naturalistic inquiry*. Beverly Hills, CA: Sage.

Maguire, P. (1985). Deficiencies in key interpersonal skills. In C. Kagan (Ed.), *Interpersonal skills in nursing, research, and applications* (pp. 117-127). London: Croon Helm.

Polit, D. F., & Hungler, B. P. (1987). *Nursing research: Principles and methods* (2nd ed.). Philadelphia: J. B. Lippincott.

Saville-Troike, M. (1982). *The ethnography of communication*. London: Basil Blackwell.

Schatzman, L., & Strauss, A. (1973). *Field research: Strategies for a natural sociology*. Englewood Cliffs, NJ: Prentice-Hall.

Shaffer, W. B., Stebbins, R. A., & Turowitz, A. (1980). *Fieldwork experience: Qualitative approaches to social research*. New York: St. Martin's.

Skipper, J. K. (1965). Communication and the hospitalized patient. In J. K. Skipper & R. C. Leonard (Eds.), *Social interaction and patient care* (pp. 61-82). Philadelphia: J. B. Lippincott.

Smith, M. C. (1984). Research methodology: Epistemologic considerations. *Image: The Journal of Nursing Scholarship, 16*(2), 42-46.

Stern, P. N. (1980). Grounded theory methodology: Its uses and processes. *Image: The Journal of Nursing Scholarship, 12*(1), 20-23.

Svejcer, A. D. (1986). *Contemporary sociolinguistics: Theory, problems, methods.* Philadelphia: John Benjamins.

Trudgill, P. (1983). *Sociolinguistics: An introduction to language and society.* New York: Penguin.

Appendix A:
Computer Software Aids for Quantitative Analysis

Listed below are a few of the most popular microcomputer software programs that are used for quantitative data analysis. They are listed in order of complexity.

ABSTAT reads and writes dBase, Lotus, and ASCII files. It is a simple-to-use, menu-driven system that will do descriptive, regression, correlations, ANOVA, t-tests, crosstabs, and other commonly used nonparametric tests.

CRUNCH is an easy-to-use, menu-driven program with tutorial that reads and writes ASCII, DIF, dBASE, and Rbase. It includes the same functions as ABSTAT but, in addition, it permits the user to calculate coefficient alpha indexes on scales and subscales and permits the printing of graphs such as histograms.

STATPAC includes the same functions as ABSTAT and CRUNCH but permits more complex analyses, including MANOVA. The printing options include graphics.

SPSS-PC+ requires a 10 MB hard disk and is mostly menu driven. It performs all the functions of CRUNCH and STATPAC.

SAS-PC also requires a 10 MB but a 30 MB is recommended. It performs all the functions of all the software programs listed above but takes a more experienced computer user.

Appendix B:
Computer Software Aids for
Qualitative Analysis

Software programs for qualitative analysis exist in several forms and are constantly being refined. The software programs mentioned here were created to aid the qualitative researcher in managing and analyzing data. These programs cannot supplant the intense work required to conduct a meaningful analysis of textual data.

ETHNOGRAPH permits coding, recoding, and sorting of text data files into analytic categories. The text can be reviewed, marked, displayed, sorted, and printed in several formats. The researcher can add contextual comments to each sorted segment.

MARTIN requires 20-30 MB and the software program Microsoft Windows, but it is a powerful text analysis program that can be used in interpretive research. This program has been tested in several sites in a number of countries. For more information, contact Dr. Nancy Diekelmann at the School of Nursing, University of Wisconsin.

Appendix C:
Computer Software Aids for
Data Presentation

The following software programs are widely available and are constantly being improved. Listed are only a few of the most popular programs.

Harvard Graphics
PFS Graph
Lotus
Reflex
PFS First Publisher
WordPerfect (WordPerfect includes some graphics and drawing features and permits shading of text in boxes if you wish to highlight data from qualitative studies; the column features make it easy to construct tables.)

Index

About the Editor

LINDA E. MOODY (Ph.D., R.N.C., F.A.A.N.) is Professor of Nursing at the University of Florida, College of Nursing. She holds an M.N. in nursing and a Ph.D. in education with a major in research from the University of Florida. In 1983, she earned an M.Ph. in health policy and administration from the University of North Carolina at Chapel Hill. She is actively engaged in theory building and nursing research. She serves on the board of directors of the National League for Nursing and is currently Chair, Council of the Society for Research in Nursing Education. She has more than 70 refereed publications in nursing and health periodicals. Recent research publications include articles in *Nursing Research* and the *Western Journal of Nursing*. Results of several nationally funded studies have been presented at the ANA Council of Nurse Researchers meeting and the Sigma Theta Tau International Research Conference. She has received competitive funding for research projects from the Robert Wood Johnson Foundation, the U.S. Department of Agriculture, Sigma Theta Tau, the University of Florida, Division of Sponsored Research, and the National Institutes of Health, (NIH). She served as co-project director of the Ph.D. in Nursing Sciences Training Program Grant at the University of Florida from 1983 to 1988. Postgraduate course work in philosophy and sociology of knowledge has prepared her to teach theory and science issues at the master's and doctoral levels. She is a member of the American Academy of Nursing and several honorary professional societies. In the summer of 1988, she was awarded a faculty research position at the National Institute on Aging, Baltimore, Maryland. International work has been done in the Soviet Union and South America.

About the Contributors

IVO L. ABRAHAM (Ph.D., R.N.) is Associate Professor of Nursing and Associate Professor of Behavioral Medicine and Psychiatry at the University of Virginia at Charlottesville, where he is also Associate Director of the Geriatric Neuropsychiatric Clinic. In addition, he is on the Consulting Staff of the Dementia Research Unit at Western State Hospital, Staunton, Virginia. Most of his research is in the area of cognition and function in dementia patients and encompasses clinical intervention as well as assessment and measurement. He is a Charter Member of the National Institutes of Health, Nursing Research Study Section (1987-1991).

PATRICIA E. BENNER (Ph.D., R.N., F.A.A.N.) is Professor of Nursing at the School of Nursing, University of California, San Francisco. She is the author of *From Novice to Expert* and the coauthor of *The Primacy of Caring* with Dr. Judith Wrubel. Both books have won Book of the Year awards from the *American Journal of Nursing*. She is currently conducting research on acquiring clinical expertise on intensive care nursing sponsored by the Helene Fuld Foundation.

JUDITH BAIGIS-SMITH (Ph.D., R.N.) is currently Director of Long-Term Care and Health Promotion at the Johns Hopkins University School of Nursing in Baltimore and was formerly Head, Family and Community Health, University of Pennsylvania, School of Nursing, in Philadelphia. She received her undergraduate and graduate degrees from New York University. Her doctoral dissertation was an example of foundational inquiry, focusing on "the idea of health," and has been cited in numerous works as an important contribution to nursing knowledge.

SANDRA L. FERKETICH (Ph.D., R.N.) is Associate Professor and Division Head for Family and Community Health Nursing at the College of Nursing, University of Arizona in Tucson. Her research focus is on the coping of reproductive and child-rearing families during catastrophic illness. She has published numerous research articles on family function and individual member health. Her advanced preparation in nursing research methodology and statistics has resulted in publications on graphic residual analysis and model building with Dr. Joyce Verran. She has served as a member of local, regional, and national grant review sections.

SALLY A. HUTCHINSON (R.N., Ph.D., F.A.A.N.) is Associate Professor at the University of Florida, College of Nursing. She teaches master's and doctoral students courses in research methods and cultural influences in nursing care. Her research interests lie in several diverse areas: chemical dependence among nurses, self-care and job stress, prehospital care, and quality of life in nursing homes. In her research, she uses qualitative methods because they provide access to human experience. She is on the editorial boards of *Image, Nursing Research, Western Journal of Nursing Research,* and *Advances in Nursing Science.* She coauthored the book *Applying Nursing Research: A Resource Book* with Dr. Holly Wilson and has written numerous chapters in books and articles in research journals. She has been a coleader of Professional Seminar Consultants trips to China, East Africa, Australia/New Zealand, and Scandinavia.

MARCIA M. NEUNDORFER is Assistant Professor at Case Western University. She received her B.S.N. at the University of Rochester in 1971. She completed an M.A. in sociology in 1973 at Case Western Reserve University as a Nurse Scientist. After caring for the frail elderly in the community as a visiting nurse, she completed an M.S.N. in gerontological nursing in 1977 at Case Western Reserve University, where she subsequently taught gerontological nursing. While studying for her Ph.D. in nursing at Case Western Reserve University, she was a research assistant for Ivo Abraham on a study of the effects of nursing treatments on the depressed aged in long-term care. Her dissertation, completed in 1989, is titled *Effects of Coping on Health Outcomes in Caregiving Spouses of Dementia Patients.*

JANICE L. THOMPSON (Ph.D., R.N.) is Associate Professor in the School of Nursing, University of Southern Maine. She received her B.A. in nursing from the University of Iowa in 1975 and her Ph.D. in nursing from the University of Utah in 1983. She teaches theory and research in the graduate program in nursing and also teaches in the women's studies program at the University of Southern Maine. Her research interests include feminist archetypal work with Khmer refugee women in the greater Portland, Maine, area. Her family includes her husband Ken and her two children, Jennifer and Jonathan.

MARY LOU VANCOTT is Assistant Professor of Nursing at the University of South Florida in Tampa. She received her diploma in nursing from Auburn Memorial Hospital School of Nursing and her B.A. from the University of Florida. Her M.A. is from the University of South Florida, where she majored in adult health nursing, and her doctoral degree is from the University of Florida, College of Nursing. She has coauthored two articles in *Nursing Research* and has completed two qualitative research studies, one of which utilized socio-linguistic inquiry.

JOYCE A. VERRAN (Ph.D., R.N., F.A.A.N.) is Associate Professor and Division Head for Adult Health Nursing at the College of Nursing, University of Arizona in Tucson. Her advanced education in clinical nursing research and statistics has lead to joint authorship on several articles with Dr. Sandra Ferketich. She is a statistical consultant for *Nursing Research* and is on the editorial board for the *Journal of Neuroscience Nursing*. Her research interests involve subjective estimation of sleep of hospitalized and healthy adults and nursing technology as it relates to organizational functioning.